Relationship Power
in
Health Care

SCIENCE OF BEHAVIOR CHANGE, DECISION
MAKING, AND CLINICIAN SELF-CARE

John B. Livingstone, MD
with
Joanne Gaffney, RN, LICSW

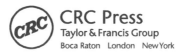

CRC Press
Taylor & Francis Group
Boca Raton   London   New York

CRC Press is an imprint of the
Taylor & Francis Group, an **informa** business

Contents

psychologists and from our personal journey, we believe that most clinicians can do a lot better, but have had too few opportunities to learn how.

Some training programs and schools have an ongoing well-intentioned effort to tackle the interpersonal domain. The time devoted, however, is dreadfully brief and the concepts are often outdated, as also seems to be true of medical education about pain (Foreman, 2013). The training in the interpersonal realm of patient care is still conceptualized by faculty members where I have worked as one more course or rotation to squeeze into the schedule. This topic cannot be taught with a silo mentality. It is most effective when interwoven throughout the clinical curriculum and with co-teaching. Programs are handicapped by selective disease-related funding and institutional barriers to change. Perhaps this text will clarify that it is fruitless to bypass interpersonal forces in health and wellness through a heavy focus on technology. Both are needed.

In recent years many new concepts and strategies have been discovered about how to establish powerful interpersonal relationships that impact outcome. They are derived from modern psychotherapy, brain biology, and the latest advances in health coaching and nursing practice. Putting them to work to improve health care seems to make good sense scientifically and ethically. To teach the new theory and skills to student clinicians also makes good sense to us—but how? To apply these new findings makes it possible to improve the quality of health care in the real world by using advances in technologies simultaneously with advanced strategies in how patients hear, learn, make decisions, change behaviors, and utilize health care. It does not need to be a choice between one or the other, nor do these functions need to be split off from each other. We suggest that both are needed within the same professional, and that the forces of relationship usually trump technology. This book is written to bring together what is known in a form that can be applied.

This project represents personal and professional values held by both of us for a long time. After graduating from the Cornell University–New York Hospital holistic-based nursing program and gaining considerable clinical experience, Joanne Gaffney decided to train in clinical social work to maintain the direct process of helping patients learn about their own healing process. She says, "Direct patient care in a healing and prevention paradigm was where my heart was and is."

I also made a shift in training. Despite enjoying success with the technical aspects of pediatric surgery, I decided to train in child development and psychiatry. I was concerned that despite my child patients having undergone excellent cardiac repairs, their social and emotional development was still dysfunctional and the anxious compensations by parents had increased their children's development delays. Also, I did not like the emotionally well-protected impersonal surgeon I was becoming.

Both of our backgrounds in doctoring and nursing have continued to play a role in our evolution as psychotherapists. Joanne Gaffney was similarly puzzled by the relationship issues in patient care. She became a supervisor for trainees in clinical social work at Simmons and since then has added training in sensory and body-based work. Both of us have supplemented our traditional medical and psychotherapy skills with many years of training in contemporary body-based approaches to personality and relationship.

Both of us started out with traditional medical care followed by traditional training in evaluation and psychotherapy of adults and children, before exploring a rapidly changing field where new concepts of mind functioning and new findings in neuroscience were revolutionizing the understanding of relationships. This revolution certainly applied to psychotherapy, but it also applied to interpersonal relationships in medical care.

The most recent motivation for this book was driven by our unique 3-year experience to redesign the curriculum for midcareer nurses doing medical health coaching in a nationwide patient support program. It started with my being asked for suggestions to improve the power of the nurse health coaching program to change health-related behaviors. I previously had worked with one of the coaching program's executives to enhance audience engagement at WGBH–PBS television. With the coaching program, I started by reviewing a sample of the interviews between the nurses and their patients. Fortunately all nursing interviews were already being audio recorded for quality control. I observed a number of repeating features of their interviews, independent of the illness or situation of the patient. For example, during the interviews when the patient's tone of voice and/or verbalizations indicated that they were experiencing increasing emotion, I would begin to hear clicking of the keyboard of the interviewer's database computer. They were starting to look up information to give to the patient. They would sometimes mutter things like, "Umm—let's see what this says about back pain." Postinterview inquiries and joint listening with the coaching clinicians revealed that when the clinician was feeling uncomfortable, using the computer helped them to decrease their tension. Other clinicians attempted to regulate discomfort using premature and false empathic talk that did not connect to the patient. The patients, on the other hand, could be heard to pull back, change subjects, or start doing things to regain their lost connection, like raise their voice volume. When this was explained, the faculty and executives got interested in enhancing their interview methods. Joanne Gaffney joined the project.

LISTENING WITH NEW EARS?

As we looked back, we asked ourselves—and you might also—why our reviews of the interviews would be any different from those of the highly trained nurse faculty members already in their program. The answers are that we have been trained to listen just below the surface of the concrete content for emotional and relational cues and for opportunities for further exploration and empathy, and that we had the confidence that our strategic framework already had been widely clinically validated. Both of us could observe the interview process on a different dimension than could the nurse faculty. The questions we asked ourselves were as follows: If the faculty and the nurse interviewers could not tune in at our level of observation, what good would it do to try to train them? Did anyone in their organization think that the interview process impacts patient outcome and therefore would be worth changing? If yes, what pathways could be successfully used to enhance their interviewing? And, what is this thing called "relationship," and how is it attained and maintained while providing or supporting specific diagnostic, treatment, and prevention services?

WHAT MADE IT POSSIBLE TO OFFER NEW PATHWAYS?

To jump ahead, we were pleasantly surprised that after discussions and joint listening to recordings with both the nurse interviewers and their faculty, they began to tune in to the new level of listening that changed their experience with patients and wanted to learn more about it. Our curriculum redesign was informed by our earlier training and considerable psychotherapy experience with medical patients. But even more important, our recommendation was guided by our training in a contemporary clinical model that had been transforming the understanding of normal personality organization. They are "Voice Dialogue and The Psychology of the Selves and the Aware Ego" developed by Stone and Stone (Stone and Winkelman, 1985) and the Internal Family Systems Model developed by Richard C. Schwartz (1995)—two models are clinically validated worldwide and are personality multiplicity models of therapy. Both models were developed by highly competent senior-level clinicians who shifted the paradigm of working with human personality. This paradigm made practical emotional sense to the nurse coaches and faculty, and they experienced a positive shift with their patients. Our versions of the work of Hal and Sidra Stone and RC Schwartz enabled clinicians in a medical setting to process and respond to emotions, beliefs, and memories in patients that are pivotal in medical decisions and behavior change.

We have been standing on the shoulders of giants—workers like Bowlby, Anna Freud, Assagioli, Damasio, Satir, Shapiro, Zinn, and more recently Learner—about emotions in decision making. Our early designs in the middle of the 2000–2010 decade and our subsequent years developing a new set of strategies and tactics for *Health Care When It Is Not Psychotherapy* would not have been possible without our direct relationships with clinicians and theoreticians like Hal and Sidra Stone (Voice Dialogue, VD), Richard Schwartz (Internal Family Systems Model, IFS Therapy), and Toni Herbine-Blank (*Intimacy from the Inside Out*, 2015). Along with the integrity of our early mentors, Sophie Freud, Avery Wiseman, Tikvah Portnoi, and Silvio Onesti, Jr., these four contemporary leaders, Hal and Sidra Stone, Richard Schwartz, and Toni Herbine-Blank, enabled us to bring to health care a fresh approach about all aspects of personality and relationships. Our basic understanding of the individual and interactive functioning of patients and clinicians is guided by their work and teaching.

OUR PROCESS

We presented to the executives and nurse faculty at the health coaching service venue how clinical research and advances in neuroscience had already begun to show that the relationships clinicians make with patients have a pivotal impact on patient outcome. The faculty asked us to help redesign their training program in 2006. At their request, I had already conducted a six-month comprehensive review of existing health psychology models since 1950. The reviews included interviews with some of the authors to be sure I was up to date. I discovered more than 100 models with different names and narrowed them to 25 that were substantively different. They were unintegrated and emanated from different specialties and corners of academia. A lot of money had been invested. We have continued to survey the field and have shared much of this information.

After two years of curriculum redesign (2006–2007), analysis of more than 100 recorded clinical interviews, and training their nurses in new approaches, a comparative controlled pilot study showed that the new interviewing strategies and tactics could in fact be learned by professionals untrained in psychotherapy. Also, a comparative patient outcome study showed that patients were more "activated" to participate in their own care through use of the new interviewing tactics.

These two pilot studies were followed by a large random comparative retrospective study conducted by other workers at the same venue of more than 174,000 patients. It showed impressive positive impacts on a number of outcome parameters, including reduction in cost of care. From reviewing their publication discussed later you will see that this retrospective study could not include recording of interviews to verify the exact nature of the nurse health coaching interventions, but there is reason to believe that our enhanced interviewing curriculum was in play. After this initial work ended in early 2008, we used unfolding research in the field to evolve a more complete, contemporary model of relational interviewing that might enhance medical and nursing student education; empower doctoring, nursing, and health coaching; and improve outcome.

Although *outcome* is one ultimate measure of our effort in health care and wellness, to us this word *outcome* means both the observable outcomes of the intervention and the subjective degree of satisfaction in patients and their clinicians. These are interacting factors. The National Institutes of Health, the Institute of Medicine, and clinicians who have been interviewed agree that the ultimate worth of increased access to care, electronic records, integrative care, patient-centered care, shared decision making, and other such items is determined by both objective and subjective outcomes.

CONTINUING DEVELOPMENT OF A NEW MODEL

After the nurse training project ended, we focused on the clinicians themselves and added tactics to help clinicians take care of their activated emotions and beliefs before, during, and after their encounters with patients. We used advancing science to incorporate and go beyond mindfulness mediation and found "clinician self-care" to be the pivotal piece which supports all processes with medical patients. Except regarding counter-transference in psychoanalysis, this domain had not been addressed in medical care. Ilana Rubenfeld, a body-centered clinical pioneer, originally wrote about this topic in 1970 (Rubenfeld, 2000). Since the Institute of Medicine (IOM, National Academy of Sciences) recommended patient-centered care, and there has been renewed talk about "the care of the patient" (begun long ago by Hippocrates, Osler, and Peabody), there continues to be little focus on "the self-care of the clinician," as recently corroborated by Sanchez-Reilly et al. (2013).

We called our newest model of interview sequencing SINHC® (Self-aware Informational Nonjudgmental Health Care). It included a clinical self-care component. Most recently I have used it to inform my co-teaching of medical students and advanced residents in behavioral medicine at Brown's Warren Alpert Medical School and Harvard Medical School's Beth Israel Deaconess medical residency program. The enthusiasm of the participants and faculty members, even with limited exposure, has been a support for this project. This is a new focus for clinical education and training.

THE CONTINUING JOURNEY

At the outset of this project we were aware of the challenge to produce a comprehensive text that supplied knowledge and also supported acquisition of interviewing kills. It would need to include a review and integration of years of polarized viewpoints across many disciplines, to include thinking systemically, and to include advances in the neurosciences.

It would be necessary to present audiovisual demonstrations so that our book would help readers to acquire interviewing skills that include simultaneous tracking of several dimensions of communication between clinician and patient. Our past experience provided a broad foundation since it included ICU/CCU nursing; pediatric cardiac surgery; child and parenting development; couples' relationship work; addiction and trauma work; psychotherapy with adults, children, and teenagers; treating medical patients with chronic conditions or in decision crisis; health educating at the United Nations Children's Fund (UNICEF) for developing countries; and teaching/mentoring in medical, psychology, and social work graduate schools. In addition, each of us has been trained in the newest strategies and tactics of interviewing and continue to hone our skills by providing direct patient care and by teaching interviewing to other professionals.

Also, we are familiar with most of the advances in health care technology and new "constructs" of care, including patient centered care, medical home, Accountable Care Organization (ACO), and shared and emotion-imbued decision making. We believe that the nursing professions—with their long-standing paradigm of healing and care of the whole patient while being informed by basic science—are one of the optimal places to begin enhancing relational aspects of heath care. The Robert Wood Johnson Foundation and the US government are already trying to expand the nursing professions. Primary care, integrative and lifestyle medicine, and health coaching are other important places to enhance relationship power.

In this volume, we have presented and integrated advances of the last 30 years in neurobiology, psychology of relationships, and training about talking with patients. We hope this project provides an impetus and a pathway for changes to occur in education and practice of health care and wellness. Italy's celebrated writer Tiziano Terzani, on his deathbed, said, "Never forget: it's not how far you've traveled, it's what you've brought back." From our long travels through the complexities of this topic, I hope we have brought back something truly useful to you.

Acknowledgments

Special thanks go to Rob DuToit, Amy Davies and Provincetown Community Television (PTV), Karin White, Mary Lou Meehan, and Joseph Vasta for understanding the goals of this project and for giving generously of themselves and their time. Loving thanks to Joanne Gaffney for truly "being with" me and the other people on this project and for keeping space for my voice.

Warm thanks and gratitude to our colleagues, advisors, and those who helped with the title and technology: Bill Brennan, Judy Forman, Toni Herbine-Blank, Ken Kaplan, Joe Martin, Silvio Onesti, Tikva Portnoi, Jenny Potter, Norm Sherry, Roy Simpson, Bessel Van der Kolk, Sarita Warrier, Richard Wexler, and Victor and Frances.

Authors

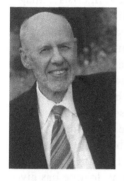 **John B. Livingstone, MD, FRSH,** is an adult, child, and adolescent psychiatrist and psychotherapist with a long-standing appointment at McLean Hospital and an assistant professorship at Harvard Medical School. For 20 years he trained clinicians from different specialties in the art and science of interviewing. He has been trained in Voice Dialogue/Psychology of the Selves, the Internal Family Systems Model, psychodynamic child and adult psychotherapy, and Eye Movement Desensitization and Reprocessing (EMDR). In addition to a private psychotherapy practice for children, adults, and couples, he periodically consults to medical schools and advanced training programs in medicine, nursing, business administration, and athletics. His interest in health coaching includes being a board member of the National Consortium for the Credentialing of Health and Wellness Coaches. Past research includes prevention of developmental deviations in children born blind and the design of an integrated child care delivery model. He is a Frances Wayland Scholar at Brown University and an honorary fellow of the Royal Society of Health (UK) for his seminal discoveries in infectious disease. He designed a trauma relief program for child victims of the 2004 Indian Ocean tsunami. For his five years of editorship of *Dialogue*, a quarterly publication on human relationships for screen and TV writers and directors, he received first prize as a medical information officer. He also has been a script consultant for PBS/Nova, Hanna Barbera, and Turner Entertainment Industries, where he appeared with Phylicia Rashad in the prime-time special *TV Violence: Parents under the Gun*. He makes his home on Cape Cod, is married to Joanne Gaffney, and has two children, two stepchildren, and six grandchildren.

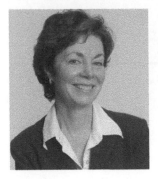

Joanne Gaffney, RN, LICSW, began her career in nursing at Cornell University–New York Hospital School of Nursing. The focus of her training was to care for patients and teach them how to care for themselves. As team leader and charge nurse, she supported a team of auxiliary personnel to participate in this goal. She also supported the family to shift in ways that supported awareness and choice. Turning her emphasis to the internal components of motivation, Joanne trained at the Simmons School of Social Work, Boston, where she became an interview mentor. She worked for several years with the challenges facing the chronically mentally ill in acute care hospitals and in the community, and in crisis management of the mentally ill in the community. She was the addictions specialist and worked with trauma patients in a large community health care center.

Joanne moved to private practice so that she could continue to train and work in ways that supported her ability to creatively help couples and individuals in reaching their goals of greater life satisfaction. She trained in the Rubenfeld Synergy method, a somatic bodily based intervention, in the Psychology of the Selves, and in Internal Family System work, becoming assistant teaching faculty in all three programs. As part of Gaffney–Livingstone Consulting, she has been an integral partner in the design of a new model of health-related behavior change and decision making and helped design the curriculum and retraining of nurse health coaches within a corporate environment. Joanne has given workshops on couples' communication skills, provided consultation to staff in hospitals, appeared on national television as a couples expert, and contributed her work to the 30-year edition of *The Ladies Home Journal: Can this Marriage be Saved?* She has been a supervisor and a mentor to individuals in both the medical model and healing model of treatment. She lives and maintains a private practice of psychotherapy on Cape Cod and is married with two children and a grandson.

Robert Du Toit (Illustrations) began painting with oils and drawing with ink at the age of 10, often inspired by Chinese paintings he saw at the Museum of Fine Arts in Boston. He received a Bachelor of Fine Arts degree from the University of New Hampshire and a Master of Fine Arts from the Parsons School of Design in New York City, where he studied with Paul Resika and Leland Bell. Post graduate, he apprenticed with a legandary frame maker, becoming a master framer and gilder, and now runs his own shop out of his studio in Provincetown, Massachusetts. An active artist since the 1980s, he has been involved in numerous solo and group shows in Boston, New York and the Outer Cape. His work can also be viewed at robdutoit.com. He has an early background in the sciences, especially biology. A student of Zen, he combines daily meditation practice as a way to further meet things "as they are." He is also a student of the Internal Family Systems model which, combined with meditation, helps deepen his relationships with others and with life. He lives in Truro, Massachusetts with his wife Janice Redman, a sculptor, and their son Alexander.

How to use this book

OVERVIEW

This guide for using the book lists the content in detail and includes instructions on how to use the video demonstrations.

The intention of this project is to provide you with the latest knowledge base of theory and strategy about the science of health behavior change, medical decision making, and the communication of information to patients. It also is to provide you with pathways to apply your new knowledge and acquire interviewing tactics. Evidence is accumulating that maintaining an effective relationship with your patients while you are performing the tasks of diagnosis, treatment, and prevention will improve outcome.

A framework for assessing the scientific status of a health theory or model is presented in the next section. Terms from this framework are used as a shorthand way to describe the research status of the various health psychology and neuroscience models mentioned in Part 2.

The book is divided into five parts. Part 1 consists of Chapter 1, an introduction, and Chapter 2, on-line links to the opening segments of three video demonstrations which are accessible later in full length in Chapter 9.

Part 2 consists of the *knowledge base*. In Chapter 3 are traditional health psychology models from the past (widely used but often of variable scientific validity). In Chapters 4 and 5 are scientific advances from the present since 1990, accompanied by supporting research and clinical evidence.

Part 3 *integrates and formulates*. Chapter 6 integrates past with present and selects items to be included in a new model. Chapter 7 formulates contemporary theory and strategy, based upon the integration. Chapter 8 contains a list of core interviewing tactics for clinicians.

Part 4 enhances the *leap from knowledge to skill acquisition*. Chapter 9 contains annotations and discussions of the three full-length audiovisual demonstrations of interviews guided by the content of Chapters 7, 8, and 9 and the on-line links to those three full-length demonstrations. Chapter 10 contains a new protocol of interviewing sequences called SINHC®. Chapter 11 contains suggestions about why and how to refer a patient to a mental health professional.

Part 5 focuses on *education and training*. Chapter 12 provides training strategies for faculty and future faculty. Health coaching is the topic of Chapter 13 and describes what it is and why it is fast becoming a modality of specialty training. Research in this field is discussed in Chapter 14 and projects are suggested.

Clarifications

A decision was made to divide *past models* from *present advances* for the purposes of this presentation. The early 1990s was chosen as the dividing timeline. Regarding relationship psychology, the paradigm shift in the view of how the human mind is normally organized took hold clinically in 1989–1990 with the work of Hal and Sidra Stone, followed by RC Schwartz. This was before the field of interpersonal neurobiology was highlighted. About the same time, fMRI brain research began to yield important findings about possible neural substrates of mind functions. Behavior change models began developing in the 1950s, and Patient-Centered Care was formulated in the late 1990s. It made sense, therefore, to use the early 1990s as our rough division of "past" (Chapter 1) from "present" (Chapters 2 and 3). There may be some overlaps, but this seemed to work best.

We wish to clarify authorship and use of the words *I* and *we*. Because Joanne Gaffney, RN, LICSW, made major contributions as the interviewer in the video demonstrations, was a principle participant in the research and training for the nurse health coaching project in 2006–2008, and was an editorial advisor for the line drawings and the overall project, the designation *with* in the authorship is appropriate. John Livingstone is the primary author of content and structure and is the *I* referred to in the text. Occasionally the word *we* is used in an editorial sense or when we specifically wish what is being said to be from both of us.

The Appendix mentions additional behavior change models, a list of patient decision aids in existence and their international requirements for design. For your information, I've listed five attributes the Institute of Medicine (IOM) suggests to guide patient centered care. This textbook takes these rules much deeper into theory and tactics. Since the topics in this book may be new territory for you, we suggest that you make liberal use of the Glossary. References give you access to publications that support what is being said and to explore new territory.

Opening statements of patients: Short audiovisual segments

For your initial video use, in Chapter 2 there is an opportunity to view short introductory sections of the three video demonstrations, the complete versions of which you will access later in Chapter 9. Our suggestion when viewing these short video segments is that you try putting yourself in the role of clinician. Ask yourself what your options of response are to the patient's opening statements and where you might head. We suggest that you speculate with the expectation that many answers will be forthcoming in later chapters. To an untrained person, these interviews may seem like ordinary conversation. As you will discover, the clinician is taking cues from her overview of the medical record and the patient's

INFORMATION TRANSFER MODELS
  Information Communication Models (ICMs)
HOLISTIC NURSING MODEL
  Scope and Standards of Practice including Barbara Dossey's work
TRADTIONAL PSYCHOTHERAPY MODELS (partially personality multiplicity)
MINDFULNESS MODEL (for clinicians and patients)
HUMAN DEVELOPMENT ATTACHMENT THEORY
NARRATIVE MEDICINE
  Includes Rita Charon's work
TRADITIONAL FUNCTIONAL NEUROSCIENCE

Chapter 4: Present advances in relationship psychology (after early 1990s): A relational context for diagnosis and treatment

These advances are compatible with the assumption that the normal human mind functions as a multiplicity of personalities and a separate capacity for self-awareness. After an orienting introduction, this chapter lists and summarizes each advance we discovered, including an assessment of their scientific status, and organizes them into the following topics:

1. Information transfer
2. Emotion regulation
3. Relationship platform
4. Emotional self-care for clinicians
5. Shift in view of mind organization
6. Role of implicit memory
7. Medical decision making is a process involving emotions and relationship, not only reasoning about facts

Chapter 5: Present advances in neuroscience (starting with the early 1990s): Possible neural substrates of mind functions

All these advances are compatible with a personality multiplicity viewpoint. After an orienting introduction, this chapter lists and summarizes each advance that was discovered, including an assessment of their scientific status, and organizes them into the following topics:

1. Learning and memory
2. Affect regulation and connections of the OMPFC, amygdala, cortex
3. Mirror neurons and plasticity
4. Neural correlates of relational attachment
5. Role of prefrontal cortex
6. Plasticity and activation of subcortical memory
7. Vagal circuitry and relationships
8. Neural substrates in decision making
9. Neural substrates of emotional awareness and mindfulness

Part 3: Building new theoretical hypotheses, strategies, and tactics for clinicians

Chapter 6: Integration of past with present advances (selections of elements to include in a new model)

After an orienting introduction, the seven psychological advances of Chapter 5 and nine neural advances of Chapter 6 are integrated with the prior models in Chapter 4. Presented are the following:

1. Concepts supported by information from Chapters 4 and 5 that are selected for inclusion in the new model are annotated as to their origin and discussed.
2. Concepts supported by information from Chapters 4, 5, and 6 that are selected for inclusion in the new model are annotated as to their origin and discussed.
3. Integrative hypotheses are discussed.

Chapter 7: Formulations of theoretical hypotheses and strategies of relational patient care

1. Updated theory is formulated in a list of six items.
2. Updated strategy and their associated tactics are formulated in a list of eight items.

Chapter 8: Tactical competencies and frameworks

1. A list of core tactical interviewing competencies translated from Chapter 7.
2. Detailed discussion of the tactics of each competency.
    a. Clinician emotional self-care
    b. Relating first to the patient's presenting personality part
    c. Relating to more than one patient personality part
    d. Responding to patients' emotions as they present, without pulling for more (not going deeper)
    e. Tracking the relational triad and seven clinical tasks
    f. Facilitating information interweave
    g. Facilitating health behavior change
    h. Facilitating decision making

Part 4: Acquiring interviewing skills

Chapter 9: Three interviewing demonstrations, links, and annotations

1. Links to three audio-video interview demonstrations approximately 18 minutes each and line-by-line annotations of tactics used.
2. Topics: Behavior change for smoking cessation (Mary Lou)
3. Information transfer in diabetes (Joe)
4. Decision making in breast cancer (Karin) (audio only; video available from authors)
5. Clinician: Joanne Gaffney, RN

Chapter 10: A learning tool to sequence strategies and tactics: Self-aware
Informational Nonjudgmental interviewing in Health Care (SINHC®)
("synch")

This chapter includes

1. A description of the strategic and tactical **sequencing of updated clinical
   interviewing**
2. Description of **SINHC®**
3. A table of the **SINHC®** process in **two tracks**: one within the clinician, the
   other toward the patient

Chapter 11: Referring to behavioral health professionals

Part 5: For faculty and others

Chapter 12: Pathways in education and training

Discusses medical and nursing school education post graduate training, and curriculum design.

Chapter 13: Health coaching

Defines health coaching as a distinct modality within health care, whoever deliv-
ers it: nurse, physician, or allied professional. Summarizes history of its development, and presents the latest developments in professional certification.

Chapter 14: Future research
Glossary
Appendix

1. Theories and Methods Reviewed in the Design of SINHC®
2. A List of Journals and Societies
3. Professionals Involved Nationally in Health Coaching
4. Institute of Medicine (IOM) Statement of 2012
5. Patient Decision Aids: A List, Resources, and Standards
6. Definitions of Patient-Centered Care: IOM and Others
7. Seven Steps and 24 Competencies of EBP in Nursing
8. Basics of the Internal Family Systems (IFS) Model

A FRAMEWORK TO ASSESS SCIENTIFIC STATUS

A systematic framework evolved as I began to study each model through a
scientific lens—the lens that assesses validity, clarifies concept, and distinguishes
between theory, hypothesis, strategy, and tactic. This topic is complex enough to
justify an entire book.

The survey of health psychology models over the past 9 years revealed
many "theories" and "models." I use quotes because many of them did not yet

appear to have the scientific status implied by their labels. You will find them described in Chapter 3. Because some medical and nursing schools and health centers continue to use them and may expect you to learn them, you may wish to know their names and something about each. Regarding behavior change, it is understandable that many different frameworks at all levels of scientific status have been formulated in different centers. At that time the science of behavior change had not fully evolved, and clinicians needed to use whatever guiding framework appealed to them for the challenging interpersonal aspects of health behavior change. Historically, behavior change models have been categorized in several different ways, for example, depending on whether the model conceptualizes behavior change as happening in distinct and identifiable "stages" (stage models) or whether it happens in a "continuum" of thinking and behaviors (continuum models). Another dimension of categorization is the degree to which they are based on any theory, one theory, or several theories. Many workers have spent great effort for years arguing these matters. The literature is filled with debate.

Regarding medical decision making, for many years it was thought that better access to evidence-based information would take care of whatever issues with medical decision might arise. Medical decision making, however, turned out to be as influenced by intra- and interpersonal psychological issues as was health behavior change. Various models of decision making, therefore, began to emerge.

Knowing that research by its very nature is a continuing process, we have done our best to categorize the scientific status of the various models mentioned in this text. You might wish to develop your own system of assessment. Psychological theories, as in theoretical physics, remain potentially untestable for a long period of time because the farther the theory departs from everyday observational experience, the more effort has to be made to design suitable experiments. Internal consistency of a theory, although reassuring, does not establish its validity. For example, both multiplicity of personality and attachment theory seem considerably closer to everyday observational experience and potentially more testable than are some of the more abstract concepts in psychoanalytic theory—although these three theoretical hypotheses have been shaped to be internally consistent.

Hopefully your initial confusion from exposure to so many heterogeneous models coming from different corners of the health world will decrease through your use of the Framework given here, the Glossary, and the summaries in Part 2 of this text.

THE FRAMEWORK consists of the following assessments

1. ASSESS whether the model or theory is one or a mixture of the following:
   a. *Theory*: A validated and internally consistent set of hypotheses (*Theory* in colloquial language, however, implies it is a guess.)
   b. *Hypotheses*: Potentially testable concepts in degrees of validation
   c. *Clinical strategy*: A conceptual operation to reach a goal
      i. Based on a set of validated hypotheses (a theory)
      ii. Based on a set of hypotheses yet to be validated
      iii. Based on themselves alone

    d. *Clinical tactics*: Observables in words and action
      i. Grounded in strategy and theory
      ii. Grounded in strategy without validated theory
      iii. Based on themselves alone

2. ASSESS the paradigm used for understanding personality organization.
    a. **Traditional monolithic paradigm** of personality organization: Views the mind as *one personality* with functional components such as conscience, cognition, beliefs, memory, emotion, and an executive function (ego), etc. The clinician relates to different functional components of one mind in order to process behavior change and decision making.
    b. **Multiplicity paradigm** of personality organization: Views the mind as having multiple dimensions or a community of *whole personalities*, each with its own consistent set of emotions, beliefs, memories, and adaptive agenda. And, the human mind as having *one* core self that is capable of awareness and making a nonjudgmental relationship with each personality "part" or "self" inside the person. The clinician relates to each personality as a person with distinct values, emotions, and functions and as the determinants of verbal and action behaviors that are activated by illness, and the processes of treatment decision making and behavior change.

3. ASSESS to what extent the model views health behaviors to be determined primarily by
    a. **INSIDE** psychological forces within people (the emotional and cognitive aspects of the person)
    b. **OUTSIDE** interactions, information, and social learning ("modeling")
    c. **BOTH**

4. ASSESS to what extent the model was originally derived from
    a. *A top-down process*: Abstract theory built downward to fit observations and to design concrete tactics
    b. *A bottom-up process*: Concrete observations built upward to theory that explains and informs strategy and tactic
    c. *A simultaneous process from both directions*: From abstract theory and concrete observation with integration and testing

5. ASSESS the type of *change theory*
    a. **Is it a stage theory?** (a category system, an ordering of categories, similar barriers to change within categories, and different barriers to change between categories)
    b. **Is it a continuum theory?** (a noncategorized system; nonlinear process)

6. FEATURES DESERVING OF COMMENT on the **quality and quantity of research** conducted on patient outcome or on professional educational feasibility:
    a. Testimonials are the sole support for validity.
    b. Repeated clinical validation (RCV) of effectiveness in a variety of conditions.
    c. Retrospective studies.
    d. Prospective studies randomized controlled comparative trials (RCTs).

e. Two cohorts were compared with the control group being "care as usual."
f. Two or more cohorts compared two interventions.
g. Three cohorts compared two interventions and a control.
h. Quality of the intervention fidelity checking was by observations or recordings with or without a reliable and valid adherence tool.
i. Fidelity was assumed from how clinicians were trained.
j. Fidelity was assumed from exit interviews of clinicians and testimonials.
k. Both the interventions and controls were recorded and checked.
l. Patient outcome was determined by testimonials of patients or others.
m. Patient outcome was determined by reliable measures and patient behaviors.
n. Statistical power of numbers used.
o. Other:

PART 1

Overview

Introductory discussion and overview

The physician who attempts to take care of a patient while he neglects their emotions and relationships is as unscientific as the investigator who neglects to control all the conditions that may affect his experiment.

Frances W. Peabody, MD
Professor of Medicine, Harvard Medical School, 1922

WHY THIS PROJECT?

You might be asking: Why a textbook on the relational aspects of patient care? Can't gaps in health care be fixed by new technology and by patient-centered integrated care systems? The answer is no. More than ever before, approaches that utilize relational attunement and people's emotions, body sensations, and beliefs are supported by research evidence in both neurobiology and relational psychology. In the past, these concepts and strategies were supported only by scattered accounts of clinical experience and research of variable quality. We now feel scientifically secure to present this degree of concrete detail to students and their faculties.

The interface between clinician and patient is always the final common pathway of health care. It is the *sine qua non* of optimal outcome. Research and clinical experience confirm it. Lack of clinician competency in relationship science contributes to costly derailment of care, unwarranted variation in treatment, stress in patients, unnecessary litigation, and clinician burnout.

At 5 a.m., only 3 hours after his postpartum patient's delivery, an obstetrician stuck his head though the curtain surrounding the new mother's bed and said something to her. Her memory 2 years later of what she had heard was, "Boy did you give me gray hairs last night!" And then he left. Most likely her obstetrician had also said something like, "Baby's fine," but she never recalled that. As a matter of fact, all of what he said during her vulnerable state dropped below her conscious radar. She did not recall the "you gave me gray hairs" comment until 2 years later in the office of a clinician participating in the neuropsychiatric evaluation of the child.

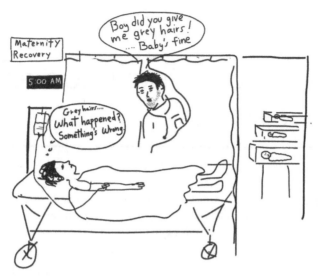

BETTER LEFT UNSAID

The clinician on the evaluation team became curious (without being judgmental) as to why she and her husband had shopped from clinic to clinic trying to find out if something was wrong with this first child, their son. She had not believed the identical negative findings of three skilled diagnostic evaluations and reviews of the birth record. Although she had buried the entire content of the obstetrician's comments, she had retained what is called an implicit emotional, body-based belief: "Something is wrong with my son." This implicit memory resulted in a persistent anxiety about the normality of when he started crawling, walking, and speaking—the child's developmental milestones. So, it was not the child who needed another visit as much as it was the parents who needed a skilled clinician to explore what was going on for them. The child's father, although less concerned than his mother and trying unsuccessfully to reassure her, was feeling frustrated. The three prior evaluations at other clinics had focused mostly on the child. At our clinic, both parents were now in focus.

Birth records showed an extra-long labor consistent with a first child, with heart rate OK, fetus in good position, and good APGAR scores. In the interview, this mother for the first time discovered memory fragments from the postpartum period (both thoughts and emotions). The interviewer, whom we observed through the one-way mirror, helped her to label and soothe her emotions about what she had heard, and her worry about his milestones. For the first time, this mother had begun to process her implicit emotional memories. In less than an hour of recall and reality checking in the attuned relational climate provided by the parent clinician she accomplished a lot. She agreed it would be helpful if, while reevaluating her son for this fourth time, the team keep in mind her recollection of what she recalled the obstetrician had said. The findings were normal and similar to the previous three diagnostics. This time, however, the normal findings were assimilated by both parents, and follow-up indicated that the shopping to different clinics had stopped.

This intervention was not about discovering key data about the child that would reassure the parents; it was about the key to the mother's concerns triggered by an untimely comment by her fatigued obstetrician who wasn't taking care of his own emotions. Whatever the OB said may have fallen on fertile ground within this mother's psychological system, and yet any such comments in those moments of poor relational connection run the risk of having a profound and unwarranted impact, including thousands of dollars in costs.

Our basic belief is that every health professional, not just the relationally "gifted," is capable of enhancing the skills required to be in tune with patients. The health psychology models developed over the last 50 years about interviewing, health behavior change, and medical decision making were built at that time upon an underdeveloped state of knowledge about human functioning. In the past decade, however, lack of modernization of these models appears due to an underuse of what has already been discovered in the fields of relationship psychology and brain biology. Separate fiefdoms of theorizing, funding, and research have dominated the field. We hope to change that. As one of our goals is to integrate a fragmented field that crosses several disciplines of research and practice, you may experience some of that fragmentation. Our advice to you is to notice any confusion and to keep going with the expectation that it will clear.

Patients and their clinicians are human beings interlocked in a vulnerable business of health, illness, treatment, birthing, aging, and dying. Yet, there is an interpersonal bottleneck in health care (IOM and NAE, 2011). Advances occurring in the last 15 years in relationship psychology and neurobiology needed to be integrated and added to the scientific knowledge base. A modern relationship engine under the hood of the latest administrative constructs, patient-centered care and patient engagement was yet to be built. A textbook on this subject was not only possible but mandatory.

At a time when medical and nursing students are expected to keep pace with an ever-expanding body of technical knowledge, this book signifies an expectation and offers a pathway to gain both knowledge and skills in yet another realm, that of the science of their relationships with patients and with themselves. Evidence-based medicine does not operate outside of the patient–clinician relationship—the final common denominator. Clinicians do not operate outside their own psychology states. There is evidence to show that the mastery of this topic cannot be seen as one more topic to add to an already crammed curriculum. It is a pervasive topic. To gain the essential skills in encounters with patients requires mentoring woven into clinical education and training over all the years by faculty already grounded in the contemporary neurobiology and relation psychology and who have mastered and can demonstrate the interviewing skills. Without this mentoring, we doubt whether the learning can take place that will positively impact patient outcomes, lower costs, and prevent clinician burnout and compassion fatigue.

Regarding the trenches of everyday medical care, mental health faculty members (including the authors) usually were not trained in contemporary health psychology. Most likely they too have some catching up to do in this realm of behavior change models and shared decision making. This textbook is for all faculty members, students, residents, and postgraduate fellows.

A main theme of this text is that the relationship dimension of patient care is now a science that can be taught and learned. The evidence is clear that information is transferred, behavior change and decisions are made across a strategic interpersonal platform between patient and clinician, and those clinicians can be trained to build that platform without training in psychotherapy. When this platform is solid, it enhances patient outcome and increases the clinician's sense of well-being. Without it, care becomes derailed. Research shows that clinicians cannot become competent in this realm without specific education and training informed by interpersonal psychological science and brain biology. New developments make training in this domain possible for the first time. This offers hope for improved patient outcome, cost containment, and increased patient and clinician satisfaction that evidence shows are unlikely to be improved solely by technological and business-driven solutions.

Observable outcomes and subjective satisfaction with health care and wellness initiatives are not only tied to the success of the procedures of diagnosis, treatment, and prevention but also to the success of three psychologically based processes within patients: assimilating pertinent information, changing health behaviors, and making sound medical decisions. Although information transfer, behavior change, and decision making were in the past thought to be primarily cognitive processes, the last decade of research and clinical observation has changed that viewpoint. Findings in the past decade indicate that the determining forces include emotions, memories, beliefs, and cognitions being processed within the minds and brains of both the patient and the clinician and include the interactional dynamics between them. All are crucial determining forces. Sometimes these forces become barriers to the goals of good care; often they are necessary components. Without emotional processing within a relationship as well as cognitive processing, enduring decisions cannot be made (Damasio, 1999; Lerner et al., 2015). Furthermore, as formerly believed, working with these forces no longer usually requires a psychotherapeutic intervention (for patient or clinician), although recent advances in relational neurobiology and psychotherapy inform this book. With proper training, nurses, primary care physicians, and others can work with these forces in the trenches of everyday heath care. That is good news for medical care and wellness projects.

We suggest that, in addition to diagnosing and treating, the role of all health care clinicians is to hold the responsibility for working with whatever the patient's personality presents and to work with their own internal coping as well. Patient outcome and cost control depend upon this approach. We are concerned that if nurses and physicians don't receive training in this domain, they will become the "technicians" of the body while others make the decisions about patient care. Unwarranted variations of care and unwarranted judgments and statements by clinicians toward patients are prevalent in our and other's recorded materials (Braddock, 2010; Livingstone, 2013). Whatever specialty you chose or have chosen, we hope this book and the demonstration videos will provide you with a pathway for gaining competency in the skills of relationship with patients and of emotional self-care. If the Accountable Care Organization (ACO), Patient-Centered Care, and Shared Decision Making become mandated practices, you certainly will need relationship-based core skills. In addition to improving patient outcome and containing cost, your possession of these skills also makes humane good sense and will add to your sense of personal and professional competency.

You are entering a culture devoted both to the science of disease and to the care and healing of the patient. There is a long-standing tradition in nursing that focuses on the interpersonal care and healing of the patient. Physicians and other scientists have made impressive advances in understanding and treating disease and in wellness preservation. The timing is right for the interpersonal side of patient care to receive robust attention—a domain that impacts patient outcome, prevention, and cost. The growing field of Interpersonal Neurobiology (IPNB) prompts a renewed focus. A clinician's relationship with patients with all its bodily and emotional vulnerability often has the elements for an attachment experience (Attachment Theory) in which implicit emotions and memories come into play (IPNB). Not to be conversant with this territory puts the clinician and his patients at a disadvantage.

Advances in neuroscience and relationship psychology have occurred and offer new guidelines for interviewing patients. Included in these advances with which you will become familiar is a shift in the concept of how the human mind and personality are organized. Several sections of this book will familiarize you with this shift in concept, a shift that makes some of the strategies of previous health psychology models outdated.

While this book gives you access to the expanding role of interpersonal neurobiology in health care, it also provides you with a pathway to learn tactical relational skills to work in an evidenced-based and cost-conscious climate, and in an expanding array of modalities, including primary care, family medicine, physician assistance, and doctor or nurse practice. Our goal has been to evolve an updated model for doctoring and nursing that contains testable hypotheses. We anticipate that this knowledge will increase over the next 10 years about linkages between neural and psychological phenomenon. At this time, we are focusing on developing specific, teachable strategies and tactics grounded in current science that clinicians can use to facilitate their patients to change behavior, make treatment decisions, and assimilate new information. In our view, this type of knowledge would be generically useful in the context of whatever overall philosophy of care one embraces—holistic, integral, mindfulness medicine, or disease-based medical models.

LOOKING FOR PATHWAYS TO IMPROVE: INTERPERSONAL RELATIONSHIPS

One morning Mullah Nasruden, the Persian folk character, was kneeling on the ground looking for something. While walking by, a friend asked what he was doing. Mullah said he was searching for his lost key. While helping him, after a short while the friend asked the Mullah where exactly he had lost his key. Mullah replied, "In my house." "Then why are we looking here," asked the friend. Mullah replied, "Because there is more light here" (Shah, 1965).

Electronic record technology and new patient questionnaires, although available, are not the only places to look for better ways to enhance patient care, improve outcome, and control costs. It may seem easier and exciting to do so, but as long as we are human beings, there is no way, as you will see from recent research, to sidestep interpersonal relationships in patient care. The increasing use of rating scales and printed patient decision aids (PDAs) and DVDs have their place, and yet they do not capture the fear in a man's eyes or the hesitation in a woman's voice or the volumes spoken by a patient's silence. Nonverbal and verbal communications and the subtle meanings behind them are essential guides for clinicians to build essential and powerful relational linkage that make diagnosis, treatments, medication adherence, decision making, and health behavior change possible.

Even management consultants believe that health care delivery is determined by individuals: "Individual behavior drives today's healthcare environment" (Thompson et al., 2010). This is not saying that patient care has not been enhanced by marvelous technological advances including integrative care algorithms and electronic records, but it turns out that they are not substitutes for the relational component. What journalist Edward R. Murrow said about international communication between diplomats is also true in health care among clinicians and between clinicians and patients: The "really critical link in the communications chain is the last three feet, which is best bridged by personal contact—one person talking to another."

Patient care is not a business, although it has business accoutrements. David Kirp, a professor at University of California said, "The impersonal strategies of the market or the transformative power of technology have not lived up to their hype" (Kirp, 2014) while speaking on improving graduate school education. We believe this is also true for the use of electronics to improve health care. Kirp again said, "It is impossible to improve professional education by doing an end run around inherently complicated and messy human relationships. The most effective approaches foster bonds of caring between teachers and their students." As we have put it, technology, although helpful, rides on the rails of the bonds of caring.

Presumably improving medical record-keeping improves care. But, when clinicians are in a duty-bound relationship with the medical record rather than making and keeping affective contact with the patient, the most powerful "conduit" is lost—the one required for assimilation of evidence-based information and for facilitating behavior change and decision making.

The relational domain of health care can no longer be viewed as an extra and dispensable. Relationships provided by telephone to a random cohort of outpatients by nurses trained in relationship has been shown to impact outcomes (Wennberg et al., 2010). The nurse health coaching training program we redesigned for a nationwide health coaching service in 2006 revised their model to emphasize contemporary interpersonal strategies and tactics. Our relational enhancement model at first concerned the management and the nurses that their coaching encounters would become so long that they could not cover their patient load. After a month of part-time training, the patient encounters took about the same and often less time. Their enhanced training gave them new keys to unlock the doors of engagement to get down to essential business. Our comparative efficacy research showed that the use of the redesign was a powerful agent to activate patients to take increasing responsibility for their own health care and wellness (Hibbard et al., 2005). We will share the nurses' testimonials in Chapter 12 on education and training. Their take-away was, "It saves time to take the time." We believed it also would save money. The large, retrospective Wennberg Study confirmed it.

The Wennberg Study published in 2010 of 170,400 patients (about half of whom were not health coached) showed that health coaching was associated with a significant decline over one year in net total costs (decline in ER use and readmissions, better treatment decisions, and medication use) associated with personal one-on-one discussions with specially trained nurses around their chronic illness, crisis decisions, and medication adherence (Wennberg et al., 2010). Much more is known now than in 2008–2010 about the relationship between patient and clinician, for example, the role that emotions play in blocking informational learning, the impact that labeling of affects has on regulation of behavior, and the powerful role played by different aspects of the normal personality. These are topics covered in Chapters 4 and 5.

Recent advances have pointed the way to new interviewing strategies and tactics that clinicians could use to work with their patients and their own emotional status in order to be effective agents of patient-centered care. It is becoming clearer how personality works and the kind of things that need to be said and when. The good news is that we no longer need to relegate gaining competency to dialogue with patients to the vagueness of "clinical experience" or "in-born talents" that "you either have or you don't." With basic education about relationships and a new type of skilled mentoring, almost everyone can make notable progress. Advances in neuroscience and relationship psychology have changed the paradigm and power of clinical interviewing and the education and training of doctors and nurses. The new strategies extend beyond what was started in holistic nursing, in the many models of health behavior change, and in updates to Shared Decision Making to include patients' values. Student clinicians have new pathways to fold specific interpersonal tactics into their diagnostic and treatment skills. Whatever the clinical task of the moment, the relationship dynamic never ceases to be important.

THEORY, STRATEGY, TACTICS

This text explains advances in theory, strategy, and interviewing tactics. The video demonstrations are designed to facilitate the acquisition of interviewing skills that are linked with the advances and to apply valuable strategies from the past.

In addition to cataloging and integrating much of what is already known and used for health behavior change and medical decision making (see Chapter 3), we address many facets of the relational side of health care which have remained unexplored in their depths despite having been recognized as gaps that hamper professional education and practice (LeBlanc et al., 2009; Zikmund-Fisher et al., 2010).

To some extent the same gaps also characterize the field of psychotherapy and a lack of collaboration between those studying emotions and relationship and those studying cognitive forces. Until recently, workers in the psychotherapy fields, as one might expect, have been using theoretical constructs heavily focused on improving symptom relief and decreasing dysfunctional behaviors. They have not been addressing behavior change and decision making in everyday health care. This is one of the reasons why so many health professionals in the mainstream remain unaware that there is an evolving science about relationships and emotions that would be useful to them. Programmatic attempts to fix problems in our health system include recommendations from the Institute of Medicine (IOM, National Academy of Sciences) such as Patient-Centered Care, Shared Decision Making, and medical home. These are good intentioned ideas, yet we suggest that in interpersonal matters they are without sufficient modern theory and strategy. Powerful engines, however, were being discovered by scientists in brain mapping and integrative research on emotions, cognitions, memory, and relational dynamics.

Medical and nursing students cannot be expected to implement patient care constructs which are not yet in the curriculum to be taught. Many students tell us they feel confused and frustrated when working with dietary compliance, smoking cessation, and decision making. Our dozens of observed interviews show that trainees turn to their usual left-brain fallback mechanisms, such as using rational discussion about compliance and turning to their database computers for evidence-based information while being out of connection with the patient they are interviewing. They are observed commonly to say things that inadvertently shame patients in an attempt to enlist cooperation after they have given up in frustration with trying, for example, to "roll with resistance," one of the recommendations from motivational interviewing. Advances in interviewing strategy and tactic are needed which while honoring motivational interviewing, use current science to move beyond.

We suggest that there are five dimensions of Patient-Centered Care that impact quality, outcome, and cost. Three of them are internal psychological processes within patients: (1) making behavior or lifestyle changes, (2) making difficult decisions, and (3) assimilating new information.

The fourth dimension is the internal process within clinicians while they are diagnosing and treating and attempting to help their patients accomplish any of the first three tasks. It is not only what clinicians are "feeling," as Daniel Elfri illustrated so well in *What Doctors Feel* (Olfri, 2013). It is how well clinicians have learned to process their implicit and explicit memories, emotions, and beliefs that determine whether Patient Centered Care can be practiced. This is the internal life of clinicians that needs attention. What are the internal mental mechanisms normally at work within the minds of us clinicians that enhance or subtract from our optimal functioning and derail our best efforts? And, what are the personal tools we can use to help ourselves both in the moment and in the longer run? Fortunately, now there are many tools, and they go beyond the mindfulness and meditation practices that have been helpful to many. We present them.

The fifth dimension of Patient-Centered Care is the interactional dynamics between the patient's personality and that of the clinician that sometimes becomes a highly energized polarizing force, to everyone's disadvantage. For example, sometimes a pressured concern of the physician is heard by the patient as "scolding." The patient may react by agreeing in order to please and to stop the scolding, but then doesn't follow through in a quiet, angry rebellion. The more the clinician pushes, the more the patient entrenches. As you will see, clinicians can be trained to become aware of such interpersonal standoffs, and to avoid them and repair them if they occur.

MAINTAINING RELATIONSHIPS WHILE ALSO DIAGNOSING AND TREATING

Just because clinicians are diagnosing or providing treatment does not mean that relational dynamics within their patients (intrapersonal) and between them and their patients (interpersonal) are placed on hold. It all is happening at once. So-called left-brain functions are activated during diagnostic and treatment processes and that can be operating but not taking over the clinician's mind. Right-brain functions are involved in processing relationships and emotions, and are the social brain that functions as the clinician's interpersonal compass. We know these different aspects of brain functioning can be balanced.

By now, you might be asking how we clinicians can facilitate the crucial psychological processes in our patients and within ourselves while we simultaneously fulfill the tasks of diagnosis, treatment planning, and treatment. In this book we answer these questions and are specific about strategy and tactic.

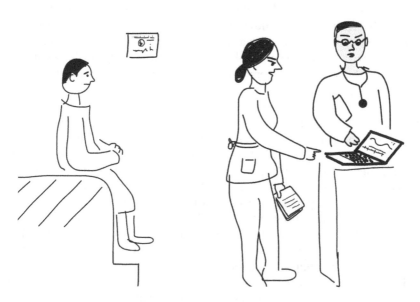

RELATIONSHIPS HAVE POWER

New time-saving administrative strategies in health care, we think, need to rest on the concrete foundation of a quantum leap in relationship science. It takes less time to build a relational foundation than many clinicians believe. By doing so, clinics and wellness programs will get "more mileage for their buck," a topic that public health professionals Bradley and Taylor addressed in their recent book *The American Health Care Paradox: Why Spending More Is Getting Us Less* (Bradley and Taylor, 2013).

Unfortunately, the use of contemporary science of relationship has lagged behind a nationwide push to implement various business-based, technical, and programmatic fixes of our health care problem—such as runaway costs, unwarranted variations in care, poor access, lack of integration, and failures to help people with chronic illness to change behavior. Patient testimonials and recorded observation indicate that clinicians more than ever before in the presence of their patients are making less eye contact and focusing more on their electronic record keeping. In 2008, an anonymous primary care physician at Harvard Medical School said, "We are encouraged to practice Patient-Centered Care (PCC) including Shared Decision Making, but what exactly are they and how exactly do we do it or teach it?" The American Nurses Association (ANA) agreed when they said that the idea of "patient-centered care has received more talk than action" (Hughes, 2011). Samples of the elements of PCC proposed by the International Patient Decision Aid Standards committee in 2009 are listed in the Appendix. As you can see, it is unfinished work in progress.

FITTING INTO THE LARGER CONTEXT OF HEALTH CARE

Our topic is but one dimension of direct health care, the relational dimension that impacts the ability of the patient to make effective use of specific services and that determine whether the clinician (physician, nurse, or allied health professional) will provide services in a fashion usable by the patient. We believe our relatively narrow topic is a powerful topic that influences the quality of life of clinicians and the willingness to embrace training in primary care and to remain in primary care practice without burning out. But we are not suggesting to look in one place for Nasruden's "lost key." The next larger context is all the rest of direct care technology and disease research, and the structure of care including care integration, information technology, and who pays. All of these are receiving attention and funding. The latest effort to reform medical care has been focused upon increasing access, integrating care systems, and fixing underinsurance—all necessary but unlikely to be sufficient if the power of interpersonal forces is lost because it is not integrated as a crucial portion of the mix.

This puts the expectations of this text (that of improving quality, outcome, and cost control through better relationship science) into a larger public health and social context. Let's be clear that to improve outcomes in the public's overall health is a larger task than improving patient adherence to prescriptions, their abilities to change lifestyle behaviors in chronic conditions, and to make effective medical decisions. And, it is more than enhancing the ability of clinicians to manage their own emotions that become barriers to patient care and their own well-being.

We recognize the overwhelming public health data showing that a significant factor of health outcome in the United States is the social determinants of heath (Bradley and Taylor, 2011). This aspect is addressed in *The American Health Care Paradox: Why Spending More Is Getting Us Less* and also in the 2013 Institute of Medicine report *Shorter Lives, Poorer Health*, which indicate that health parameters of U.S. citizens are much lower when compared with population segments with the same demographics in other industrialized nations (for example, middle-class income, similar ethnic backgrounds, and education). The social and nutritional determinants of health outcome continue to receive much less attention and funding in the United States—despite double the expenditures ($3,000 more per person in US dollars adjusted for purchasing power parity in 2009) and the significantly poorer health of Americans (ranking 25th) with similar demographics compared within 34 industrialized nations. The largest context of our topic is the *health* of our citizens, as defined by the WHO, "a state of complete physical, mental, and social well-being."

Decreasing care fragmentation, improving medical decision making and behavior change, and creating "medical home models" cannot alone offset the social determinates of poor outcomes and high costs. These are matters of government priorities. For these to change will depend upon awareness of our citizens; despite the huge amount of money we spend on direct medical care, we are not getting the healthy outcomes that many other countries enjoy. Just as schools were an entry point for the public health campaign against measles, diphtheria, and polio, we suggest that medical care and schools remain an underused entry point for enhancement of wellness. Both clinics and patients can be made more aware of the social, nutritional, and environmental causes of our poor health outcomes. "Made more aware" no longer means placing brochures and posters in the waiting room. It means to weave the public health information into the relational aspect of the care itself. The argument going on about cutting back on yearly medical checkups is a case in point and an idea that seems "penny wise and pound foolish." Both children and adults can benefit from well-visits to well-trained primary care health providers, as this is where wellness is maintained, especially with children, teenagers, and parents. Schools and their staff members are not trained or designated to be health facilities or health providers. We are not suggesting that they should be. The federal Departments of Education and Health and Welfare were separated long ago under the law, and many in Congress believe that the U.S. Department of Education could be eliminated. Those in Congress and some physicians who remain unclear about the value of yearly health checkups and the value of the school nurse are said to be misinformed and misguided (Dugdale, 2015).

Health behavior change then, in this book, is not just about the clinician facilitating the lifestyle change required in diabetes and cardiovascular disease. It includes public health initiatives *which include ongoing relationships*, not only informational booklets. This cannot be added to the responsibilities of practitioners or of school nurses, as currently trained and funded. But politics and government so far seem unable to initiate these changes efficiently. Shifts in individual and public attitudes, including health care professionals and their organizations, can, however, create pressure for increases in nutrition and wellness initiatives and increased social service expenditures rather than increased spending exclusively in the direct care arena.

Our topic only fills conceptual and educational gaps in the Patient-Centered Care model and its application. Also, we know that this project will be looking in only one place for the "lost key" unless it broadens the impact of relational science to the topic of wellness. The scope of our topic is health care and wellness. This phrase embeds the **WHO's** definition of *health*. If clinician's are willing and trained to make it so, the increased access to medical care promoted by the Patient Protection and Affordable Care Act and its inevitable iterations will become a public health entry point to enhance wellness in families and communities. This would go beyond clinicians' offices and hospitals. Health care could be designed to have a more powerful impact on the societal determinants of health outcomes such as nutrition. We recognize that clinicians cannot remedy the spending imbalance between health care and wellness services, but they can keep their perspective that the high cost of U.S. medical care is not mainly within medical care; it is about preserving wellness (Bradley and Taylor, 2013).

This book gives a broader meaning to the term *health behavior change*. It goes beyond changing lifestyle in chronic conditions. It includes health-related behavior change toward wellness—an area already known to primary care medicine and health coaching and where innovations are usually welcomed.

Pertinent history

Worldwide, in the past 20 years, considerable amounts of money and intellectual capital have already been expended to improve methods of health behavior change and medical decision making. We decided to share with you some history and the historical tensions between the various stakeholders. Otherwise, you may be surprised during one of your own projects to discover some standard you wish you had known about ahead of time. For example, the IOM sometimes hands down standards of practice that impact you because Congress listens to them. Or if you decide to create a patient decision aid (PDA), you may be asked to comply with rules such as the International Standards for Decision Aids (IPDAS). You can find reference to these in the Appendix.

Earlier changes in clinical training and practice

Douglas D. Bond, MD, Dean at Case Western Reserve (1959–1966), the first psychiatrist and psychoanalyst to be Dean of a large medical school, worked to modify medical education curricula. He was concerned that medical students were losing the personhood that motivated them to start medical school. He wanted to see if the ability of medical students to stay connected with their emotions like sadness and fear and if their capacity to be empathic could be maintained and increased throughout their clinical years. This was his effort to improve patient care in all of medicine. We view medical and nursing students as coming from their relational lives in high school and college, and perhaps some family tragedy during those years, entering professional school in touch with their feelings and with varying motivations. Revealed by our own personal journeys, from listening to our classmates and from conversations with current health profession students, the motivations have remained the same mixture of wishes: namely, to relieve human suffering, scientific interest and curiosity, and some degree of "this is one good way to earn a living." College and high school usually presented opportunities for nurturing personal psychological abilities to be with emotions, to be in intimate relationships, and to reveal vulnerability in sports—the capacities required for engaging patients. Focused on medical school, Bond's hypothesis was that these abilities were quickly submerged early in medical school by the immediate experiences of dissecting dead bodies, followed by cutting up organs, followed by a highly technical journey through biochemistry and other subjects and exams requiring heavy use of their left-brain functions. Douglas Bond wondered how to preserve and even improve over four years whatever ability existed in the entering medical student to be connected to their own emotions and those of their patients. These days, neuroscientists would call it an effort to "preserve social brain functions." Bond's work initiated some changes, such as being immediately assigned to spend part of their week following a well-grounded family practitioner. Changes in many medical school curricula continue to reflect his and other's ideas about this issue.

Enter technology, evidence-based information, and Shared Decision Making

Meanwhile, from 1965 to the present, in the halls of mainstream clinical care and academic cognitive psychology, the prevailing thinking has been that the waste in time and money in the direct patient care sector could be solved by increasing active patient involvement and improving the information base of informed consent for treatment. One of the biggest cost items needing remedy was identified as unwarranted variation in treatment. Physicians at Harvard and Dartmouth medical schools hoped that solutions would be realized by improving the quality of and access to evidence-based medical information and by increasing the sharing of information between physician and patient—"shared decision making" it was called. They were viewing the task, however, as primarily cognitive. Also, information technology, electronic records, and care integration were thought to be major pathways to a solution. This pathway, as important as it was, also narrowed the exploration for causes and skewed available research funding to cognitively driven projects. In some circles there continued to be little awareness of what has been missing, namely, a unifying integrative theory about emotions, cognition, and relationships and a set of validated strategies and tactics that could be taught. We believe that insufficient cross-discipline collaboration was one of the reasons for the missing pieces.

Several years of research in the science of medical decision making in the early 2000s had been conducted by the group in Ottawa (O'Connor and Edwards, 2001) before they realized that in addition to cognitive sharing evidence-based information that was pivotal in Shared Medical Decision Making (SMDM) were what they called the patient's "values and preferences." Their initial approach to including values and preferences in their protocol was to simply ask the patient or to give them a questionnaire, rather than use a skilled exploratory interview and check the inter-observer reliability. Meanwhile, psychologically trained clinicians working elsewhere in medicine were in doubt about the validity of approaches that used what a patient might say to a relative stranger on a questionnaire. Clinicians who were doing psychotherapy already knew that people's conflicting values and preferences don't settle out until they are facilitated to become aware of implicit emotional memories (Badenoch, 2008; Cozolino, 2010; Siegel, 2011). We were discovering that to make stable decisions, patients needed reliable information both from the *inside* of their minds (the different sets of values, emotions, memories, relational needs from different aspects of their personality) and from the *outside* (evidence-based information and the reactions of loved ones to their situation). Some workers associated with the group in Ottawa began looking at how dyadic relationships might impact decision making (LeBlanc et al., 2009). We discuss this dimension in later chapters.

Enter information transfer and emotions

For the first time, research was beginning to show that the emotional status of patients impacts the quality of information transfer, and to indicate new tactics to mitigate communication barriers. Many clinicians who had good access to evidence-based information discovered that their patients misconstrue what they say and don't assimilate what they hear accurately. The word *informed* in Informed Medical Decision Making (IMDM) promised a lot. A well-supported foundation was created in Boston to address the need to improve access to updated evidence-based information on a continuous basis. It was called Foundation for Informed Medical Decision Making (FIMDM, "fim-dim"). This group from Harvard and Dartmouth medical schools created an institution in Boston that gathered evidence-based information on many conditions and treatments and shaped it so patients could assimilate it. FIMDM began to create a series of PDAs in collaboration with a nationwide health coaching service, Health Dialog Inc. At the time of their major thrust, the role of the *patient's* emotions in information transfer and decision making was underappreciated. The role of the *clinician's* emotions was off everyone's radar except for psychotherapists and a few social psychologists associated with the Decision Science Lab at Harvard's Kennedy School (Lerner et al., 2015), neither of whom were part of FIMDM. The work of Lerner's group in the political and social sciences was in isolation from the remainder of decision making research and from behavioral medicine.

The role of emotions and relationships in effective information transfer was not (and still is not) a sufficient part of the conversation in the development of PDAs. This hurts those well-intentioned projects that foster the role of information as a prime goal while not giving the other human forces (emotions and relationship) a central place in their models. The assimilation of information is an interactive process involving cognition and emotions and relationship factors— all three. At this writing, the concepts and the skills of information transfer are not being widely taught in the training of physicians, nurses, and allied professionals (Jordon and Livingstone, 2013).

More of the same

Research was still showing persistent unwarranted variation in treatment across the country and showing that information transfer between clinician and patient was not optimal. Many centers competed, using models such as Shared Decision Making (SDM), Shared Medical Decision Making (SMDM), and IMDM. SMDM and IMDM in many circles seemed to overlap, but both implied that evidence-based information (on disease, treatment choices, and risk) was to be "transferred" and "shared" between clinician and patient. A course evolved in SDM and the curriculum was trademarked. During this time, however, surveys revealed that application of shared decision processes by doctors and nurse providers was sparse (Braddock, 2010). There are recent publications about the barriers to implementation (Friedberg et al., 2013). From our discussion with some of them, it seemed that providers who still didn't have access to PDAs had "too little time" to gather the latest evidence-based information and to meet with patients to share. The underlying message was that there was no training to navigate the territory of mutual sharing, and providers felt too uncomfortable to do it.

Enter more and more patient decision aid booklets and DVDs

As you will see from the list in the Appendix, a great deal of money and effort was spent creating PDAs in print and DVD form. It became an industry. Different centers began developing their own versions. One of the biggest efforts, as we have said, was funded by collaboration between FIMDM, Health Dialog, Inc., and third-party payers including Medicaid. They began producing PDA programs on conditions, like angina, breast cancer, and diabetes. Some of their PDAs were the main source of evidence-based information that existed. The downside was that the PDA programs were not available to providers or the general public. They were only available via Health Dialog to patient members of insurance companies that had contracted with Health Dialog to provide health coaching services.

So many enterprises began to create PDAs that a committee was formed in 2003 by workers in Canada and the United Kingdom to establish International Patient Decision Aid Standards (IPDAS). Ostensibly it was to protect the public and yet it seemed to have a competitive agenda. Many of us counseled against imposing such standards because it was premature until more study was done about the interplay of relationship dynamics, emotions, and cognition on the design and patterns of use of PDAs. Such research has been sparse. FIMDM in collaboration with Health Dialog produced about 30 useful PDAs. They are listed in the Appendix.

Challenges and barriers to implementation of Patient-Centered-Care (PCC)

As PCC, an ideal promoted by the IOM and ANA, was evolving, the biggest challenge was to build a science-based engine under the hood of this shiny new patient-care automobile. It took several years before anyone noticed that one thing was missing—despite the "symptom" that PCC and SDM were sparsely used by practitioners in their everyday medical care (Zikmund-Fisher et al., 2010). It was discovered that for practitioners to apply these ideal constructs required understanding of a psychology of personality and relationship that did not yet exist. There were many pleas for more research on the psychological aspects. Some research was done but seemed dominated by a cognitive paradigm despite what was already known about the role of emotions and relational dynamics.

In many ways medicine had prompted itself to practice ideas (PCC, SMDM, IMDM) without having widespread clarity about core theories, strategies, and tactics. This was an understandable result of political pressure and of the involvement of many different scientific specialties including primary care medicine, neuropsychology, nursing, clinical psychology, social psychology, experimental psychology, public health science, decision scientists in business, economics, government. This cross-disciplinary atmosphere was coupled with the fact that people in these specialties seldom were reading each other's publications and were not attending each other's scientific meetings.

For example, not until 2013 did the special interest groups (SIGs) on the psychology of decision making within the Society of Behavioral Medicine and the Society of Medical Decision Making (SMDM) start attending each other's scientific meetings. There is still too little cross-discipline collaboration between these scientists and several other groups, including decision scientists studying the role of emotion in decision making and psychotherapists working daily with patients over their medical decisions. Now the Society of Behavioral Medicine is playing a somewhat larger role toward integration of knowledge but still seems isolated from contemporary findings. The SMDM was created in an attempt to bring together specialists in many fields with that common interest. As one of their journal reviewers, I observed that the topics submitted for publication were heavily determined by the politics of funding from the public health and cognitive psychology arenas—important to include but not to the exclusion of psychology of emotions, interpersonal dynamics, and brain biology.

Increasing pressure to use incomplete models

For a while, rumor from Congress and NIH had it that several of the behavior change models and shared decision making might become practice requirements on which insurance payment would depend. It was unclear whether the pressure to implement was coming from the proponents of the models, from the IOM, or from members of Congress responding to special interests. This was premature, since 25 of the best of these models were unintegrated, incompletely validated by research, and without contemporary understanding of interpersonal psychology and neurobiology. These were disparate islands of study spread throughout academia that did not have sufficient understanding of each other's work. The good news was a trickle of publications indicating that collaboration had begun between principle developers of Motivational Interviewing (Miller and Rollnick, 2002) and Self-Determination Theory (Deci and Ryan, 1985).

Other possible causes of unwarranted cost were being overlooked. For example, the "demand" referred to above may be driven by normal patient anxiety to which clinicians yield because they have not been trained to mitigate anxiety in their patients. Also, "overtreatment" may occur because clinicians do not know how to soften the anxiety within them which drives overtreatment. A new type of "R&R" was needed: Research first, and then Remedy.

CURRENT SITUATION

Despite the avowed importance of all these topics, we could not locate a comprehensive textbook or a training program for doctors and nurses that made use of the last 15 years of advances in relationship psychology, interpersonal biology, and human development. Our survey did not reveal one text that informs the teaching of contemporary theory, strategy, and interview tactics suitable for the brief interpersonal encounters of health care. There seem to be no one-on-one interviewing demonstration videos. There continue to be enough statements about what should be done but little strategy or updated training as to how. The pervasive mentality of "information above all" continues to neglect the influences of the patients' beliefs, values, emotions, and memories and the influences within clinicians triggered by their vulnerability. A shortfall continues in funding and skilled researchers in these realms.

For research design, we did not find an intervention adherence scale for checking the fidelity of relationship-based interventions in medical care. This hampers prospective efficacy research.

Regarding the status of PDAs, you will see from the impressive list in the Appendix of topics on which decision aids were created that a great deal of money and effort was spent. They are important topics. The science of using the PDAs is missing. Their development continues at a slower pace, and updating all of them is a priority. As far as we know, currently they remain underused.

PCC, SDM, SMDM, and IMDM continue to evolve in somewhat separate fiefdoms. The IOM, without being specific as to theory and strategy, still recommends that health care embrace PCC, Medical Home, and SMDM. A new model designed by us for health coaching became available in 2013 called Self-aware Informational Nonjudgmental Health Coaching™ (Livingstone and Gaffney, 2013).

It is hard for us to understand how, without a textbook and without faculty skilled in this aspect of patient care, the gaps in this domain would ever be filled—the gaps that we believe will continue to negatively impact outcome, costs, and professional well-being, no matter what else is changed.

Throughout this volume we address when and how to interweave psychologically based processes of patient care into the concrete procedures of prevention, diagnosis, and treatment.

This process scientifically grounds the practice of mind-body medicine, holistic nursing, physician assistance, and health coaching. We hope the content of the coming chapters will provide you with fresh motivation and will help dislodge the log jam in understanding and teaching about relationships in health care.

Getting started: Patients' opening statements

VIEWING OF PATIENTS' OPENING STATEMENTS

Now is a good point for you to review the opening segments of the three demonstration interviews, the complete renditions of which you will access in later chapters. The beginning of interviews is the most powerful opportunity to start building the relationship platform, which facilitates everything else that needs to happen to reach your clinical goals of care or prevention. You may wish to listen several times so that you can imagine yourself in the room as the interviewer. Below we tell you something about each patient that the interviewing clinician knew before starting so that you are closer to the clinician's level of information.

As you read the next chapters about theory, strategy, and tactics of interviewing, you will have the beginning of each interview to keep in mind. You could speculate as to what your opening choices of direction might be, before you view in the full demonstration the choices that our clinician made.

BEHAVIOR CHANGE: INTRODUCTORY INFORMATION ABOUT MARY LOU (SMOKING)

This is a 67-year-old woman who has been smoking cigarettes since age 10, whose mother died from COPD. She has been told the risk factors by her doctor and has used nicotine patches, gums, and oral medication to try to quit. Her primary care physician has referred her to the nurse health coach in the practice to help her stop smoking.

This video may be accessed at: http://goo.gl/WNtjnK

Writing down your plan

After viewing the opening statements, you could write down what you would say next, based on some strategy and theory, if you have one, and your intuition.

We expect that your initial answers will shift and more answers will emerge as you read on about theory and strategy. Notice any reactions you may have to the diagnosis and his or her situation.

INFORMATION INTERWEAVE: INTRODUCTORY DATA ABOUT JOE (TYPE II DIABETES)

This is a 55-year-old man who has recently been diagnosed with type II diabetes and whose mother died at age 56 from complications of diabetes. His primary care physician has referred him for health coaching to help alter his lifestyle not only because of the new diagnosis but also because this man suffers from several other chronic conditions (osteoarthritis of hip and knees and cardiovascular disease). He has not been making use of evidence-based information the physician repeatedly has given to him.

This video may be accessed at: http://goo.gl/OrjXc5

Writing down your plan

After viewing the opening statements, you could write down what you would say next, based on some strategy and theory, if you have one, and your intuition. We expect that your initial answers will shift and more answers will emerge as you read on about theory and strategy. Notice any internal reactions you may have to his situation diagnosis.

MEDICAL DECISION MAKING: INTRODUCTORY INFORMATION ABOUT KARIN (BREAST CANCER)

This is the first interview between a hospital outpatient oncology social worker (C) trained in relational science (health coaching) and a patient (K) who, 5 days before, heard she has breast cancer. Her physician had already told her plentiful evidence-based information about treatment choices.

This video may be accessed at: http://goo.gl/vPivTx

Writing down your plan

After viewing the opening statements, you could write down what you would say next, based on your intuition and any theory and strategy you might already know. We expect that your initial answers will shift and more answers will emerge as you read on. Notice any internal reactions you may have to her situation.

PART **2**

Knowledge

3

Past health psychology and neuroscience (prior to the early 1990s)

It ain't what you don't know that gets you into trouble. It's what you know for sure that just ain't so.

Mark Twain

INTRODUCTION

Many concepts believed to be true from 1950 to 1990 about behavior change, decision making, and information communication do not fit recent scientific findings and observed realities of how people function. Some aspects of the old, however, are worth preserving, and we have incorporated them in our model-building. For example, one condition for successful information transfer is to shape information to the educational level and cognitive style of the target audience.

We recommend paying close attention to this chapter and Chapters 4 and 5 because they contain pieces of the puzzle used to build new strategies and tactics for Patient-Centered Care in Chapters 6, 7, and 8.

The world of health psychology models used in medicine and nursing has been divided into three realms: behavior change, decision making, and communication of information. These realms have been treated as if they are distinctly separate entities, and the communication topic was seen almost exclusively through a cognitive lens. Emotions, if considered, were seen to be a hindrance to rationality that needed to be side-stepped. As you will see later, in fact, these three realms of clinical activity interact and depend upon common psychological processes that involve emotions, beliefs, cognitions, and memories of past experience.

Focusing on the personhood of the patient is not new. Sir William Osler (1849–1919) and Francis Peabody (1927) wrote on the subject. The detailed scientific theory, strategies, and interviewing tactics for doing so, however, are quite new, although intermediate models in nursing made a robust start (Dossey, 2009).

It always has been difficult even for experienced clinicians to facilitate patients to make enduring changes to health behaviors and make stable medical decisions. Clinical experience, rote methodologies, or computer programs have been disappointing approaches to improve this area of practice. We now view this domain as basic relationship science in doctoring and nursing that can be taught.

Before introducing you in Chapters 4 and 5 to the many scientific advances, here we summarize 10 models selected from our survey of several dozen models created since 1950 which were and still are used in medicine, nursing, and health coaching. We have called them *prior models*. Many of them are about behavior change, decision making, and holistic nursing. Others present concepts from the various other realms, such as mindfulness medicine, which lend valuable concepts relevant to interviewing processes in health care. In general, a huge amount of intellectual and financial capital has been invested on these models over the years.

You may be asked still to use portions of these past models in your clinical work, for example, for smoking cessation, eating disorders, or lifestyle change, to use the updated Motivational Interviewing model first created in 1989, or for a patient with a high-risk decision crisis to use a Shared Decision Making protocol. As you will see, some of the strategies from these older models are integrated into the new model building in Chapters 6 through 8. We hope that by using this text you will be able, on your own, to update older models if you are given them to use.

We believe the priorities of Congress, governmental agencies, and funding sources have determined the focus of research attention for the last 65 years. Public health concerns about TB, smoking, and alcohol abuse drove the agenda early on. Later, other health issues took the spotlight, such as noncompliance with medical recommendations, prevention of hepatitis and AIDS, and more recently the discovery of unwarranted variation in treatment and the lifestyle changes needed for costly chronic conditions such as diabetes, heart disease, and arthritis. The work, therefore, had a public health and disease-model focus and the solutions have tended to be externally applied without much attention to inner and interpersonal psychological forces.

Understandably, health professionals began to apply in other domains of medical care those health models already being used in the public health approaches to the addictions. This was done despite incomplete efficacy research. They used what was available. Also, the vast experience in psychotherapy with health behavior change was not made part of the conversation in general medical care. This was a loss. There seem to be three reasons for the latter: the strategies and tactics from psychotherapy were not translated for use outside a psychotherapy context; clinicians and researchers were from many different disciplines working in isolation; and Western culture had a bias that rational thinking (the cognitive realm) was the only tool for controlling emotions and the "unpredictability" of relationships.

To permit you to make easy choices as you read, first the models are listed along with occasional comments. Some sections are titled "Going Deeper," in which each model is discussed as to its nature and scientific status with citations to references. This allows you to return to these topics as needed without interrupting the flow of the book toward something new.

HEALTH-RELATED MODELS IN USE

Below is a list of models about behavior change, decision making, and other topics of importance. A model was chosen because it is pertinent to strategy-building for patient care, and because it is either popular or some efficacy research was conducted on it. The models are grouped by their primary focus, for example: health behavior change, medical decision making, health communication, standards of patient care, theories or practices regarding human development, coping, and growth. The order of the list is without implication as to their validity.

A more complete list of existing models of behavior change is located in the Appendix. Our sincere apologies to the proponents of theories, methods, or models we have omitted. Please refer to the Framework (p. xxxii) for how I have assessed their scientific status. Also, you may find the Glossary helpful.

List of models

SEVEN SELECTED BEHAVIOR CHANGE MODELS

Motivational Interviewing (MI) A *continuum* model of *strategies and tactics* in the *monolithic* paradigm

Transtheoretical Model and Stages of Change (TTM-SOC) A *stage* model of *strategies* in the *monolithic* paradigm

Self-Determination Theory (SDT) A *continuum* model of *to-be-validated hypotheses* in the *monolithic* paradigm

Self-Efficacy Theory (SET) A *continuum* model of social learning theory

Health Belief Model (HBM) A *continuum* model

Precaution Adoption Process Model (PAPM) A *stage* model of *strategies* in the *monolithic* paradigm

Theory of Planned Behavior (TPB) A modernized theory of reasoned action

FOUR DECISION MAKING MODELS (all *monolithic*)

Shared Decision Making (SDM)

Expected Utility Calculations

Statistical Aids and Decision Analysis

Clinical Intuition

INFORMATION TRANSFER MODELS (all *monolithic*)

Information Communication Models (ICMs)

Communication Guide for Parents and Pediatricians

HOLISTIC AND INTEGRAL NURSING MODEL (*monolithic*) Scope and Standards of Practice

TRADTIONAL PSYCHOTHERAPY MODELS (*monolithic*)

MINDFULNESS MODELS (*monolithic*)

ATTACHMENT THEORY OF RELATIONAL DEVELOPMENT (*monolithic*)

NARRATIVE MEDICINE (*monolithic*)

TRADITIONAL FUNCTIONAL NEUROANATOMY

SEVEN SELECTED BEHAVIOR CHANGE MODELS

Motivational interviewing (MI) (Miller and Rollnick, 2012)

At the time it was introduced in 1988, MI was a refreshing change in the field of behavior change toward strong consideration of the relationship between clinician and patient. In the view of many workers, Rollnick included, the model has many useful features yet has been in need of more theory about intrapersonal dynamics and clearer interpersonal tactics. I think that random, controlled, *comparative* efficacy research with fidelity checks of the interventions are also important to add.

Originally supported by the Australian drug and alcohol agencies, for many years it was the only interpersonal model for interviewing addicted people. MI changed the treatment of addiction to a more personal and nonjudgmental dynamic between clinician and patient. More specifically, MI contained a framework of strategies (listed below) called by the proponents "an amalgam of interactional elements used systematically" which clinicians found helpful as a guide to move away from the confrontational and moralistic interactions and threats of negative consequences prevalent at the time in behavior change practice.

Although MI applies many elements used for 50 years in traditional psychoanalytic therapies and Rogerian psychotherapies (both are also **monolithic** models), the model shaped them to facilitate behavior change. Miller and Rollnick did this by using an interpersonal context of communication, which elicits the person's thinking about reasons for and advantages of making a change in health-related behaviors. In our view, this is primarily a cognitive pathway to change, while making use of empathy to support the patient to think differently about their addictive desires and behavior. How the empathy tactic is actually used by clinicians is open to question.

It put the **external** relationship behavior of the professional with the patient at the center of behavior change. It was a **continuum model**, which assumes that features of the **external** interaction, for example, the use of empathy and rolling with resistance, will determine the timing of internally driven behavior change. Later in its evolution the authors incorporated a **strategic stage model**, TTM-SOC, which defines a linear set of stages through time. (See Glossary and also TTM-SOC below.)

The MI model recommends using **eight motivational strategies**: (1) giving advice, (2) removing barriers to change, (3) providing choices, (4) decreasing desirability of the status quo, (5) practicing empathy, (6) providing feedback, (7) clarifying goals, and (8) active helping (e.g., reminder calls). It offers **five intervention principles** to be applied in an "adjusted recipe used at decisive moments": (1) express empathy, (2) clarify and develop discrepancy (present behavior that doesn't fit their stated goals), (3) avoid argumentation, (4) roll with resistance, and (5) support self-efficacy.

The various interpersonal tactics a clinician might learn and use to perform these items effectively was not clarified or demonstrated. How clinicians are to go about applying the eight MI strategies and five intervention principles (how

The transtheoretical model is also known by term *stages of change.* There is a popular book, *Changing for Good,* by Prochaska et al. published first in 1994.

Originally supported by the Australian Drug and Alcohol Office, TTM-SOC was helpful to many counselors who wanted some way to be strategic with trying to evoke change and with tracking "change" process for people with smoking cessation in psychotherapy. It provided a structure of procedure where there was none. That makes it a welcome heuristic, not a validated theory. It was eventually paired with MI and broadly applied, for example, in programs involving exercise, AIDS, and mammography utilization (Rakowski et al., 1996). The model's Stages of Change are as follows:

Pre-contemplation is the stage at which there is no intention (in thought) being paid to changing behavior in the foreseeable future. The proponents say that many individuals in this stage are unaware or under-aware of their problems.

Contemplation is the stage in which people are aware that a problem exists, are thinking about overcoming it, but have not yet made a commitment to take action.

Preparation is a stage that combines intention and behavioral criteria. Individuals in this stage are intending (thinking) to take action in the next month and have unsuccessfully taken action in the past year.

Action is the stage in which individuals modify their behavior, experiences, or environment in order to overcome their problems. Action involves the most overt behavioral changes and exhibits commitment of time and energy.

Maintenance is the stage in which people work to prevent relapse and consolidate the gains attained during the action stage. (For addictive behaviors this stage extends from six months onward.)

The stage of change is assessed by conversations or questionnaires with the patient. Our analysis of sound recordings of clinical encounters that use SOC illuminates the inconsistency with which clinicians assess the stage their client or patient is in. Medical students in their behavioral health rotations continue to be asked to learn these stages but say they are confused when the patient's process of successful change does not follow them.

Self-determination theory (SDT) (Deci and Ryan, 1985, 2002; Ryan and Deci, 2000)

This is one of the most comprehensive attempts at modeling the process of motivation to change. It is quite confirming of contemporary theory that Ryan and Deci, working at the University of Rochester, New York, sensed that the mind seemed to be "compartmentalized" in a fashion different than the id, ego, and superego of psychoanalysis. They saw it as compartments of "beliefs"—a cognitive concept to be sure—but on the edge of a multiplicity concept of mind which Carl Jung was also positing. Now many workers (Assagioli, 1975; Schwartz, 1987, 1995; Stone and Winkleman 1985, 1989; Rowan, 1990) view that the compartments are not just beliefs but are "full personalities," *each* with its distinct set of beliefs, emotions, behavioral tendencies, historical memories, and role within the person's personality. This view of personality organization is supported independently by literature and the arts, observations from a huge psychotherapy experience. It makes sense that Ryan and Deci independently observed something similar.

SDT, although still basically based on a monolithic paradigm of personality, brought a much-needed emphasis on internal psychological processes of motivation to behavior change theory. It is more grounded in existing knowledge and theories in human psychological development than most other health psychology models in the list in the Appendix. Ryan and Deci's theory had the status of not-yet-proven hypotheses and a few not-yet-proven strategies for improving internal motivation without specific tactics of application. Their basic theoretical assumption is that "the most enduring and robust motivation to changing behavior is an internal psychological matter in a dynamic relationship with external variables." They give examples of what they mean (Deci and Ryan, 2002).

The proponents of SDT have focused on internal motivation and what strategies might promote it. The theory, SDT, is shy on interviewing **tactics**. They posit that all behaviors lie along a continuum ranging from those that are externally regulated to those that arise from self-regulation. Ryan, a clinical experimental psychologist, Deci, a social psychologist, and Geoffrey Williams in the Department of Medicine at University of Rochester, have produced a voluminous literature and are influential in theoretical and research domains in health care, education, forensic work, and sports. Historically these workers began by focusing on filling conceptual/theoretical gaps existing at the time about the psychology of change and motivation more than they were attempting to formulate clinical strategies and tactics to help people change, as did SOC and MI.

SDT, when contrasted with SOC and MI , is a **continuum** theory (see Glossary) of behavior change focused strongly on factors internal to the individual and the relationship between internal and external experience. For example, Ryan and Deci conceptualized that there is a continuum of motivation to change a behavior ranging from *external motivation* (for example, external rewards and external negative consequences could motivate change) to *internal sources of motivation,* which they call *autonomy or self-regulation* (for example, one's internal values and sense of competency could motivate change, making it an internal self-esteem issue). They make distinctions between what they view as the most powerful and stable form of internal motivation called *identification,* defined as a truly self-determined, autonomous self-regulation based on positive personally valued outcomes, and a type of internal motivation called *introjected motivation* controlled by self-esteem-related contingences, which they believe is a less stable and "ambivalent" in nature. Whatever distinctions they were implying need further research and development to become validated hypotheses of a comprehensive theory of behavior change.

Ryan and Deci did described **strategies**. There are two major pathways specific to SDT which they hope will promote change: *autonomy support* and *competency support*. Their idea is to support clients to use the *internal* sources that they can bring to the situation like "following internal tendencies and needs" related to the following:

Motivation: affective and cognitive aspects
Autonomy: freedom from external control

Connectedness/relational: experienced by both parties
Competency: experienced, perceived, and gaining new skills
Reflective capacities: mindfulness of what is blocking

The latter has been one of their main interests. They also recommend reducing external barriers to change in the family and health care system.

These strategies are clearly stated, are on a reasonable level of abstraction as strategies, but would benefit greatly from translation into specific observable tactics that can be learned and validated for efficacy in comparative studies. The tactics, for example, at to how a clinician would provide competency support in an interview with a patient, are not elaborated or sufficiently specific. The skills of these observable tactics could be taught to, and learned by, health clinicians.

We do not believe formulaic tactics are effective, for they run the risk of not being attuned to the patient. There is a level of specificity, however, that can be used flexibly and personally while still remaining adherent to the strategy and theory to which it is linked—as we will discuss in Chapter 8. It would need to be demonstrated in interview recordings with different types of patients.

Ryan, in a personal communication in 2009, stated that "cognitive aspects have been overplayed in the field of behavior change." We agree with him and expressed that in addition to cognitions, we had discovered clinically that the role of emotions and relationships are pivotal. We also encouraged his group to integrate cognitive, emotional, relational, and cultural dimensions in their theories and research. We suggested that they extend what they call "compartmentalization of the mind" from compartments of "belief" (a cognitive viewpoint) to compartments of "full personalities" (each with a different set of emotions, cognitions, beliefs, memories). There are several ongoing SDT application projects in various disease and problem entities, utilizing health counselors whom they have trained. They monitor their delivery for the sake of internal fidelity checking and for supervision and training. They measure SOC but do not find it useful.

Some theoreticians and experienced clinical interviewers think it is challenging to imagine how the seemingly vague interpersonal tactics of MI could be used with validity to enhance SDT theory and strategy (Markland et al., 2005). We believe MI would be enhanced more by use of the theory from SDT than the opposite. On the other hand, most SDT strategies about behavioral motivation would be enhanced in both theory and tactics—by applying personality multiplicity theory and the strategies and tactics of both the Psychology of the Selves (Stone) and the IFS model (Schwartz). You will find a discussion about integration of models in Chapter 6.

Self-efficacy theory (SET) (Bandura)

Albert Bandura was born in Canada, a social psychologist at Stanford, a leader since the 1960s in the school of social cognitive theory, and a proponent of social learning theory. His work on SET has been vigorously applied in the real world of health care by Loreg (2006), Lenz and Shortridge-Baggett (2002), and others. The SET approach is focused on **internal**—mainly the cognitive determinants of behavior. It is in a **monolithic paradigm of personality**, was evolved **both bottom up and top down,** is a heavily researched **continuum theory,** and is a set of **strategies** of intervention *without* comprehensive clinical interviewing tactics.

Historically, this almost exclusive emphasis by Bandura on the role of internal "thinking" as a determinant of behavior in general, and health behavior in particular, was driven by an opposition to the operant conditioning of behaviorist psychologists. The latter believed that thoughts were separate entities from behaviors and an unnecessary deviation from their positive reinforcement intervention strategy, the operant conditioning paradigm of the behaviorist movement. This conditioning approach is still in exclusive use with mixed success in some venues, for example in some residential programs for children with developmental behavior disorders. However, Bandura believes that people's assessments of self-efficacy are the main determinants of behavior and are the outcome of "reflective thoughts" about an experience; that is, the power of the experience depends on how it is processed and the meaning put on it (Bandura, 1997). His book (Bandura, 1997) gives you access to a body of work starting in 1963.

When compared to psychodynamic/psychoanalytic theory, which tended until the last 15 years to emphasize internal emotional and cognitive processes, social learning theory and self-efficacy theory was a construct focused on external social influences and internal cognitive determinants of behavior, but shy on giving emotions, relationships, and past history sufficient attention. Contemporary theorists, including psychoanalysis, would now say that (1) the determinants of behavior are multifaceted (emotions, beliefs, memory, body sensations carried by personality), internal and external, interpersonal and interactive in a dynamic system, and (2) interventions are powerful when they reflect this systemic understanding.

SET is not just about what people **think** about their efficacy. The proponents included additional dimensions: their expectations of outcome, their short- and long-term aspirations, and their perceived personal and situational impediments to behavior change. But, self-efficacy is seen as the *biggest determinant* of how people make their choices to act. Bandura posited that the self-efficacy a person perceives within themselves contributes to their performance over and above their skill development. Those workers who view the mind as one monolithic entity and who assess "perception of self-efficacy" by asking their subject a series of questions will think the answers are the valid answers. But, those who understand that people normally have ambivalence about changing behavior find that different personality parts drive ambivalence and that different parts of the personality of one person have differing assessments of that person's efficacy. All are true in a sense. If the research interviewer is not trained in interviewing in a multiplicity paradigm, the results would not have the necessary reproducibility and validity (Chapter 14).

Regarding clinical strategies, Bandura described a series of strategies which he believes promotes health behavior change. He grouped a cluster under the heading of "self-efficacy enhancers," which, taken individually, have been used clinically for many years before SET but not called anything special. Some people find this categorization helpful for teaching and structuring interviews. Bandura

(1996) stated that he was searching for explanatory cognitive mechanisms that would foster the creation and implementation of modeling influences for interventions. He described four subprocesses of modeling, and with one of them, motivational processes, he described three types of incentive for motivation: direct, vicarious, and self-administrated. SDT, developed later, has a similar ring.

All of the detailed heuristics of SET are useful theory for some workers even though **beliefs** are a primary focus and **modeling** is a primary intervention. Bandura's idea of a tactic of application of his modeling strategy, for example, Anna Freud who introduced the concept of Developmental Lines which she observed to be universal and not based on modeling (*The Anna Freud Tradition*, 2011).

Although SET is a masterful and voluminous set of abstract concepts about cognitive subfunctions and social learning mechanisms, which was an important balancer of theories then and now, we will be integrating other significant determinants of health behavior evident from clinical observation and research, such as emotions, childhood memory, internal interactions between parts of the personality, and relationship dynamics.

Health belief model (HBM)

The HBM was developed in the 1950s, before Bandura's SET, by social psychologists (Hochbaum, 1958) working in the U.S. Public Health Service because of poor utilization of free TB screening programs. Later it was applied to people's responses to symptoms and diagnoses of illnesses. HBM is an **internal** belief-based, **continuum** model of health behavior change, and in a **monolithic** paradigm of personality. It is basically a confluence of various *social learning theories* that posit that **reinforcements and consequences** are the major determinants of behavior, not physiological drives and cognitive-behavioral theory. The theory posits that behavior is a function of the subjective and expected value of an outcome. They call it a "value expectancy theory."

In 2004, Victor Strecher, a PhD in health behavior at the University of Michigan School of Public Health (Streacher et al. 2008) frequently recommended (like Rosenstock et al. had in 1988) that the concept of self-efficacy (Bandura, 1997) be added to the HBM model's five operating concepts in order to help it fit lifestyle change programs aimed at such unhealthy behaviors as smoking, overeating, and a sedentary lifestyle. This gave HBM six determining factors in behavior change related to how people **think**: (1) perceived susceptibility, (2) perceived severity, (3) perceived benefits of an advised action/treatment, (4) perceived barriers, (5) cues that promote actions (education, media, etc.), and (6) perceived self-efficacy. *Perceived susceptibility* is thought by HBM to be a particularly strong determinant of health behavior.

This model has been elaborated into a colorful and complex flow chart. This does not alter that fact that it embraces both a cognitive and a monolithic paradigm of the mind while being shy on emotions and relationship factors. We see major flaws in the model itself and in the research. Put simply, even if a conscious belief can be statistically correlated with a given health-related behavior, an alternative explanation of cause and effect is that both that belief and that behavior are observational derivatives of a set of underlying, observable, internal factors operating in a biologically driven systems context. This would make contemporary neurobiological good sense. Workers associated with HBM are Becker (1974), Janz and Becker (1984), Rosenstock et al. (1988).

Precaution adoption process model (PAPM) (Weinstein et al., 1998b)

This is a **cognitively based stage** theory, in a **monolithic** paradigm, about individual preventive behavior. The proponents posit that a series of stages is moving along a continuum of thinking and action between ignorance and completed preventive action. They believe that different interventions are needed, depending upon the stage a person is moving toward. The model was first tested in people willing to test for radon in their homes. They used an algebraic equation to come up with a number that stands for the likelihood a person will adopt such a preventive action. Any intervention that increases the value of the number is considered to increase the chance that the person will take action. Interventions are assessed in this fashion. It has been applied to prevention programs in hepatitis C (Hammer et al., 2003) and osteoporosis (Blalock et al., 1996).

This model adds two new stages to TTM-SOC (summarized earlier). They distinguish between people who are unaware of an issue, stage 1, from those who know something about it but never actively thought about it. Also, people who have decided not to adopt the precaution (in stage 4) are differentiated from those who are not taking action because they have not yet given it serious consideration. All these refinements presumably come from their interviews and questionnaires of subjects they tested. They also identified a variable that seemed to influence whether people proceed through the seven stages, for example, *perceptions of personal vulnerability* seemed crucial to move from stage 3 to stage 5. *Situational obstacles* were seen to influence moving from stage 5 to stage 6—adopting the preventive behavior.

It is hard to know whether it would be useful for health professionals to think in stages and whether clinical researchers would be successful identifying specific and universal variables that facilitate moving from stage to stage within one health condition or one health situation. When this type of heuristic seems helpful, we hope those who find it useful will do the efficacy research that is needed.

We question the current value of pursuing this cognitive, stage approach, since there may well be new opportunities to hypothesize and conduct research on a broader dimension—a dimension that integrates cognitions, emotions, relationships, and childhood experiences, and is likely to be testable in many personalities across many health conditions.

Theory of planned behavior (TPB) (Ajzen, 1991)

TPB, a modernized version of Theory of Reasoned Action, is a social cognitive **hypothesis** (as yet to be fully tested) that people's intentions and attitudes are the immediate determinant of behavior, and that intentions (assessed in a **mono-lithic** paradigm) are determined jointly by attitudes toward the behavior and perceived social pressures to engage in the behavior. Ajzen (1991) sees *beliefs and the thinking system as primary determinants of behavior* and do not deal with the role of emotions and relationships. This model is a good example of theory evolved from an abstract **top-down** process. The key component to this model is behavioral intent, guided by three considerations: (1) beliefs about likely outcome, (2) beliefs about normative expectations of others and motivation to comply with those expectations, and (3) beliefs about factors that may facilitate or block performance of the behavior.

One proponent, Martin Fishbein, PhD, who died in 2009, became the founding director of the Health Communication Division of the Annenberg Public Policy Center at University of Pennsylvania and was focused on populations, theoretical matters, measurements of attitudes and values, and consumer psychology. The other proponent of TPB is Icek Ajzen, PhD, is a cognitive–behavioral social psychologist at the University of Massachusetts, Amherst.

Their orientation is that systems of beliefs are the major determinants of behaviors in populations of people. Followers of this model have devised a questionnaire for assessing and weighing beliefs of populations, for example of people with a particular disease. Their descriptions of theory and strategy are intellectual, intricate, and mathematical, requiring the learning of a specialized elaborate language, some of which seems motivated by the hope that better validity would be attained through precise detail. Hale, Householder, and Greene (2002) believe that this model was developed out of frustration with use of the SOC and other behavioral research which downplayed the influence of beliefs and intentions. Their interventions are at a social level, for example, using mass-delivered social persuasion. Interpersonal **strategies and tactics** are not within the domain of this model. You may hear of this model when public health issues about behavior change are discussed.

FOUR DECISION MAKING MODELS

a. **Shared Decision Making (SDM)** (for patients and clinicians)
b. **Expected Utility Calculations** (for clinicians and patients)
c. **Statistical Aids and Decision Analysis** (for clinicians and patients)
d. **Clinical Intuition** (for clinicians primarily)

Shared decision making (SDM)

THE TOPIC

To create an "informed and value-based partnership" between clinicians, patients, and their loved ones is an important ideal. The implementation of this idea takes a deeper scientific understanding about human personality and relationships than many who promote SDM previously imagined.

SDM is a high-profile topic in patient care, and it spans both sides of our time definition of past and present. It was being "designed by committee" since before 1990 and was created as an ideal without an interpersonal or intrapersonal psychological component. Sharing of credible information and making decisions was thought to be a relatively straightforward process between doctor and patient. It was thought that evidence-based information and rational reasoning by patient and clinician together would provide a positive outcome. The fact that interpersonal dynamics and emotions are a necessary aspect of the process (not just the aspect that blocks it) was not considered, despite the September 1848 brain damage case about Phineas Gage, The American Crowbar Case (Harlow and Martyn, 1868), Damasio's subsequent work on decision making (Damasio, 1994, 1999), and research by Jennifer Leaner at Harvard's Kennedy School Decision Lab showing the pivotal and necessary role of emotion in decision making (Lowenstein and Lerner, 2003).

Initially it was believed that better access to more credible information would reduce unwarranted variations in treatment and bring better outcomes. This belief has declined somewhat. A laudable campaign was launched by the Boston-based Foundation for Informed Medical Decision Making (FIMDM) and others to accumulate and update evidence-based information about all the major diagnostic and treatment choices patients were making, for example, whether to have a prostate specific antigen (PSA) test and whether to take the radiation or surgical route for prostate cancer. Increasing public and professional access to credible information was needed but, as you will learn, was necessary but insufficient to realize the ideals of SDM.

The Institute of Medicine (IOM) of the National Academy of Sciences set the tone in the famous report *Crossing the Quality Chasm: A New Health System for the 21st Century*. It defined patient-centeredness as "providing care that is respectful of and responsive to individual patient preferences, needs, and values, and ensuring that patient values guide all clinical decisions" (IOM, 2011). This sounds very nice, but the question remained as to how to accomplish that. Some clinicians see shared decision making as the pinnacle of patient-centered care (Barry, 2012).

Despite the theoretical and strategic incompleteness of SDM, practitioners are encouraged currently by the IOM to apply its two elements: (1) the patient is invited into sharing and learning the same evidence-based information to which their clinician has access and is encouraged to discuss it, and (2) the patient is asked for their personal values and preferences regarding choices in the decision. As you will see, both elements are more psychologically based than they at first appear. For example, regarding the first element, sharing information with patients does not mean they will assimilate and use it, even if they might nod their heads in affirmation. Even when the information is matched to their intellectual style, assimilation is still determined by the patient's degree of psychological receptivity. As you progress in this book, you will see that emotions and inner conflict block assimilation of information, and that this can be remedied by a clinician with training. Chapters 6 and 7 and the interview demonstrations and annotations of Chapter 9 cover more of this topic.

The second element, including the patient's values and preferences, is a more complex arena than is information transfer. Although in later chapters this aspect will be discussed at length, stated briefly, normally people's major subpersonalities hold quite different values and preferences (Schwartz, 1995). One could ask,

"Which values are *the* ones to use in making the decision?" The answer is that all of them need to be considered. For both clinician and patient to accept quickly that the patient has found his or her "true" values and preference is a misleading notion. Clinical observation shows that it saves time for patients to first explore their mixed emotions and mixture of values, especial if they conflict, rather than somehow selecting what to give voice to and have that be taken as an enduring truth. The clinician must be willing not to pressure the patient to find an answer. For example, our voluminous collection of recorded clinician–patient encounters of experienced clinicians demonstrates that, despite having been trained in the concepts and given a list of the SDM elements to apply, when they start talking with a live patient, they quickly discover gaps in their interpersonal training. Their own feelings get in the way. Their own preferences and attitudes leak through. They describe their attempts to implement SDM as frustrating, confusing, and uncomfortable.

This experience supports our opinion that the SDM strategy and training programs need more interdisciplinary development. We hope this text provides a new pathway for that.

CURRENT SCIENTIFIC STATUS

Through the lens of our framework, SDM (and its iterations) is a set of operational **cognitive** strategies that evolved from the bottom up in a **monolithic** paradigm of personality. Emotions are not processed even when considering patients' values. It conceptualizes the decision process as a **continuum**—except that a stage model was created for adults of lower literacy (McCaffery et al., 2010). (Check back in this chapter to the section on "Seven selected behavior change models" if you want clarity this issue.) SDM, although it is seen as an individual matter between provider and patient, is shy on psychologically informed relationship theory, strategy, and interviewing tactics. We believe SDM is in a **midstage of evolution**, not ready to be successfully rolled out, and for this reason is underused (Zikmund-Fisher, 2010). Despite this, we have listed it as a prior model because of the national and international pressure for clinicians to apply its two basic elements mentioned above. Elwyn et al. (2012) more specifically outlined the steps clinicians can learn. Among the 12 authors of this publication is Stephen Rollnick, one of the creators of Motivational Interviewing.

REVIEW AND DEVELOPMENT

We are sharing more details of this complex history to lower the risk of your getting caught up in repeating it, and also so you will recognize the names of the models you may use.

Until the late 1980s medical decisions were made by clinicians inside their heads or in discussion with colleagues, and then advice was given to the patient. Clinicians tried to "settle" most concerns or questions voiced by patients by representing the "facts." This was a system that some called paternal. The doctor had the knowledge, and the patient yielded to that. The holistic nursing movement, however, left us a different model of care (Dossey, 2009; Bark, 2011). Paternalistic-style medical care began to be replaced over the past two decades by patient participation. Not only did patients begin to gain increased access to their medical records, but a trend began that encouraged physicians to actively involve their patients in medical decisions affecting them. Informed consent became an issue. Physicians and many nurses, however, had no training to navigate this territory.

This expectation of patient participation was supported by comparative research on the use of decision aids (O'Connor et al., 2003), which showed that patients who are informed and involved in their health care demonstrate enhanced decision making across several outcome measures without an increase in the duration of consultations. The outcome measures included reduced decision conflict, reduction in indecision, increased question-asking during consultation sessions, and increased patient satisfaction.

Also, expectations of patient participation were prompted by the concern over the discovery of unwarranted costly variations in treatment (O'Connor et al., 2004). O'Connor and Llewellyn-Thomas stressed a need to confirm "the feasibility of building and sustaining patient decision-support systems that improve decision quality." The question is, "quality for whom?" This work addressed important external public health issues but was not focused on the internal psychological and relational dimensions upon which at least some aspects of quality depend.

Led by Professor Annette O'Connor, a University of Ottawa doctor in nursing who established the Ottawa Health Decision Center, a movement started in 2006 to include the "patient's values" in SDM. Perhaps more than her group realized, this addition implied a more sophisticated and psychologically driven process between clinicians and patients. To mitigate the complexities of human psychology, it is understandable that many workers tried straightforward approaches for including patients' values—such as, "Just ask the patient" or "Use a questionnaire." Unbeknownst to the developers of SDM at that time, research in the specialties of interpersonal neurobiology and relationship psychology was showing (and continues to validate) that human decision making involves many interacting forces that are a necessary aspect of the process (see Kahneman and Tversky, 1979). These interacting forces include a patient's implicit and explicit emotions, memories, values, rational thinking, and the interpersonal dynamics between clinician, providers, and loved ones. Little research was conducted to assess whether the patient's answers to a simple question or a questionnaire are likely to yield the same values as would be discovered from a skilled interview. In any case, the covert message to the patient was to negate conflict. Furthermore, as you will see in later chapters, it is not the discovery of "the answer" that is pivotal; it is the mental processes within patients that are fostered during a skilled interview that are crucial to the patient's internal decision making. These mental processes include better regulation of emotion and better assimilation of the evidence-based information they have heard but not yet taken in.

Driven by the imperative to contain cost while maintaining care quality, the administrative elaboration of shared (and informed) decision making outstripped the search for underlying science and the research. For example, Norway's Oslo University Center for Shared Decision Making and Collaborative Care in 2011 began making a strong contribution to research (Ruland et al., 2013). Yet, leaders in the field have been unable to describe the core conceptual ingredients and the competencies needed by providers to apply an idea to which almost everyone ascribes. Before deciding what the internal and interpersonal psychological processes might be behind the words *informed* and *shared*, an abundance of funding spurred a national and international administrative roll-out. For example, in Sidney, Australia, McCaffery et al. (2007) developed a rigorous framework for facilitating shared decision making among adults with lower literacy.

The meaning of the term *shared* continued to be debated. We have become part of that discussion. The idea was to share with the patient the evidence-based information the clinician possesses so that they can make a decision together. What *together* meant was unclarified. This was one of the earliest meanings of the word *shared* in shared decision making. If the goals did not include improving care and lowering cost, just telling patients the information—whatever the result—could be called shared decision making. But, when "sharing" has the goal of influencing human behavior, it is another matter. Many scientists are aware that a deeper story needs to be understood and told. As one researcher said, "Wish it were that simple, but it is not. Many of us in this field have now realized that much more than communication theory and cognitive theory is involved." An insightful mass media colleague said to me: "I may have all the information possible, but I still have to make a decision."

The focus in mainstream health care shifted in 2008 to "engaging the personhood" of the patient. The hope was to reduce cost while improving the quality of the interpersonal side of care. The topics of attention included how to engage patients to change their health behaviors, the discovery of costly unwarranted variations in treatments for the same conditions, an increase in litigation and burgeoning of informed consent, and an increase in diagnostic and treatment choice from an explosion of evidence-based knowledge, for example, the PSA test in prostatic cancer and choices for treatment of breast cancer and cardiac angina. Engaging patients in their own medical decision process became the prudent thing to do. *Patient engagement* became a buzzword, but again, the theory on how this could be accomplished was not crossing over from relationship psychology and interpersonal neurobiology to mainstream medicine, public health, and cognitive psychology. Historically the external mechanics of decision making remained a primary focus, although most everyone in the center of the field had a sense that they somehow were not getting to the core mechanisms. Some kept saying new research studies needed to be done about engaging patients, while what was already understood on this topic in other circles was not being used. Our observations of recorded encounters between clinician and patients and the experiences of thousands of psychotherapists working with both individual people and couples including medical clinicians indicated that health decisions usually involve interpersonal relationship dynamics and emotions, beliefs, and memories in both patient and clinician. This is no surprise to those professionals who are in the daily practice of successfully engaging people to work on their relationships. It is a surprise to those focused mainly on the treatment of disease.

Historically, researchers in many specialties were working on ideas in isolation from each other. For example, special interest groups (SIGs) on the psychology of decision making existed for more than five years within both the Society of Medical Decision Making and the Society of Behavioral Medicine. They had not attended each other's scientific meetings until we prompted attendance to happen a few years ago. You will see that this field is still on an uphill journey of collaboration between disciplines. Another example of the isolation is that Jennifer Learner's work starting in the 1980s, which measured the physiological component of emotion, showed that emotions present in the decider were a pivotal force in how and what decision was made, regardless of the information they possessed. She became the founding director of the Decision Science Lab at Harvard's Kennedy School of Government. The experimental work in that lab is still not a significant part of the conversation in the field of shared medical decision making (Lerner et al., 2015 and personal communication; Livingstone, 2009a).

Consideration of the role of emotions in decision making is as sparse in SDM as it is in the field of behavior change. Lerner writes: "In economics, the historically dominant discipline for research on decision theory, the role of emotion, or affect more generally in decision making rarely appeared for most of the twentieth century, despite featuring prominently in influential eighteenth- and nineteenth-century economic treatises" (Loewenstein and Lerner, 2003). The case was similar in psychology for most of the twentieth century. Even psychologists' critiques of expected utility theory focused primarily on understanding cognitive processes (Kahneman and Tversky, 1979). Research examining emotion in all fields of psychology remained scant (Keltner and Lerner, 2010).

The process of "sharing," according to communication theory, at first meant that the information had to be translated into forms that matched the cognitive abilities and style of most patients, and that a clinician needed to take the time to shape and discuss the information. What interpersonal strategies would go into that time-sensitive discussion were never clarified. Supporting this, informal studies in education had shown that the assimilation and retention of information told to parents of schoolchildren was quite poor and was often distorted until teachers learned first to process parental emotion-based concerns (Personal Consultations to schools, 1975–1978).

SDM had become a worldwide topic with the creation of several societies, journals, and scientific meetings in the United States, the United Kingdom, and Europe. Said to be motivated by ethics, it was also heavily motivated by the goals of improving outcome, lowering cost, and litigation control. In the United States it has become a central element of Patient-Centered Care promoted by the IOM and in the code of ethics of the ANA. The term *shared decision making* was built upon an increasing interest since the 1970s in patient-centeredness and patient autonomy in health care interactions (President's Commission, 1978). If you are new to doctoring and nursing, you may have little awareness that for over the past 20 years medical decision making has evolved into a multimillion-dollar policy, administrative, research, and public health business.

Too few regulatory teeth were built into the care system, however, to back up the rights of patients to be included and consulted. Peter Drier's experience indicated this gap in 2014 (when he received an uninsured $117,000 bill from an out-of-network surgeon) as reported in the Sunday *New York Times* in 2014 (NYTimes, 2014). Yet clinicians and hospitals were being encouraged to involve patients to share in medical decisions. To protect the providers and hospitals, patients were asked to sign consents stating that they had been "fully informed." But providers and hospitals were not expected to guarantee for patients the nature and costs of treatment nor were they legally bound in most states to inform patients about the involvement of additional physicians and services at their expense.

The term *shared decision making* has metamorphosed into Shared *Medical* Decision Making (SMDM) and *Informed* Medical Decision Making (IMDM), depending on who was promoting it. The length of this summary reflects this state of affairs and our awareness that this domain is likely to become central in your professional life. As your career unfolds you may notice that as twenty-first century interpersonal science seeps into mainstream medicine, the challenge will be to integrate, unify concepts, apply, and teach then, and to update faculty.

PATIENT DECISION AIDS BECAME A BIG INDUSTRY

Time allotted by insurance companies devoted to office visit discussions was getting shorter and also many clinicians did not have time or resources to stay fully updated on all the evidence-based information available. This was resolved by creating presentations of facts about disease and treatments and giving it to patients and their families. The "Patient Decision Aid" in print and later in DVD became a big industry. A foundation devoted to acquiring a steady stream of updated evidence-based information on the value of diagnostic procedures, conditions, and treatments was formed.

Beginning in 1989, Boston-based FIMDM, in collaboration with a Boston-based health coaching service company (Health Dialog, Inc.), began developing carefully crafted patient decision aids (PDAs) for patient consumption through their insurance companies and by 2008 had developed more than 30 in print and DVD. They are regularly updated (see the Appendix). Since the funding to produce and distribute them came via insurance companies for their own members, the general availability for patients and physicians has been limited. Patients who have used them report their unique usefulness. We are quite familiar with all of them. Patients are relieved to have information in one place, which is presented for their consumption, in print and DVD, and is evidence-based. A list can be found in the Appendix. Here are three titles to give you some idea: *Treatment Choices for Coronary Artery Disease, Living with Diabetes: Making Lifestyle Changes to Last a Lifetime*, and *Is a PSA Test Right for You?*

Also, O'Connor and her group in Ottawa became leaders in the development of decision aid technology and by 2008 had made available evidence-based information on more than 200 diverse conditions (https/decisionaid.ohri.ea).

Because of the rapid proliferation of PDAs, Elwyn et al. (1999) made a recommendation in the *British Medical Journal* that a set of international standards be used for PDAs. In 2005, Annette O'Connor and an international group developed and codified International Patient Decision Aid Standards (IPDAS) and a checklist (www.ipdas.ohri.ca). Of medical shared decisions they said, "The best choice involves matching which features matter most to a person with the option that has these features. To make a good decision, you need an expert on the facts (e.g., a health practitioner) and an expert on which features matter most (e.g., the patient) and a way to share their views with each other in ways they prefer." These guidelines made general good sense at the time, but they were not able to define either (1) the psychological science for helping patients to discover within themselves "which features matter most," or (2) the interpersonal strategies that the patient and practitioner could use to "share their views." As you will see, both of these domains are sensitive to the emotional status of both the clinician and the patient, and to the dynamics between them. These factors determine of outcome. This book now helps to define these matters so they might become part of the education and training of clinicians.

Workers who focused on the psychological dimension, including us, believed it was premature to be setting standards and creating a checklist in 2007 when sufficient theory about medical decision making and use of decision aids had not been evolved and tested. I counseled against standards but recommended that temporary guidelines be created and research be started. By 2009, decision science still had not supplied answers. Hillary Bekker (2010) of the University of Leeds, UK, said, "Adhering uncritically to the IPDAS checklist may reduce service variation but is not sufficient to ensure interventions enable good patient decision making. Developers must be encouraged to reason about the IPDAS checklist to identify those component parts that do not meet their intervention's purpose."

In 2009 Angela Fagerlin, a specialist in risk communication at the University of Michigan, published an editorial about the development and use of decision aids. She said, "Little is understood as to which design elements contribute to better decision making or whether different design elements affect people differently based on their individual characteristics—and how DAs affect patient–physician communication—and there is the timing component" (meaning, from whom does the patient receive the decision aid and when?). Funding was not readily available for research, and good hypotheses to test were sparse.

We agree with Fagerlin (2009) and have made patient–physician communication a consistent thread throughout this book. Developing science is confirming that this "communication" is not solely a cognitive matter; it is a matter of two or three people (patient, loved one, clinician) in a dynamic relationship that requires that clinicians learn specific skills. The action of giving patients PDAs as print, DVD, or interactive access on-line—no matter how well designed—does not mean that "shared" decision making will occur.

Nonetheless, physicians nationwide were encouraged in 2010 to start practicing shared decision making and using decision aids. In 2011, the IOM of the National Academy of Sciences set the tone in the famous report *Crossing the Quality Chasm: A New Health System for the 21st Century* (IOM, 2011). It defined patient-centeredness as "providing care that is respectful of and responsive to individual patient preferences, needs, and values, and ensuring that patient values guide all clinical decisions" (IOM, 2011). In 2013 the IOM convened a committee of experts to examine the quality of cancer care in the United States and formulate recommendations for improvement (IOM, 2013).

BRANDS OF MEDICAL DECISION MAKING YOU SHOULD KNOW

Originally, as a symbol that evidence-based information should propel a patient's decision process, the word *informed* had been emphasized by FIMDM, who called the process *Informed* Medical Decision Making. To symbolize the goal of vigorous patient participation, the word *shared* was added, probably by O'Connor's group. So then it was referred to as Informed Shared Medical Decision Making. Words, however, did not solve the gaps in theory, strategy, and interviewing tactics.

ORGANIZATION NAMES

In 2014, FIMDM merged with Healthwise and became the Informed Medical Decisions Foundation (IMDF). (See http://www.healthwise.org or IMDF.org for more information.) Health Dialog Services Corporation and their 38 PDA programs are now owned by Rite Aid. Also, a joint conference is held yearly by the International Society for Evidence Based Health Care and the International Shared Decision-Making Group (ISDM-ISEHC2015.org). The Health Foundation in the UK in 2009 prompted the implementation of shared decision making. Angela Coulter, in her review, cited international initiatives in Australia, Germany, The Netherlands, and the United States (Coulter, 2011).

The names Shared Decision Making and Informed Medical Decision Making have remained prominent as what seems to be the same general process within patient-centered care. Regardless of how it is defined, the concepts were endorsed early on by the U.S. Department of Health and Human Services and the IOM in 2001, and by the IOM again in 2011. SDM, in the generic sense, became a required part of the Affordable Care Act, Section 3506, which states, "Program to facilitate shared decisionmaking" (Patient Protection and Affordable Care Act 2010. Public law 111-148. Sec. 3506). By 1997, Shared Decision Making was a registered trademark of the Foundation for Informed Medical Decision Making in Boston. It was listed as re-registered by Healthwise in 2012. The term has been used generically for years and that continues in its various iterations.

When the inclusion of the patient's "values" was introduced into SDM in about 2004, unknown to many workers, this addition changed the playing field from one of information transfer to one that also requires increased attention to the interior psychology of patients and the interpersonal dynamics between patients, clinicians, and loved ones. Because workers in SDM who were without relational psychology training believed that not enough was known about the psychology of patients and their values, they recommended more research. Professionals in other fields already knew a great deal about the personality dynamics of medical decision making but were not writing about it and were not being asked to contribute.

TRAINING IN SDM

A new curriculum for clinician training in SDM was proposed (Livingstone, 2009a). The stakeholders were interested but not ready to embrace change. Although this has not yet been realized, the evolution of SDM changed the education and training requirements to apply SDM and required closer collaboration with contemporary relationship psychologists and interpersonal neurobiologists. This is happening slowly. This dimension of SDM is addressed thoroughly in this book. In Chapter 9 you will find line-by-line annotations of the recording of an interview about the decision process, which is not the SDM of the past.

Medicine and nursing have been in a period of finding theory, strategy, and tactic to fit the administrative imperatives of SDM and patient engagement. Viewing it as good care, some holistic nurses, health coaches, and psychotherapists working with medical patients are training in the principles presented in this book. We hope this project helps support an increase in interdisciplinary collaboration within the field of shared decision making.

Now we are moving on to other decision making theories, most of which were created in economics and business administration and later applied to health care.

Expected utility calculations (for clinicians and patients)

The clinician and patient are expected to choose between alternative treatments by surveying all options and their consequences and estimating (cognitively) the utility and probability of each. The treatment with the highest expected benefits (utility) is chosen. For some people, this approach fulfills the criteria for shared decision making, that is, clinicians provide data on alternatives and consequences, and patients attach numbers or values to the potential benefits and harms; they decide. Gigerenzer (2007) says that there is no proof that expected utility calculations are the best form of medical decision making.

Statistical aids and decision analysis (for clinicians)

Complex statistical aids were created, for example, the *Heart Disease Predictive Instrument* (Green and Mehr, 1997). These seem to be more popular among clinicians than are expected utility calculations. Gigerenzer thinks, however, that the majority of clinicians do not understand them and stop using them, leaving them only with "clinical intuition," which is unconsciously biased by geographic traditions and liability control (Gigerenzer, 2007). He proposes using intuition (gut feelings) combined with "rules of thumb" (Chapter 4).

Clinical intuition (for clinicians and perhaps patients)

This is a process driven by an unknown mixture within the clinician (and sometimes in patients) of ideas, emotions, relationship obligations, self-protection, and a variable use of good rules of thumb. But a problem is that it is mostly going on outside of awareness and without transparency for either the clinician or patient. Intuition as a solo approach is thought to be unwise by us and by Gigerenzer (2007).

INFORMATION TRANSFER AND COMMUNICATION

Information "communication" and the interpersonal matter of "information transfer" is a necessary component of both health behavior change and medical decision making. We are unable to find health psychology models of information transfer similar in detail to those about behavior change and decision making or models that addressed the interpersonal dynamics in information communication. Most of what exists seems to be in the state of cognitive description derived from clinical experience and public health projects. Most clinicians and researchers agree that this domain needs more comprehensive psychologically based theory and strategy. This book responds to that need and describes a new strategy called "Information Interweave™."

Information communication models

There are dozens of information models in communication, marketing, and public health. Mostly, they do not focus on interpersonal information transmission and assimilation involving individual people and what that process involves. Education and marketing have addressed some of the issues but focus primarily on the cognitive dimension. The disadvantage of all these models is that they tend to omit the role of relationship bonding and emotions in the process of communication of new information, despite the fact that educators of children know about this aspect, and corporate America knows that "sex sells" products.

Health care has made some use of communication theory for shaping information to match the patient's culture, education, and intellectual style and has been a component of decision making and behavior or change. There has been very little research on health-related information transfer and its specialized aspects, except on the gross level of electronic information transfer from clinician to clinician. In 2013 Laura Kreofsky, a certified professional in health information management in a business paradigm, proposed to establish nationally an electronic connection of patients and families to their health care providers as a method of increasing patient engagement and consumer satisfaction (Kreofsky, 2013). This might be effective if it were within the context of a well-managed continuing personal relationship, rather than as a cost-saving substitute for personal relationships. Just because electronic media are used does not mean that it can't build in a relational component.

Ann-Louise Caress (2003), a lecturer in nursing at University of Manchester, UK, addressed this interpersonal issue with a double-blind peer-reviewed article, "Giving Information to Patients." She reiterates that knowledge alone does not change health outcomes (Scherer et al., 1998; Gibson and Pick, 2000) and goes on to say that patients may not understand what they are told or the links between the information and their situation. The article is organized as nine items called "Time Outs," with each one giving advice, for example, on the level of not assuming that just because someone speaks another language that they can read it, or finding a setting without noise intrusion and interruption. Although Caress's advice may give a student some basic ideas, the articles does not cover how training programs might help students decrease the intrapersonal and interpersonal dynamics that are common barriers to effective communication with patients. This may be work in progress.

Although not solely about information transfer, a rigorous physician communication skills training study by Lesley Fallowfield and team at the

University of Sussex, UK, was conducted in response to observations of problems in communication competency of senior clinicians providing cancer care (Fallow Fied et al., 2002). Involving 2407 patients and 160 oncologists at 34 cancer centers, they studied the efficacy of intensive three-day training in communication skills assessed by video recording of interviews using a random, controlled design. Course content included structured feedback, videotape review of patient interviewing, role-play with simulated patients, interactive group demonstrations, and discussion led by a trained facilitator. Primary outcomes were observable improvements in the key communication skills they selected. For example, the trained group showed a reduction in closed leading questions, an increase in combinations of open and focused questions, more appropriate responses to patient's cues, more empathic responses, and an increase in summarizing information mainly by senior level clinicians. They used a moderate level of statistical analysis and showed that "modest but potentially meaningful change in key outcomes are measurable three months after training." One portion of the study engaged participants to work on interview tasks they found particularly difficult. The author believes that if the teaching methods are acceptable and effective, busy doctors will attend. The doctors apparently asked for more and were disposed to recommend the course to colleagues.

Although we prefer to review their video recordings through our own lens and would probably select additional key interpersonal skills to measure, this study is worth reviewing for any group planning medical school or in-service training in basic communication skills to physicians and nurses. The study has certain design elements that are similar to our own comparative controlled pilot study of the impact of workshops and mentoring on the interviewing skills of midcareer nurses doing telephonic health coaching. Their study has entered another phase, and we anticipate more findings.

Our past analysis of recorded interviews showed that experienced and well-trained nurse-health coaches and health educators who were quite aware of all these items still failed to prepare their patients' psychology for the information they provided them and failed to soften their own discomfort with hearing patients' fears—a discomfort that compelled them to supply more and more information in an untimely manner (Livingstone and Gaffney, 2013). The nurses were surprised by hearing sequences in their own recorded interviews, were encouraged to get curious about what was going on for them at those moments, and learned new ways to take care of themselves in-the-moment so that they were not *behaving toward* their patients.

As you will discover in subsequent chapters, we have added concepts to this field by observing that the information patients require for their processes of behavior change and decision making emanates from two sources: *from the inside* of the patient's mind (memories, beliefs, emotions) and *from the outside* supplied by (1) their loved ones (including facts, beliefs, and emotions), (2) information from their clinicians, and (3) patient decision aids.

Fear has been tried as strategy of persuasion in health communication. Hannah Arendt said, "Fear is an emotion indispensable for survival." Edmund

Burke said, "No passion so effectively robs the mind of all its powers of acting and reasoning as fear." Both are true.

Some prior models of health communication use fear-based strategies. Over the last half-century, a substantial amount of research has been done on the influence of fear on persuasion. A multitude of theories and models of fear-appeals, also known as "cognitive mediating processes," have been derived from this research. The goal of each of these has been to conceptualize the influence of fear on persuasion so as to better understand how to employ it in addressing the public on a number of social and health issues. Some people believe it is effective. The public campaign on smoking cessation, however, that told the public that if they smoke they will have a long and painful death and showed them gruesome photographs, did not boost smoking cessation. You might imagine how little positive effect would be gained by specific warnings of diabetic patients with the risk of future complications, such as amputation, heart attack, stroke, kidney disease, blindness, and problems with infection and wound healing.

In our opinion, fact-related fear and an empathic attuned relationship must be paired together. Let's alter the word *fear* to *concern*. There is an optimal level of concern, and this can be best monitored for that person within an empathic, attuned relationship. Prompting fear in patients without having a relationship to process the emotion is counterproductive. It runs the risk of activating protections within the personality that are so strong that they become barriers to enduring behavior change and conscious decision making (for example, stubborn teenager-like responses). There appears to be an optimal amount of concern within people that prompts courage and adaptive behaviors.

Healthy communication: A guide for pediatricians and parents

In 1996 the American Academy of Pediatrics published for their pediatrician members a handout for parents on communication with their child composed by Dr. Livingstone when he was adviser to the Institute for Mental Health Initiatives (IMHI) (Livingstone, 1996). It emphasized generic elements of healthy communication that were known at that time, namely: (1) being a good listener even when the child is upset and it can't be fixed; (2) showing empathy in the form of appreciating his or her feelings "for their own sake," even if the parent disagrees with what is being said; (3) being a good "sender" happens after being a good "listener" and requires that the tone of voice match the words; (4) setting an example by using words of feeling and "I" statements when sending; (5) using feeling words to share what is felt rather than using behavior, for example, screaming and sarcasm are verbal behaviors. (In a re-write in 2015, I would recommend that parents first put oxygen on their own emotions before talking to their child.)

Some of the prior models list tactics for clinical use; others have little. Only a few of the theories have tactics tied to theory and strategy; many are tactics that float free. We believe it is important for research testing to derive tactics from consistent strategies based on a theory—so that there is linkage between theory, strategy, and tactic in research design.

HOLISTIC AND INTEGRAL NURSING MODELS

This field is important enough to include here, although integral and holistic nursing are not focused solely on patient-centered care, health behavior change, decision making, information transfer, and clinician self-care. The field does embrace all these topics as important. Advances in the fields of relationship psychology and neurobiology (Chapters 4 and 5) are not in conflict with holistic and integral nursing practice. Rather, they inform it and would be a significant enhancement to holistic curriculum development when the goals of faculty include that trainees acquire updated specific interpersonal skills that can be documented by recorded patient–nurse interviews.

Holistic nursing

In 2009, Dossey and Keegan published the fourth edition of their handbook, *Holistic Nursing: A Handbook for Practice* (Dossey, 2009). In 2006, holistic nursing was recognized as a specialty by American Nurses Association (ANA), and a fifth edition of the handbook (735 pages, 36 chapters) came out in 2007. In addition, a 136-page volume of practice standards, *Holistic Nursing: Scope and Standards of Practice*, was published by the AHNA and ANA (2013).

These two publications contain plenty of good advice for all nurses and physicians. It is one of the most comprehensive menus in existence about the general ingredients of professional practice of the care of the whole patient within the larger health care system. Osler in 1892 and Peabody in 1927 would each have been pleased to read them and also to read what Tresolini and Pew-Fetzer (1994) wrote on what they called "relationship-centered care."

Scientifically speaking, however, these writings are not so much based yet on validated theory, strategy, and clinical tactic as they are comprehensive reviews and points of view. They present a philosophy and the goals of embracing a holistic scope of practice. Rather than presenting a testable clinical model, Dossey's book is useful in that it contains a comprehensive survey by various authors of practically every topic possible in health care, including basic elements of all the traditional psychotherapies. It is so comprehensive and inclusive that it would not have been possible to go into more depth than was done. The handbook, therefore, functions as a much-needed menu to familiarize the uninitiated with the scope of the field and mainly to initiate curriculum development for faculty. To reach the level of specificity needed to evolve a skill-based curriculum, faculty and practitioners would need to go deeper into the evidence-based research and theoretical literature. There are some items of interest that need to be mentioned.

For example, in Stuart-Shor and Wells-Federman (2009), there is an exercise to promote empathy. First the authors define empathy as "the ability to take into consideration the other person's perspective." There now are new definitions of empathy. No distinction, however, is made between empathy and compassion or mention of the issue of feeling so much that the listener nearly becomes the other person. The latter is a common phenomenon that blocks the connected relationship needed for the patient to experience empathy. The exercise indicates that they get the general idea, yet they see empathy primarily as a matter of gaining cognitive control. Now we know much more about how to facilitate an interviewer to be empathic, and it involves their own inner relationship with their emotions and body. It matters a great deal to the patient.

Here is their stepwise approach to empathy, for your information. Other outlines from their model are contained in the Appendix.

- Stop (break the cycle of escalating, awfullizing thoughts). Take a breath—release physical tensions, promote relaxation.
- Reflect—Emotionally, how do I feel? (angry, hurt?); What are my automatic thoughts? What are the thoughts and emotions being expressed by the other person?
- Choose—My feelings are hurt but I choose not to react defensively. I choose to listen actively to the other person's response and will try to understand that person's perspective, using the phrase: "You sound (emotion) about (situation)."
- Their discussion is more promotional of an integrated holistic philosophy. However, the authors do say, "What people learn depends upon their mood or feeling at the time of the experience."

Our comment in 2015 is that these steps might be helpful for the clinician who is not strongly triggered. When clinicians get triggered, the point is that they can't "stop," and they can't "choose to actively listen." They are emotionally blended with a personality part and are often unware of it. Perhaps you might prove that to yourself by observing your relationship with an intimate partner. This event of getting emotionally activated happens to everyone and often—and for internal reasons regarding vulnerability. This makes sense. An updated self-strategy and set of tactics has been needed and now have been developed and been proven by research to be effective (Schwartz, 2013; Herbine-Blank et al., 2015; Livingstone and Gaffney, 2013). We present strategy in Chapter 7 and the tactics in Chapter 8.

As indicated by Bernadette Melnyk et al. (2009) and Carol Baldwin et al. (2008) from their work at Arizona State, holistic nursing embraces *evidence-based* practice. Regarding coverage of *behavior change*, their emphasis, including smoking cessation, mentions some of the models already summarized in this chapter such as Motivational Interviewing. Not covered are models of decision process and Shared Decision Making.

The topic of *mind-body* is covered in Chapter 30 in *Holistic Nursing: A Handbook for Practice*, "The Psychophysiology of Body-Mind Healing" by Genevieve Bartol and Nancy Courts from the University of North Carolina (Bartol and Courts, 2009). They quote work from Dan Siegel and conclude, as we also do, that the "research data overwhelmingly document the importance of mind-body relationships. However, there are still many unanswered questions." Their particular focus, however, within these questions is, "Does the mind exist after physical death? Does the soul survive death of the body?" We pose a very different set of questions in alignment with our scientific goals, those of developing testable hypotheses and clinically useful strategies and tactics.

About *information transfer*, Bartol and Courts describe and embrace the Santiago Theory of Cognition, which has been criticized by many. One point in the theory with which we agree is, "Emotions are not just an accompaniment of perception and behavior, but are an inherent part of this domain." They do not focus-in at the level of our particular interest which is how clinicians can help patients process their emotions and whether emotions felt by the patient determines the quality of his or her cognitive functions.

Regarding *clinician self-care*, under "Nurse Self-Care," they say, "Holistic nurses engage in self-assessment, self-care, and personal development, aware of being instruments of healing to better serve self and others. They endeavor to integrate self-awareness, self-care, and self-healing into their lives." No one would disagree with this. How to accomplish these goals, however, was not stated in this book, and whatever theories and strategies for doing so that existed at the time are not referenced.

About *practitioner–patient relationship*, the text embraces the Theory of Human Relatedness, which, according to Hagerty and Patusky, consists of four stages of relationship and four social competencies of the practitioner that are "vital for relationship" (Hagerty and Patusky, 2003). They list this series of items and define each; for example, under stages of relationship, they list *connection* and define it as: "Connection means there is active involvement with another, associated with enhanced comfort and wellness." Under the four social competencies, they list *reciprocity* and define it as: "Reciprocity is a positive aspect of relationship in which there is perceived equal exchange between parties." The level of abstraction of these items is too high to inform specific interviewing tactics for skill training.

Despite its inclusiveness, understandably in the field of holistic nursing in 2007 the knowledge and skill gaps relevant to practicing patient-centered care were similar to those in mainstream medicine, psychology, public health, psychotherapy, clinical social work, and health coaching. The high level of abstraction of content in this book gives the student a general picture of how they are supposed to conduct themselves—without clarity as to the pathways to achieve this. In doctoring and nursing the pathway to clinical conduct has traditionally been left to "clinical experience."

Integral nursing

In the section entitled "The Theory of Integral Nursing" in *Holistic Nursing: A Handbook for Practice,* (Dossey, 2009) embraces and goes beyond holistic nursing and organizes multiple phenomena of human experience into four perspectives, which they call Individual Interior (personal), Individual Exterior (behavioral and physiologic), Collective Interior (shared cultural), and Collective Exterior (systems). The proponents say they examine values, beliefs, assumption, meaning, purpose, and judgments related to how individuals perceived reality and relationships from the four perspectives. They believe that an integral worldview helps to open dialogue between nurses and other disciplines. The goal appears to be to decrease fragmentation in the nursing profession and supply a comprehensive map as a basis of dialogue and action and is open to use the existing theories we present elsewhere in this chapter. Although the goal of integration of a fragmented nursing field makes sense to us, consider the current status of this concept, rather than as a scientific theory, to be a set of unproven hypotheses and a helpful construct to help the thinking and actions of nurses as professionals to be integrated. Neither the theoretical nor strategic basis for their grouping of the elements into their four perspectives is clear enough to teach. For example, they separate "personal" (psychological) from the "behavioral and physiological" when modern science has discovered the inseparable, bi-directional interactions between these forces. The organization for their map may send the message that it is really possible or advantageous to separate the personal internal forces from those of behavior and the body. They have included the cognitive items like values, beliefs, meaning, purpose, and judgments but omitted the forces of "emotions" from their list of considerations. They use the word "intentional" when a lot of people and groups function outside their awareness. To understand the value of this worldview, it would help to see examples of its specific applications and advantages over systems theory and mindfulness. In 2014, Melnyk, Dean of The Ohio State University Nursing Program, published 24 competencies for nurses (Melnyk et al., 2014). You will find her list in the Appendix.

TRADITIONAL PSYCHOTHERAPY MODELS

Traditional fields of psychotherapy were not ready or inclined to contribute strategies and tactics to medical care practice in the trenches. Although they had clinically validated certain principles which medical interviewing can still use with advantage, workers developing the prior models of behavior change and decision making made too little use of proven strategies from psychodynamic psychotherapy and medical liaison psychiatry. This happened for several reasons. The strategies were not translated into ordinary language. They were imbedded in processes of long duration not suited to medical care. Cross-discipline collaboration was sparse. And finally, physicians and public health professionals outside mental health believed that the concepts and tactics of psychotherapy applied only to "psychopathology."

A case in point was my conversation in 1971 in Paris with Paul Vesin, MD, a world-renowned public heath pediatrician at International Children's Center, an organization of WHO and UNICEF. He said, "What would you as a child psychiatrist know about the normal, everyday life of children in schools and communities? Don't you treat disturbed children in hospitals?" I thought, "How could that be his view—even in France? After all, child, adolescent, and adult psychotherapists spend every day talking with people who are not severely mentally ill and who struggle with their health, school performance, and medical care." At that time, Dr. Vesin and others had little awareness that normal child development and communication of health-based information to parents and teachers was the foundation of a child psychiatrist's work. As we began to know each other, Dr. Vesin's view changed, and he invited me to become an editorial advisor for their health information publications to developing countries. The point is that sophisticated workers in public health, cognitive psychology, and medical model-building were at that time and are still now unfamiliar with the relational principles of psychotherapy that were applicable in health care. Working collaboratively helped then and would help now.

Several traditional psychotherapy models should be noted since some of their principles are particularly useful to mainstream health care: psychoanalytic psychodynamic (Freud, Klein, Winnicott), Rogerian-client-centered (Rogers, Kohut), systemic family therapy (Minuchin, Bowen, Satir, Haley), Reichian (Reich), and Gestault (Perls). It should be said, however, that although relational principles for years had been clinically validated in psychotherapy, they were not understood through an interpersonal neurobiological lens until recently (Badenoch, 2008).

In his detailed and well-balanced review of all these models, Louis Cozolino, professor and clinician from Pepperdine University, Los Angeles, on close analysis of practice concluded that among all of the models, "Intellectual understanding of a psychological problem in the absence of increased integration with emotion, sensation, and behavior does not result in change," and also noted that "the primary focus of (all) psychotherapy appears to be the integration of affect, in all its forms, with conscious awareness, and cognition" (Cozolino, 2010). In their current state of validation, these psychotherapy-related principles can be translated and embedded with advantage in new processes for interviewing medical patients. Now, most of the psychotherapies emphasize that the "relationship" between therapist and patient is a crucial element, and lately that "attachment" is a crucial element. Although there is much data that relational therapy works, the nature of the therapeutic element within relationships has been the subject of much discussion. The importance of *being with* the patient to discover pivotal clinical evidence has been reemphasized recently by Gordon Harper et al. (2015).

As you will see from Chapters 4 and 5 on advances, more light has been shed on this topic of looking in the right places, particularly since the disposition of the therapist's emotional state and attachment theory both have been universally embraced in the therapy world, including by psychodynamic theory.

MINDFULNESS PRACTICE MODELS

Regarding mindfulness practices for clinician self-care, in the 1970 Jon Kabat-Zinn, now professor emeritus at University of Massachusetts Medical School, was responsible for starting a stress reduction clinic and mindfulness meditation course in a hospital setting (Kabat-Zinn, 2007). Ronald Epstein, a physician in family medicine at University of Rochester, and Herb Benson, a physician at Harvard affiliate Beth Israel Deaconess Medical Center, for years have promoted and trained physicians in this approach. In 1999 Epstein wrote, "Mindful practitioners attend in a nonjudgmental way to their own physical and mental processes during ordinary, everyday tasks. This critical self-reflection enables physicians to listen attentively to patient's distress, recognize their own errors, refine their technical skills, make evidence-based decisions, and clarify their values so they can act with compassion, technical competence, presence, and insight." He explains that mindfulness cannot be explicitly taught, but can be modeled, and should be considered a universal practice in relationship-centered, evidence-based medicine. Kabat-Zinn's work is seminal and is about "paying kind attention, on purpose, without grasping onto judgments, to whatever arises in the mind from moment to moment." Dan Siegel, a pediatrician and child psychiatrist at UCLA, wrote about the subjective experience that clinicians can facilitate in their patients through the practice of mindful awareness (Siegel, 2011).

ATTACHMENT THEORY IN HUMAN DEVELOPMENT

Attachment theory has been validated by observation and research on children and adults for many years. Attachment is defined by many as "a lasting psychological connectedness between human beings." Longitudinal studies have been conducted, and hundreds of articles and books have been written about this well-validated, ubiquitous phenomenon of attachment between people. The hospital care of children and adults is universally impacted by the phenomenon. Inge Bretherton (1992) at University of Wisconsin authored an extensive review of the theory and history about John Bolby and Mary Ainsworth (Uganda Project), and Eric Erickson and Grossmann reviewed the literature on longitudinal studies about attachment (Erickson and Kurtz-Riemer, 2005). Attachment has been embraced by psychology, neuroscience, social science, and the general public, as a fundamental core principle of human relationships throughout the life cycle, and led to the formulation of separation distress/anxiety and later to the steps of mourning described by Kubler-Ross. "Loneliness is bad for you" say McLean Hospital Harvard-affiliated physicians Richard Schwartz and Jacqueline Olds (Olds and Schwartz, 2010). This concept is supported by a review in 1988 by James House at University of Michigan that social isolation is associated with premature death (House, 1988). Genomic biologist Steve Cole at UCLA in 2007 said loneliness alters the expression of genes associated with the immune system. These findings point out the biological underpinnings of attachment theory in psychological development (Bolby, 1969). Damasio (1999) pointed out that the body is the key to awareness of emotions. In subsequent chapter we show how attachment theory is applied in our new model of communication in healthcare relationship.

NARRATIVE MEDICINE

The work of medicine (doctoring and nursing) rests on the clinician's ability to listen to the stories that patients tell, to make sense of those often chaotic narratives of illness, to inspect and evaluate the listener's response to the story told, to understand what those narratives mean, and to be moved by them.

Rita Charon, MD, PhD
Primary Care, Columbia University
College of Physician and Surgeons

Rita Charon (2001) in *Narrative Medicine: A Model for Empathy, Reflection, Profession, and Trust*, responding to the increased mechanization of medicine, has enhanced the human side of medical care by "making genuine contact with patients through storytelling." This is an important focus. She states that narrative medicine leads to more humane, ethical, and effective health care (Alcauskas and Charon, 2008). We agree that listening to a patient's narratives is essential and also would take it further in 2015. We would add that a robust way to accomplish this is to listen to the narrative of *each* personality part that has been activated by the patient's health situation. And, we also emphasize that the nature of the clinician's responses to what he or she is hearing is what determines the patient's likelihood of changing a behavior and making a stable medical decision. As you read on, you will see that Drs Hal and Sidra Stone, Richard C. Schwartz, and Rita Charon, working separately, have embraced the importance of narrative in their patient care, and that this strategy is standard practice in our model as well.

TRADITIONAL ANATOMICAL AND FUNCTIONAL NEUROBIOLOGY

Fernando Augusto, a Rhode Island-based psychologist and IFS-trained psychotherapist, reviewed interpersonal neurobiology (personal communication, 2011), and Frank Anderson, a physician–psychiatrist–psychotherapist who specializes in neuroscience and psychopharmacology, reviewed neurobiology pertinent to psychological trauma (personal communication, 2012). Their review of basics is useful here. In Chapter 5 you will find a discussion of advances from neuroscience that are relevant to our focus on patient care and an updated version of functional neurobiology that has accumulated since about 1990.

Working separately, Fernando and Anderson (personal communication, 2013), outlined traditional entities and functions of the CNS from before the 1990s. They associated anatomy with function in the following ways:

Brain stem—heart rate, breathing, degree of alertness, sleep, fight–flight–freeze
Limbic—affect, attachment, memory, making meaning; includes amygdala–hippocampus–hypothalamus
Cortex—experience dependent; *right*: perception, nonverbal, autobiographical; *left*: linear, logical, factual, language
Insula—awareness of body-based emotions
Anterior cingulate—coordinates memory and emotion
Prefrontal cortex—an integrator that links all of the above

4

Present advances in relationship psychology (after early 1990s): A relational context for diagnosis and treatment

The real act of discovery consists not in finding new lands, but seeing with new eyes.

Marcel Proust

This chapter contains seven sets of new findings in relationship psychology that are relevant to our focus on the core fundamental tasks of Patient-Centered Care (PCC). We show you a list of the advances with comments about their scientific status, then discuss each advance, then illustrate two frameworks that place the advances into a health care context, and finally present a section on specific advances in the field of nursing. All the advances in this chapter are within the scope of an emerging field called Relationship Psychology and Interpersonal Neurobiology (IPNB) (Siegel and Solomon, 2013). Although currently heavily informed by interpersonal clinical psychology integrated with emerging concepts in neurobiology, we anticipate that as neural measurement tools advance, IPNB may play a major role to integrate research studies focused on intrapersonal emotional functions and relationship behaviors with those focused upon neural functioning. We recommend Van der Kolk's book (2014) as a resource on this topic.

SEVEN ADVANCES IN RELATIONSHIP PSYCHOLOGY

Each advance below is stated as a hypothesis. Each of these hypotheses is in a different stage of evolution and scientific validation. We have discussed them in the section "Going deeper into each advance." As a group, these advances impact the following elements of patient care: relational attunement, compassion, and empathy; clinician emotional self-care; affect labeling and regulation; health behavior change, contemporary view of personality organization; role of emotions in decisions, the body holds memory; transfer of information; implicit memory reconsolidation; perceptual learning, and shared decision making.

1. **Information Transfer:** People who are experiencing intense emotions are unable to recall with accuracy or completeness (short or long term) the new information supplied at that time. This advance is a hypothesis supported by repeated observations of parents and medical patients. No comparative controlled trials were located.
2. **Emotion Regulation:** Assigning a verbal symbol to felt emotions (affect labeling) softens the intensity of the emotion within that person. This advance is a widely used hypothesis supported by repeated observations from multiple sources during clinical encounters in health care, psychotherapy of all types, and sports coaching.
3. **Relationship Platform:** The relational attunement between clinician and patient enhances information transfer, decision making, changes in patients' behaviors, and transformation of beliefs, emotions, and memories. This advance is a hypothesis supported by repeated observation of clinicians with patients, and by comparative controlled research.
4. **Emotional Self-Care for Clinicians:** Clinicians who have acquired an ongoing internal method to soften their inner reactions to their patients' behaviors and illnesses are able (1) to reaccess their capacity to be empathic and psychologically present with their patients in order to facilitate behavior change and decision making, and (2) to regulate those verbal and action behaviors toward patients, which behaviors are primarily designed to protect their own feelings and inadvertently harm patients and increase costs. This is a hypothesis supported by reliability-tested comparative controlled pilot studies of recorded health care interventions, and by abundant clinical observations by physicians, nurses, allied professionals, and psychotherapists.
5. **Shift in View of Mind Organization:** The human personality operates as a multiplicity of separate interacting personalities (as a community of "parts") not as one unit (monolithic paradigm). This perspective increases the power of the above two advances: relational platform-building and clinician self-care. This view of mind organization is a hypothesis supported (1) by repeated observations from multiple sources: medical care, theater, literature, psychotherapy, sports, negotiation, and (2) by outcome findings in health care and psychotherapy of patients with a variety of chronic bodily illnesses and mental health conditions.
6. **Role of Implicit Memory:** Interviewing that brings about implicit memory reconsolidation is reported to be a successful strategy for facilitating change and symptom relief. This is a hypothesis supported by recorded and repeated clinical observation and by comparative controlled research trials.

7. **Medical Decision Making Is a Process Involving Emotions and Relationship, Not Only Reasoning about Facts:** During decision making by clinicians and patients, weighing pros and cons of available information is overshadowed by both explicit and implicit emotions, beliefs, relational needs, intuitions, and rules of thumb. This is a hypotheses supported by recorded clinical observation, a few controlled research studies, laboratory studies isolated from relationship factors, and many clinical trials.

GOING DEEPER INTO EACH ADVANCE

In these discussions we present the psychological advances without mentioning the possible correlations with the neuroscience advances, which you will read about in Chapter 5. One reason for separately introducing the advances in each field is to avoid conflation of the research coming from these two distinct, yet related, domains. The nature of interplay between these topics becomes clearer in Chapter 7, where we formulate new theory and strategy, and in Chapter 9, where we describe and you witness in the videos how the two domains overlap in real-life interviews. We cite here and in Chapter 5 a limited number of the dozens of research studies in order to simplify the complexity of the field and maintain a focus. What we have not discussed can be found by reading the references. In Chapter 6, we integrate past traditional with many of the current advances.

Information transfer

The block in assimilation of information is remedied by processing of the patient's emotions in a relationship.

No passion so effectively robs the mind of all its powers of acting and reasoning as fear.

Edmund Burke (1720–1797)
Irish and British statesman, supporter of the American Revolution

Fear is a prime blocker of information assimilation for patients. Waves of fear are an aspect of ongoing experience for patients during encounters with clinicians, whatever their degree of awareness and however kindly their clinicians behave. The clinician can periodically reduce this block to information assimilation by using certain effective interviewing skills. We discuss the strategies and tactics for this later on, and the videos demonstrate them.

In the past, information transfer has been treated as if it is primarily a cognitive task, while many clinicians and program directors were discovering the contrary (Livingstone and Wexler, 2007). The cognitive paradigm in the field of public health education and communication had dominated theory and strategy and understandably has been carried over into direct patient care. The forces of emotions, memory, belief systems, and relationships were left out of all the former strategies (Patient-Centered Care, shared decision making, behavior change models, holistic nursing, narrative medicine) for transferring evidence-based information to patients. No publications or research about relational dynamics and emotional aspects of this topic could be found. Two clinical examples are given here.

The first example is how emotions generated in the present by the clinician can cause information transfer blockage.

A consulting chief thoracic surgeon walked to his desk without a "hello" or making eye contact with a new patient and said, "What are you doing next week? We need to schedule you." You might imagine the fear, confusion, and whirl of thoughts that were triggered in the patient and how most of the evidence-based statistics pro and con surgery that the surgeon began spouting fell on either deaf or distorting ears. This is not an uncommon blockade of the information transfer needed to foster shared decision making about treatment choice. The patient consulted another medical center. A shared decision was made with the second consultant to check if there was blood flow across the pulmonary A-V malformation that had been identified, and there was none.

The events in the second example you have already read about in Chapter 1 to illustrate how clinician self-care and well-conducted clinician–patient relationships are essential cost savers. We mention it again here to illustrate how emotions from distant past events can blockade information transfer in the present.

This is the story about the postpartum mother who was impacted by what she heard her obstetrician say, namely, "Boy, did you give me gray hairs last night." What she believed she heard in a semiconscious and vulnerable state became and remained an implicit emotion-charged memory. Despite the pediatrician's reassurances, she and her husband had taken their 18-month-old child to the big medical centers for three identical evaluations which included reexaminations of the birth record and the same exam elements including an EEG. All the evaluations had been normal, yet a worry that something was wrong with her child persisted and kept driving the motivation to obtain another evaluation. The facts of the repeated evaluations and the companion reports were not assimilated. During this fourth evaluation, a skilled, curious interviewer helped the mother recover the implicit memory that was linked to her ongoing fear that her newborn son was not fully intact. After she and her husband had processed their emotions and were reassured effectively, they were able to assimilate the identical normal findings from this fourth evaluation. They stopped shopping from clinic to clinic. Her husband was able to appreciate his wife's emotions and how her concern got started, instead of trying to reduce his wife's anxiety and his own with the facts from three expensive evaluations.

Regarding public health precautions of parents about measles vaccinations, Peter Coy reports that dramatic images and narratives given to parents about children with measles that intended to motivate parents to vaccinate actually decreased the parent's intent to vaccinate. The article states, "People are pretty good at coming up with reasons to continue to hold the beliefs they already hold. Insulting and disrespecting people's beliefs only hardens their perspective" (Coy, 2015). We have also observed in recorded interviews that persuasion and reasoned pressure creates a hardening push-off between clinician and patient. Another interpersonal route needs to be developed.

Exit interviews of patients after clinical encounters (and of parents after parent–teacher conferences) indicate that when the professional starts the session by providing informational data, very little is recalled and with much less accuracy than when the session begins with the professional listening to and connecting with whatever emotions and concerns the patient has on board. Paying attention to presenting concerns is a necessary preparatory step. This type of failure of information transfer persists even when the information being provided is well matched with the patient's cognitive style and educational level. Also, our studies show that because the nature of the information often triggers additional emotions in the patent, these reactive emotions also need to be processed as they arise during the information provision phase of the interview. Our information transfer research indicates that the clinician needs to be processing the patient's emotions and beliefs before and during the provision of information—in a relationally attuned fashion. We call this approach "Information Interweave™" (Chapter 6), which focuses on an *interpersonal process*, rather than to use the common term *information transfer*, which refers to a goal.

Emotion regulation

Affect-labeling also facilitates interpersonal *verbal sharing* while experiencing *some* of the emotion. This is a tactic promoting *implicit memory reconsolidation*—an additional downregulator of emotions—as compared to *verbal behaving* the emotion toward another person which disrupts relational connection.

You are probably familiar with statements like, "I felt that he did not listen to me." Pause a moment to realize that this statement expresses a thought, but the "feeling" has *not* been shared. Feelings are usually one word and often experienced in the body—such as sad, angry, hurt, relieved, etc. If a skilled interviewer was told this, she might reply, "I hear you. So when you think someone is not listening to you, could you check on what feeling you may experience—checking your body—what word would describe that?" With this kind of guidance, the sender usually finds the word or words that are right for them, like "frustrated" or "hurt" or "annoyed." Each of those words is a symbol or label for an affect, and it seems to impact where in the brain it is processed. Find more on this in Chapter 5 on neuroscience. The act of labeling affects is not only for accurate communication to another person but is for the benefit of the sender's brain and mind. It softens the intensity and calms down their bodily sensations.

Recorded interviews of nurse health coaching repeatedly confirm this. Labeling a feeling, when done properly, doesn't escalate feelings; it lowers the risk of behaving it and keeps the other person engaged. This tactic and the strategy behind it was one of the major items in our curriculum for nurse health coaching (Livingstone and Gaffney, 2013).

Toni Herbine-Blank (2015) nationally-recognized lead trainer in couples therapy and developer of the curriculum *Intimacy from the Inside Out*®, has demonstrated in live interactions for years the value to relationships of putting words on feelings and locating where they show up in the body of the speaker. That process reduces the risk of expressing feelings toward the partner as verbal and action *behaviors*, which usually trigger the relationship partner.

The kindergarten teacher says, "Use your words" (instead of action), and it is never too late for adults to do the same, so that they can have choices about how they behave. Some studies, however, indicated that affect regulation was not associated with affect labeling. They were studies done in laboratories, using questionnaires—but outside the context of an interpersonal relationship. We believe that the foundation of the efficacy of affect labeling may be the relationship platform. Observation supports this, and continuing behavioral and neuroscience research will tell us more. The clinical testimonials are overwhelming, yet we could not find a comparative controlled clinical study that tests this hypothesis. Some laboratory behavioral research negates the association of affect labeling with emotional regulation. So far many studies have too many design flaws to be useful clinically. For example, a study by Black (2013) attempted to attribute the mechanisms of emotional regulation observed in mindfulness work to the affect labeling that takes place within mindfulness therapy. There was an indirect association with a mindfulness process. The laboratory condition they used to simulate affect and measure labeling was so far removed from the relationship context of mindfulness work and the conditions that usually surround affect labeling that it was difficult to assess the findings. The affect labeling condition was that the subjects were asked to label an affect from looking at pictures of faces—not from feeling it. We believe that this type of laboratory study attempts, understandably so, to control variables and measurable conditions, yet it is at the expense of research designs that are meaningfully linked to clinical and real-life experiences with emotions.

Relationship platform

How clinicians can establish a relational platform can be learned and no longer needs to be consigned to the vague entities of "clinical experience" and "innate talent." The success of both attachment-based models of psychotherapy and interpersonal biology indicate that relational attachments are transformative when empathic room is made for the activated and disassociated past memories.

What we used to call *alliance* many years ago we have broadened to call *relational platform*. This implies more than an alliance or an agreement as to goals. Relational platform implies something solid upon which other processes rest and depend. It is an attuned, reciprocal relationship within which awareness, compassion, and empathy exist and where judgments are noticed, explored, and helped to soften. The three videos demonstrate it.

Later we present a self-directed process for clinicians (see "Clinician Emotional Self-Care" in Chapter 8) to learn to be affectively present to establish a relational platform—neither too detached nor too activated by emotion—so that being present is possible. The work of Bolby, Ainsworth, Main, and Wallins, who modified the Freudian model to one of relationship (right-brain/relational interventions), supports the understanding that relational affective connection and attachment are crucial to optimal functioning throughout life for everyone. Wylie and Turner (2015) emphasized that individual internal processes of mindfulness, along with attachment relationships, help generate an internal and secure foundation.

As a result of her growing interest in IPNB, Bonnie Badenoch (2008) authored a book and became one of the founders of the nonprofit organization Global Association for Interpersonal Neurobiology Studies (GAINS), a group that fosters application of IPNB in all walks of life. She is editor-in-chief of the *GAINS Quarterly* publication.

HISTORICAL PERSPECTIVE ON RELATIONSHIP PLATFORMS

Early in my staff-ship as a newly graduated fellow in child and adolescent psychiatry, I was given a project to check the medical record system of our clinic to see if they reflected the care being given. What jumped out at me from the reviews was that many children and parents who came for diagnostic evaluations had already been to several other clinics. A lot of questions popped up for me. Where we doing something perceived as that different? What was unsatisfactory at the preceding clinics? How could we be their last stop? I wanted to explore the factors involved—including that the clinicians might need to find new ways to engage patients.

A review of records showed that the factual results of previous evaluations compared to our evaluations were nearly identical. So I wondered, why did some of the families stop with us? Were we doing something different on some other level? I discovered several hunches ("hypotheses" in science parlance), none of them tested. In our clinic parents were seen for several visits separately from the child. In the notes I reviewed, parent interviews included explorations of the emotions and beliefs of parents in response to their child's trouble and often not directly connected to the child diagnostic questions. It was a "meeting the parents where they were," as parent interviewer Ms Portnoi would say. The goals, reservations, fears, and mistrusts of each parent were well articulated. This approach to parents was not by administrative design; it was the insight of Tikva Portnoi, a Smith College faculty member and director of clinical social work at a Harvard affiliate medical center. She believed that parental alliance was crucial to coordinating any child psychiatry case. I practiced the ability to put my diagnostic agenda about the child on a back burner initially while focusing on engaging parents. That engagement was like the platform for the entire evaluation. It seemed to make little sense to gain diagnostic accuracy about a child if the parents couldn't assimilate the results or follow through on our recommendations. We discovered that results about children had to be presented to parents with whom a relationship had already been established and in ways that made room for their ambivalence and expression of emotion. With the child, the same strategy was needed—relationship-building with her or him at whatever age and in whatever form worked. Regarding a plan, there is no point of parents being in one "place," and the child or teenager being in another. I recall our staff conferencing, which was interspersed into a four-hour-long interviewing process. We could really care about the child *and* both parents, about their uniqueness and their pain. It bonded the staff together for a 10-year-long project of practice, teaching, and research.

Long story short: what started as a records review turned into the design of a multidisciplinary evaluation clinic in Boston, the first of its kind in the country to integrate pediatrics, neurology, child psychiatry, clinical social work, and clinical psychology (Livingstone et al., 1968). We had the full support of the chief of service, Silvio Onesti, Jr, whose work is referenced below. A comparative research study showed that we became the last stop for many families, overall costs to our families were low in comparison to failed treatment plans, and several other centers adopted the same model in child health (Portnoi and Livingstone, 1973; Livingstone, 1981). It probably wasn't the model of team integration that was most powerful, although enjoyable. It was the attention paid to gathering data via a relationship, building psychologically based relational alliances, and also obtaining comprehensive diagnostic facts about the child—all three. This combination propelled a process toward sound treatment choices, which were shared between patients and our staff and the referring professionals—Shared Decision Making, 1968-style, before the phrase was coined.

CURRENT EXPERIENCE WITH RELATIONSHIP PLATFORMS

The Accreditation Council for Graduate Medical Education (ACGME) in 2012 embraced the idea that medical graduates should be knowledgeable about both established and evolving behavioral science and "competent in interpersonal communication skills that result in effective exchange of information and communication with patients and their families."

A recent publication by psychiatrists from the Group for Advancement of Psychiatry (Harper, 2013), including Drs. Gordon Harper and Silvio Onesti, Jr., remind us of the diminishing use of relationships between clinician and patient, even in psychiatry. The experience of psychotherapists is that a *diagnostic category* does not provide sufficient information to guide treatment. These concerned authors from leading medical schools say, "Data from interaction with patients are increasingly marginalized in psychiatry, even as interactional data have an increasing role elsewhere in health care. Data from the clinician's engagement *with* the patient, including appreciation of how the patient feels, differ from observations *of* the patient. Although data obtained from relationships are an essential component of the clinician intervention, their use has been decreasing in recent years." They note that categorical diagnoses "reinforce reliance on data *about* the individual patient, as opposed to relationship-based data." We notice also that patients take on the identity of their diagnostic category—"I'm a bipolar" and "I'm an ADD," often said by teenagers and adults in my office. This keeps them from getting in touch with their feelings and thoughts about themselves and their illness, and often is an attempt to mitigate shame.

INGREDIENTS OF RELATIONSHIP PLATFORMS

The degree of connection and synchrony that is possible for each person in a relationship is influenced by early attachment patterns (Siegel, 2011, 2013) and the growth that has occurred since then.

One of the advances in neuroscience presented in the next chapter provides hope for change in this domain at any age. The attachment-based therapies (Schwartz's Internal Family Systems Psychotherapy and the Stones' Voice Dialogue and Psychology of the Selves) emphasize that the combined experiences of relational attachment and of mindfulness are a powerful combination to foster optimal psychological growth. The relationship evolves between clinician and patient. It is the foundation upon which rests the common clinical tasks of health care and wellness, including taking a meaningful history; exploring current concerns, values, emotions, beliefs; transmitting new information; facilitating behavior and lifestyle change; and providing decision support. The goals of a clinical relationship could be stated as building trust and safety from being shamed, judged, abandoned, or violated in some way, for example, not being told the full truth about your illness.

The basic neurological substrate of a relational platform, as discussed in Chapter 5, is an emotional brain-to-brain linkage. That our brains are social organs was emphasized by Anette Karmiloff-Smith et al. (1995). The *basic psychological ingredients* of relational platforms with which most workers agree are captured by the following phrases: affective connection, body awareness, attunement; resonating through sounds, speech, and movement that connect; being in synchrony (Siegel and Hartzel, 2003; Cozolino, 2013; van der Kolk, 2014).

An important advance regarding building a relational platform is the observation that during an interview or encounter between clinician and patient, when the clinician respects and relates to the presenting personality part of the patient at the start, the initial presentation usually relaxes, and a vulnerable emotional "voice" starts to appear. The clinician can then get in tune with that vulnerable part also, without generating overwhelming affect intensity. This double attunement deepens the relational platform and sense of safety.

RESEARCH ON ESTABLISHING A RELATIONSHIP PLATFORM: A HYPOTHESIS FOR THE FUTURE

A current hypothesis derived from the research to date is as follows: When clinicians make attuned relationships with *both* a presenting protective part and a vulnerable part of their patients, the accomplishment of the other tasks is enhanced, namely: information transfer, behavior change, decision making, and adherence to recommendations. It turns information transfer into "interweave" and assimilation. It helps behavior changes to endure. It makes decision making more stable and with less remorse. Chapter 7 discusses this, and the recorded interviews linked to Chapter 9 demonstrate the interview process.

Nurses who learned the relational skills to attune and to be compassionate and empathic with their patients' dominant presenting part and later with their vulnerable personality parts (including the affects and beliefs and memories) were better able by following this strategy to facilitate patients to take active responsibility for their own health when compared to those nurses who coached using the traditional models (see Chapter 3) without having had specialized skill training in this domain. These outcome results were from one random comparative controlled trial using a valid outcome measure, Patient Activation Measure (PAM; Hibbard et al., 2004; Livingstone and Gaffney, 2008). Replication and broadening this research would help validate further the hypothesis stated in the above paragraph.

RELATIONSHIP PLATFORM AND THE ROLE OF EMPATHY AND ATTACHMENT

About implementing these elements in medical care, when at Jefferson Medical College, Steven Klasko, MD, MBA (CEO of USF Health and Dean of the Morsani College of Medicine at the University of South Florida in Tampa) wrote: "It's doable in 2012, but you have to want to do it. Doctors don't buy into any change. Because we look at it from our point of view, and we believe we are right. If I ruled the world, for the next three years, I would put money into changing the DNA of healthcare one doctor at a time" (Marchese, 2014).

Feshback (1978), Waal (2009), Goleman (1995), and Ekman (1989) have written about empathy. Most workers now agree that people may mean two different things by the word *empathy*. *Affective empathy* is the feelings we get in response to another's emotions, and *cognitive empathy*, or perspective taking, is our ability to recognize and understand others' thinking. If researchers do not specify, it is hard to know what they are meaning. Much has been written about the human and social value of empathy, for example, Richard Davidson, John Medina, Paul Ekman, the Ashoka Foundation's Start Empathy Initiative, and Playworks. We have found many times that despite what people call this relational process, we need to hear it and see it for ourselves to know what interpersonal process they are talking about.

Norma Feshback in the 1960s was one of the first to study normative development of empathy in children. She now believes that many in psychology and medicine still conceptualize empathy as social comprehension and cognitive role taking. She goes on to say, "But from my perspective, it is not compassion or caring, but empathy may mediate compassion or caring. It is not social comprehension or cognitive understanding, but both processes may be fundamental to empathy. Perhaps research on mirror neurons will help us" (a recent personal communication from her home in California).

The Institute for Mental Health Initiatives in Washington, DC, decided to enhance the development of empathy in television audiences, based upon social learning theory (modeling behavior). For 10 years they supported my part-time project to help writers and directors in the creative community to portray empathic relationships for their characters, especially as a pathway to adaptive ways to regulate interpersonal hurt and anger. Aspects of the project included periodic conferences with leading actors, writers, executives, and members of Congress and a quarterly publication, called *Dialogue,* for the creative community. We defined *empathy* as a combination of feeling into the other's experience without becoming the other person, and cognitive understanding of the other's viewpoint without having to be in agreement. One of my take-aways from that project was that there were many opportunities in a script that could portray interpersonal empathy, even by "strong" action-bound men, once the writers understood the strength required to own emotions and to speak them rather than to behave them. The types of scenarios we changed to verbal expression were the standard expressions of anger in teenagers of slamming the door, leaving the room, and then perhaps hearing the car burn rubber. Just as effective—and even more engaging for their audience—was to have the teenager express anger verbally and effectively toward his or her parents without calling them names. Writers had little notion of how to script these important aspects of their dramas, and actors had only a narrow repertoire from their own teenage memories but loved this new approach.

Helen Riess, founder of the Empathy and Relational Science Program at Harvard Medical School affiliate Massachusetts General Hospital, teaches about the power of empathy in medical relationships and developed a "neuroscience-based empathy training program." Although she does not provide us with her operating definition of empathy or her specific teaching tactics, for her there is an affective component. In describing her program she says, "We weren't teaching doctors what to say, but more how to be and to be responsive to picking up patients' cues and clues about their emotional states." She says her training teaches physicians to ask about "not just the chief complaint but also the chief concern." She and colleagues conducted a systematic review and meta-analysis of randomized controlled trials for possible impact of patient–clinician relationship on health care (Kelley et al., 2010). Their stated goal was "To determine whether the patient–clinician relationship has a beneficial effect on either objective or validated subjective healthcare outcomes." They found only 13 RCTs that met their eligibility criteria—that the patient-clinician relationship was "systematically manipulated" and that the health care outcomes were objective, such as blood pressures and pain scores. They excluded studies on routine physicals, substance abuse, or mental health visits or when the outcome measure was patient satisfaction. Using a random-effects model, the estimate of the overall effect size was small ($d = 0.11$), but statistically significant ($p = 0.02$). They concluded that the studies showed a small but statistically significant effect of patient–clinician relationship on outcomes. They note that few trials met their selection criteria and none were specifically designed to test the effect of the patient–clinician relationship on health care outcomes. It is not clear to us what observational relational criteria were used in the studies surveyed. The authors suggest that more research be done on this topic.

Also, Riess and team (2011) pilot tested the effectiveness of their empathy training protocol with 11 otolaryngology residents. Results showed that a brief series of three empathy training sessions significantly improved physicians' knowledge of the neurobiology and physiology of empathy, as well as their self-reported ability to empathize with patients. They said, "A trend toward increased patient satisfaction was observed." Although this encourages more research, the need for improvement in research design remains clear. Knowledge about empathy does not necessarily help develop the skill. Self-reporting has proven to be an inadequate indicator from our supervision of therapy trainees and from recorded observations of nurse health coaches who possessed plentiful knowledge about empathy but couldn't perform it well. Also, from comparing self-reports with direct observations of interviewing in my training of child mental health clinicians, self-reporting is very different from what is observed, including observations by the same clinicians who, soon after the clinical encounter, observed a recording of their same session (Livingstone, 1968, Team Clinic). The differences were significant between their recall and their observations of the same session.

The method of asking patients after the session may not yield the same results as direct observations of their psychic or neural experiences during the relationship encounter. Often, the affective and implicit memory trends of a session and nonverbal and physiological responses both tend to remain outside the awareness of trainees. When doing empathy research, we prefer also to include directly observed nonverbal indicators as to whether the patient has experienced empathy in the relationship with a clinician since anecdotal evidence points to those indicators as being most directly linked to concrete outcomes such as behavior change, pain relief, and adherence to recommendations.

There are a considerable number of professionals who now embrace the use of empathy in health care. These include Linda Efferen, MD, FCCP, chief medical officer at South Nassau Communities Hospital in Oceanside, New York; Ruth Malloy, PhD, managing director and global head of leadership and talent at Hay Group in Boston; Jeffrey Spike, PhD, professor at the McGovern Center for Humanities and Ethics and director of the campuswide ethics program at the University of Texas Health Science Center at Houston; Stephen K. Klasko, MD, MBA, CEO of USF Health and dean of the Morsani College of Medicine at the University of South Florida in Tampa; and Jennifer Potter, MD, associate professor of medicine Harvard Medical School. What is meant by *empathy* regarding the cognitive and emotion-based processes between people, however, continues to be discussed by contemporary relationship therapists (Hendrix, 1988; Schwartz, 2013; Herbine-Blank et al., 2015) and by developmental psychologists who conducted child developmental research on empathy (Feshback, 1978).

If research is to be replicated, it matters that researchers and clinicians are consistently clear about the range of interpersonal observables being assessed and the definitions being used. Our conclusions about the cognitive and emotion-based aspects of relationship are discussed in Chapters 6 and 7. We will discuss in Chapter 7 that there are opposing research priorities being lived out all over medicine, including psychiatry, **between** the clinical power of information from being with patients (and its revival) **and** the clinical power of data about patients, i.e. technology, categories, protocols (and its expansion) (Harper et al., 2015). Obtaining "data" from patients is not the main feature in our view of being *with* the patient. The clinical power of being *with* the patient is that emotional and cognitive processes progress in the safety of an attuned relationship between patient and clinician, resulting in affect regulation and the tolerance required for making changes in behavior and tough decisions. Research issues pertinent to this domain are discussed in Chapter 14.

Nursing also has paid robust attention to education on empathy. Brunero, Lamont, and Caotes in 2010 (Brunero et al., 2010) reviewed the efficacy of empathy education programs in nursing. The studies included were required to have measured the effectiveness of empathy training in postgraduate and/or undergraduate nurses. The included studies incorporated both qualitative and quantitative methods and were published in peer-reviewed journals. Of the 17 studies that met inclusion criteria, 11 reported statistically significant improvements in empathy scores, versus 6 studies that did not. The authors conclude, "Models of education that show most promise are those that used experiential styles of learning." However, the definition of empathy and the methods of measurement again were design issues, and they impact the ability to replicate the studies.

The newest findings on empathy and attachment suggest, however, that more than being taught to show empathy, students of medicine and nursing can learn to uncover what keeps getting covered over within them that would allow them to be empathic, with psychological safety. We have observed that whatever researchers mean by empathy and whatever are the attempts to teach it, most clinicians have more empathic ability than they are able to safely access within themselves. During their lives and their medical training, much is covered over by an increasing need to protect their own vulnerable emotions activated by seeing so much illness, by carrying big responsibilities, and by aspects of the learning culture. This is not a new understanding. What is new is a theory that explains the dynamics of how this cover-over happens and that leads to strategies and self-directed tactics most clinicians can use to remedy it. Going deeper into clinician emotional self-care is the next topic.

Emotional self-care for clinicians

Clinicians who have acquired a reliable internal method to soften their inner reactions to their patients' behaviors and illnesses are able (1) to reaccess their capacity to be empathic and psychologically present with their patients in order to facilitate behavior change and decision making, and (2) to regulate those verbal and action behaviors toward patients, which behaviors are primarily designed to protect their own feelings but inadvertently are sometimes harmful for patients and increase costs.

After the recent Boston Marathon bombings, one of the ER doctors treating children replied to a news reporter: "You just keep working at it without stopping or feeling, and when you're done, the feelings flood in and overwhelm. I have to somehow take care of myself before I can talk to the parents, but how do I do that?"

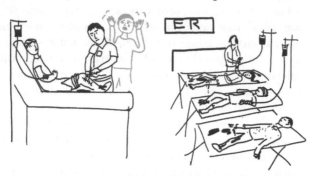

CLINICIAN SELF-NEGLECT

Nancy Sowell, who organized a research study using the Internal Family Systems (IFS) model of psychotherapy with rheumatoid arthritis patients at Harvard-affiliated Brigham and Women's Hospital, described clinician self-care well when saying, "If I am feeling anxious about my patient's medical condition and self-destructive (health) behaviors, my effectiveness as a clinician is diminished. As I begin to work, I help my protectors (parts) know that I am here with them and with my patient—I subtly communicate with my own (personality) parts" (Sowell, 2013).

In the analysis of several hundred recordings of patient–clinician interviews we found that clinicians almost always said and did things (like starting to look up information on their computers) that blocked the formation of an attuned relationship with the patient or disrupted the affective connection and ability to empathize. In the subsequent inquiries with the same clinicians, they realized that their disconnection from the patient's process and from themselves was driven by the dominance of their own emotions and concerns at that point in the interview. They noticed that they had been emotionally triggered by something the patient was saying or by memories coming up in their minds. This type of reaction can be remedied by emotional self-care.

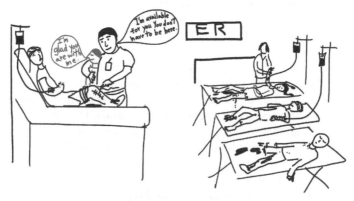

CLINICIAN SELF-CARE

PALLIATIVE MEDICINE AND CLINICIAN SELF-CARE

Clinician emotional self-care began to evolve in the field of oncology and palliative care (Meier et al., 2001). Simultaneously, quantum leaps in emotional self-care were developed and being practiced by psychotherapists (Stone and Winkelman, 1985; Schwartz, 1995). These two tracks needed to be integrated. The term *emotional self-care* as we use it here means the psychological process by which clinicians work within themselves (both in-the-moment and as an ongoing practice) on the emotions, thoughts, memories, and body sensations that normally become activated during their encounters with patients and often block attunement with patients. More specifically, self-care consists of the strategies and tactics clinicians can learn to use within themselves to manage their own emotional reactivity and to stay in relationship with their patients. Although historically, emotional self-care has not been a salient feature in the training of health care clinicians, except in oncology, mindfulness practices are used by some clinicians and are found helpful. And, neural correlates of both mindfulness and labeling of affects have been discovered, and you will find them in Chapter 5. A helpful collaborative review was published from University of Texas, Dana Farber/Harvard, Mayo Clinic, Baylor, Duke, Yale Cancer Center, Stanford, and Palo Alto, VA, titled *Caring for Oneself to Care for Others: Physicians and Their Self-Care* (Sanchez-Reilly et al., 2013). Meir had already described, "professional loneliness, loss of professional sense of meaning, loss of clarity about the goals of medicine, cynicism, hopelessness, helplessness, frustration, anger about the health care system, loss of a sense of patients as human beings, increased risk for burnout and depression" (Meir, 2001). Continuing in 2013, Sandra Sanchez-Reilly et al. still found a lack of adequate self-care professional training of medical students, residents, and fellows to recognize and deal with their own unrecognized, unexpressed, and unexamined emotions. The accreditation standards for American and Canadian medical schools (Liason Committee on Medical Education) do not specifically identify self-care or other related areas. The search by medical schools for remedies was also motivated by the findings of others (Drybyc, 2010), that clinicians' unprocessed emotions are associated with "important patient-related outcomes like medical errors by physicians, lower patient satisfaction, longer post-discharge recovery by patients, unprofessional conduct, and less altruistic values." What was called "compassion fatigue" was written about in the Psychosocial Stress Series (Figley, 2002) and by Wright (2004). These authors had described symptoms in clinicians that "mirror post-traumatic stress disorder," including hyper-arousal, avoidance, and reexperiencing memories of stressful clinician encounters.

In addition to the gross symptoms and behaviors mentioned above, this textbook deals with the not-so-obvious verbal and action behaviors of clinicians that impact patient outcome that have been recorded and observed in our work. We found no published curriculum in medical or nursing schools on this topic. Based upon several randomized trials on the effects of mindfulness-based interventions for health care clinicians, nursing, and medical students, the self-care training and education for medical learners proposed by Sanchez-Reilly et al. (2013) included mindfulness meditation and reflective writing as two methods to enhance self-awareness. Their article is one of the first publications to list competencies relevant to self-care. Without specifying how, their list clarifies what clinicians should be able to do, such as "process own emotions in a clinical setting; demonstrate respect and compassion, demonstrate capacity to reflect on personal attitudes, values, strengths, vulnerabilities, and experiences [in order to] to optimize personal wellness and capacity to meet the needs of patients." This sounds very good, but how to apply it was not clarified.

SELF-DIRECTED EMOTIONAL SELF-CARE USED BY PSYCHOTHERAPISTS

For the first time, psychotherapists have discovered an effective pathway to work with their own emotions and beliefs from moment to moment during a session with their patient—what was traditionally referred to as *countertransference*. The biggest shift in strategy of clinician emotional self-care came with the development by Richard Schwartz of the IFS model (see later, Shift in Mind Organization). Contained within this model of psychotherapy is the most clinically proven, scientifically grounded method we have discovered for emotional self-care. Not just theory and strategy, it illustrates tactics. Aspects of the IFS model have given thousands of IFS psychotherapy clinicians an effective, new power to work within themselves that uses mindfulness and goes beyond it to directly care for emotions and memories within and also the protective armor that may get behaved toward patients (for example, countertransference reactions like disconnectedness and lack of interest masquerading as therapeutic neutrality, or overintellectual explanations used by the therapist to defend against his or her own triggered feelings masquerading as therapeutic interpretation, or overidentification and protective advice-giving).

In the past, some form of mindfulness meditation has been the main approach. This tactic makes use of the breath and goes beyond mindfulness. Through the multiplicity lens, however, a new entity gets added. The addition is the therapist being in an internal relationship with each separate personality within him- or herself. This has a powerful, calming, and regulatory impact. Psychotherapists have discovered the usefulness of accessing this capacity to explore and take care of their own emotions and thinking as they work with their patients—especially when they are triggered by their patient's verbal and action behaviors. Some psychoanalysts and psychodynamic therapists have seen this approach as a new power to work with countertransference (Kaplan, 2014 and Onesti, 2013, personal communications).

In health care the protective armor includes judging, scolding out of frustration, pulling back your presence, providing more information, blaming the patient for perceived clinical failures, and abruptly giving over the care of patients' emotions to another professional. Carrying too much vulnerability or continual struggling with strong internal protectors are causes of *compassion fatigue*. Based on the self-care skills of IFS, I successfully designed a self-care routine for rowing athletes and their coaches to add to their general mindfulness practices. Here, we propose a self-directed routine (see Chapter 8) for clinicians as a new pathway to apply the recommendations made in the article cited above by Drs. Sanchez-Reilly and Morrison.

We hope you can understand that the clinician's ability to self-care is a *sine qua non* for optimal care of any patient. Presence of a core nonjudgmental awareness potential capacity within people is now confirmed by thousands of psychotherapists worldwide. This has changed the IFS professional's role from being primary to becoming a secondary facilitator and safe relational container for the patient's own inside work. This is different from the Voice Dialogue session for which the professional maintains the role of external facilitator. The role as external facilitator is also used occasionally in IFS psychotherapy—being called "direct access."

The health care clinician, however, always is making a "direct access" relationship with the medical patient's personality parts. Whereas for that same clinician's emotional self-care, that clinician is accessing his or her own core self to make the aware relationship with his or her own personality parts—not unlike the self-directed process between IFS therapy sessions.

Both IFS and Voice Dialogue seem to be advances beyond the clarifications and interpretations of traditional psychotherapy of the past and implicit emotional memory reconsolidation of the present when conducted in a monolithic paradigm.

EMOTIONS DOCUMENTED IN MEDICAL PRACTITIONERS: IMPACT ON CLINICIANS AND PATIENTS

It is no secret that doctors struggle with their own feelings. In her recent book *What Doctors Feel: How Emotions Affect the Practice of Medicine*, Danielle Ofri (2013), from New York University School of Medicine, vividly described her own thoughts and those that other doctors experience during their medical practice. Here is how the inner thinking sometimes goes: "Suddenly I began to feel unsure of myself, what did I know about office-based medicine—. I could feel the pressure like a barometric surge. This patient clearly wasn't going to back down. Well, damn it, neither was I. If she thinks she can railroad me just because I'm the new doc in town." An IFS-trained clinician would hear the different personality parts that have been activated in these clinicians.

Those familiar with human personality would see the likely dynamics here as the doctor protecting herself from a sense of failure. Nothing is wrong with getting triggered by a patient; it is what the clinician does with it on the inside of themselves and outside of them as behavior that determines how the relationship with the patient unfolds. Interestingly, Ofri reports that low "empathy scores on the cognitively oriented Jefferson Scale of Empathy" (Ofri, 2013) may predict which specialty the student chooses (primary care vs. radiology). But, it does not predict that a medical or nursing student cannot learn the tactics of emotional self-care and how to be empathic—that "something" that we are going to be talking about and demonstrating.

The ability to be empathic is compromised in clinicians who have not been trained in contemporaneous emotional self-care? Recorded interviews and informal observations indicate that clinicians are *relationally* compromised when they are interviewing or examining a patient if *in the moment* they have no effective way to step back from their own strong affective and cognitive reactions to their patient's behavior or to their own emerging memories. What is compromised is their ability (1) to remain connected with their patient, a prerequisite for becoming attuned and empathic, (2) to facilitate the openness required to obtain history and explore values and preferences in a valid fashion, and (3) to regulate their reactive verbal and action behaviors toward the patient so as not inadvertently to destroy trust and do psychological harm. Compromise of these three competencies is found to block the clinician's power to facilitate health behavior change, support conscious decision making, and transfer new information effectively. The impact on care quality has been noted by many workers.

Cheryl Regehr and her group (2014) said, "A significant proportion of physicians and medical trainees experience stress-related anxiety and burnout resulting in increased absenteeism and disability, decreased patient satisfaction, and increased rates of medical errors." They concluded that interventions in programs incorporating psycho-education, interpersonal communication, and mindfulness meditation were associated with reduced stress and "*may* contribute to lower levels of burnout" in physicians. From our initial experiences with already well-trained nurse health coaches from 2006 to 2008, their learning of enhanced relational interviewing skills through mentoring made a marked difference in their reported and observed stress levels as heard in recordings (Livingstone and Gaffney, 2013). As you will see, the new self-care model being developed here adds specific tactics of emotional self-care skills useful in the moment and as ongoing practice that are designed to include and go beyond mindfulness meditation.

SHAME AND CLINICIAN EMOTIONAL SELF-CARE

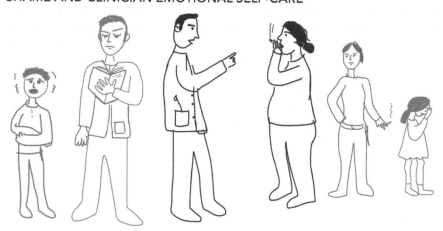

SHAMING PATIENTS IS A PARTS ISSUE

The painful feeling of shame and the protections against feeling it are observed to be a common occurrence in medical care on both sides of the clinician–patient relationship. The seminal work by Brené Brown (2010, 2012), a research professor and doctor of social work at the University of Houston—10 years of research on shame and emotional vulnerability—has helped everyone to better understand. Brown (2012) said, "Vulnerability is the core of shame and fear and our struggle for worthiness but it is also the birthplace of joy and creativity, of belonging, and of love—we learned to protect ourselves from vulnerability—from being hurt, diminished, or disappointed—by putting on emotional armor and acting invulnerable when we were children." Brown believes it is essential for people to expose themselves "to a wide range of feelings in order to combat shame, break down the walls of perfectionism and stop the act of disengagement that separates many from themselves and others." The new tactics of self-directed Clinician Emotional Self-Care presented in Chapter 8 seem to allow this to happen safely thereby preventing protective internal armor from completely taking over again and again.

In *Emotional Cannibalism: Shame in Action*, Martha Sweezy and Ziskind (2013), a psychotherapist, teacher, and researcher at the Harvard Medical School affiliate Cambridge Health Alliance, explains the intrapersonal and interpersonal dynamics of shame. She asserts that all clinicians without realizing it experience shame in many circumstances. Doing a good job is a high priority for clinicians. When I have done something wrong and I am thinking, "I have *behaved* badly," *guilt* is the feeling that comes up. When I have done something wrong and I am thinking, "I *am* a bad, flawed person," *shame* is the feeling that goes with that. The underlying sense that makes the feeling of shame so painful is that the person is identified with a personality part who thinks he or she is unworthy, will not be included, and is alone. The mind sometimes turns judgment and guilt into shame. Also, people are shamed by others ("You should be ashamed of yourself!"), and they also shame themselves on the inside. Observations have shown that shame is hard for people to regulate because often they have been shamed in overt and covert ways much of their lives by parents in a misguided attempt to socialize them and by teachers who mistakenly believe shame and fear of it motivates children and graduate students.

Often you may hear clinicians make statements to patients that in essence say, "What's wrong with you? You *know* what to do, but you don't do it" (take your pills, stop smoking, change diet, etc.). These types of statements shame the patient for behaviors that are caused by the patient's inner protective system, which needs processing with a clinician, not shaming. For example, a protective system would block adherence to a nutritional program that threatens relational ties linked to their family's culture of eating, of which the patient is not yet aware. Shaming the patient does not propel a process of change.

Judgments and shaming occur in many subtle forms. Why do clinicians do this? Our recordings of clinician interviews and inquiry of the same clinicians show they are trying sometimes to regulate their own feeling of frustration with lack of progress and, below their conscious radar, are trying to keep shame of failure away from their door. Why is it so difficult for clinicians to stop themselves from saying these things? Contemporary psychology knows some answers and some remedies.

Clinicians shame others, it is observed, in order to downregulate their own feelings of shame. Whether conscious or not, shame activates the sense of a risk of being abandoned. As hard as they may earnestly try to manage these behaviors toward patients, it is an exercise in futility unless the clinician is given an opportunity to learn how to regulate their shame *from the inside*. Continuing to shame and blame others only increases the tendency to self-shame. Many clinicians are helplessly caught in a cycle of shame. It is now clear that competency at emotional self-care is required to break out of this painful cycle.

It is clearer that the way people try to regulate their shame gets them into more trouble—that is, into a cycle of shaming and feeling shame. For example, here is how the cycle can develop. If a clinician as a youngster witnessed the peripheral vascular complications of diabetes in a loved one (an amputation), he/she will have protections against the reemergence of the same level of fear buried within. This will block empathy and the ability to tune in to what his diabetic patient may need. The protections against re-experiencing the same level of fear will unconsciously drive behaviors of the clinician, such as anxious scolding of the patient to follow the regimen. Outside the clinician's awareness, this extra pushing of the patient may activate aspects of the patient's personality that work against cooperation. Then the patient gets blamed for being resistant or difficult, and the clinician feels more frustration toward the patient of which he secretly feels ashamed, etc.

EMOTIONAL STATUS OF STUDENTS AND STRATEGIC CHALLENGES FOR FACULTY

Helpful for the third-year medical school slump was the Robert Wood Johnson Medical School's Humanism and Professionalism Program, a series of discussions with faculty facilitators about their stressors and the challenges of maintaining humanism. However, when any clinician is triggered by a patient or a faculty member at any point in their career, all the humanistic good intentions, much like in a marriage relationship dynamic, appear to be covered over by default mechanisms of self-protection. These are well-honed inner survival forces that trump good relational intentions.

Dyrbye (2010) emphasized medical student stress. Minnesota medical students now spend a full year working and living in a rural community. The assumption behind this program and others is that the environment of medical training is the main cause for the disappearance of empathy in physicians in training. We and others find that external experience is only one contribution, which if fixed, may improve things somewhat. The internal dynamics of the clinician, however, make a significant contribution. The good news is that now we know new pathways to educate and train in this domain. In reality, contemporary psychotherapists who work in health care when it is not mental health find that students and practicing clinicians faced with a lot of vulnerability in their work life all have the potential to handle better the emotions that bubble up from their past. For example, many clinicians attempt to bury them with mindfulness only to find them reappearing and affecting their behavior. When we mentored nurses in small groups by reviewing with them their recorded clinical interviews with medical patients and helped them focus on what was coming up inside of them, they were able to gain some specific self-care skills that included mindfulness and went beyond it to inner dynamics that they were able to soften.

Some workers believe that "mindfulness" works well as a self-care strategy for students. The question remains as to how student clinicians can gain this skill. Ronald Epstein at the University of Rochester's Departments of Family Medicine and Psychiatry stated, "This critical self-reflection enables physicians to listen attentively to patient's distress, recognize their own errors, refine their technical skills, make evidence-based decisions, and clarify their values so they act with compassion, technical competence, presence, and insight." He recommends that mindfulness is a link between "relationship-centered care and evidence-based medicine and should be considered a characteristic of good clinical practice." He states, however, that mindfulness "*cannot be taught explicitly*; it can be modelled by mentors and cultivated in learners" (Epstein, 1999). Evidence accumulated since 2000 shows however that student clinicians and practitioners can explicitly learn self-directed tactics of emotional self-care that go beyond mindfulness and that work well. (See Chapter 8, "Tactical Competency 1.")

Shift in view of paradigm of mind organization

The human personality operates as a *multiplicity* of separate interacting personalities (as a community of "parts") not as one mind (monolithic paradigm). There is increasing consensus that each distinct personality within one person is a mental "document" containing its unique set of emotions, memories, beliefs, behaviors, and bodily sensations and has an adaptive role in the personality system.

Often you may hear people say things like, "I don't know what got into me," "I just wasn't myself that day," "A part of me doesn't want to go; on the other hand—," "Why did I ever buy this car?," "I don't even know who you are anymore," "I was so stupid to do this." These comments reflect people's everyday experiences with distinctly different parts of personality and their partial awareness of them. Literature, film, and theater are filled with examples of the same phenomenon. The multiplicity paradigm posits that the existence of distinct and separate personality parts explains these common experiences and that it also explains and reveals a remedial pathway when health care patients shift behaviors and change their minds. For a *New York Times* article, Vatican Revisits Divorce (January 25, 2014), random people were interviewed by Italian journalists. One person said, "I am thinking about annulment. I would like to remarry someday. There are little parts of me that regret that I wasn't married at church. But then that other side of me thinks this is ridiculous; there's been divorce as long as there's been marriage." Almost everyone has a sense that parts are at work within them. With interviewing, each part of Ms Puglio might have a distinct set of emotions and beliefs, and a distinctly different history of her childhood and their adaptive role in her childhood. Jon Schwartz and William Brennan (2013) wrote a book for lay people, *There's a Part of Me*—. It explains personality parts and tells stories to illustrate them. Schwartz is a clinician in Oregon and Brennan is an Emmy award-winning TV writer and producer.

PERSONALITY MULTIPLICITY, EVIDENCE FOR EMBRACING IT, AND HOW IT WORKS

The concept of multiplicity of mind is not new (Minsky, 1986; Wright, 1986; Rowan, 1990). If over millions of years you were designing a mind and brain system for survival, wouldn't you think it advantageous for people to possess minds that were wired for many whole personalities available for different functions and circumstances?

Antonio Damasio (1994, 1999), a neuroscientist working separately and simultaneously with the psychologists Hal and Sidra Stone and Richard Schwartz, proposed the hypothesis that supports the concept of personality multiplicity. He said that humans have survived biologically by having a huge repertoire of alternatives and duplications of thinking and feeling, "since the brain holds and retrieves knowledge in spatially segregated rather than integrated manner, they (each) require attention." The later hypothesis about the brain's program supports observation in everyday life experience and the clinically validated discovery that the mind has many replications of personality each with their own "program," that is, with varying sets of emotions, beliefs, and version of memories of our childhood experiences. This sounds like biological adaption at its best. These functionally different programs are called "personality parts" by Richard Schwartz and are called "selves" by Hal and Sidra Stone. Interviewing a part or a self is a convincing experience of their separate existence within one mind and also of the adaptive role each plays for that person's choices, decisions, accomplishments, and pleasures. It explains the complex behavior patterns and relational dynamics of humans and their behaviors when they are ill.

John Steinbeck noticed that we don't function as one mind; so did the actress. Steinbeck (1941) said in his book *Sea of Cortez*, "…but the atavistic urge toward danger persists and it is called your adventurer. Your adventurer feels no gratification in crossing Market Street in San Francisco against the traffic. Instead he will go to a good deal of trouble and expense to get himself (and you) killed in the South Seas." Throughout his writing he shows us personality archetypes and multiplicities, for example, Doc and Mack in *Canary Row* (Steinbeck, 1945) and Tom Joad in *Grapes of Wrath* (Steinbeck, 1939). To us, in addition to being a signature of Steinbeck's writing style, this way of writing is a reflection of his astute observations of normal human personality. Mariska Hargitay (Olivia Benson, *Law and Order*, NBC TV), when asked by James Lipton (Actors Studio) about her acting method, said, "I have a box here within me [pointing to her core] that contains all kinds of characters that I can pull out when I need them." TV comedian Kevin Nealon said, "Although I've been married for 15 years, I have a wandering eye—that looks at women and says, 'hey baby how would you like to come back to my place for a drink?', and then my lazy eye says, 'sounds like a lot of work.'"

Our recorded material indicates that the concept of multiplicity explains common everyday occurrences from which no one seems to be free. The main solution within the multiplicity paradigm is the practice of becoming conscious of what is going on within. The monolithic or unitary sense of personality is a hypothetical construct that reflects only a person's main personality part—the only person they believe they are—that is, until another part shows up and surprises them. Cyril Connolly, the British editor, said "it may seem safest to stick with one consciousness, but multiplicity has a way of making its presence felt. Freud referred to the techniques one uses to keep one's unwanted consciousness away as defense mechanisms. And, sometimes people characterize these other ways of thinking as a different *self*. After all, why not explore the labyrinth, since we are all serving a lifetime in the dungeon of self" (Connolly, 1994). Rather than a "dungeon," we observe that self-awareness and curiosity result in shifts toward experiencing inner calmness, clarity, and relational ability.

Western culture has preferred a unitary view of personality, although many other cultures explore different aspects of the self. As we have said, multiplicity of personality is not a new observation. In the past, however, personality parts have been noticed by professionals mainly when there is a severe disorder of their inner regulation. A disorder results when parts of the personality have become extreme and take over the consciousness of the person—completely shifting from one persona to another. The story of Dr. Jekyl and Mr. Hyde is a classic description of two contradictory personalities in one person, and the films *Three Faces of Eve* and *Sybil* heightened public awareness, but incorrectly also caused some people to worry that they had a disorder if they noticed another personality within themselves.

Although the concept of multiplicity of mind is not new, what is new is the universal observation (1) that each personality part is a full personality—like a person—within one mind, and serves an adaptive purpose which becomes clearer as they share their thinking, and (2) that personality parts (some call them "selves") are willing to be interviewed by a nonjudgmental person and have a unique narrative to share. Also new is the observation that no matter what we have suffered we all continue to possess a capacity in our "core" for awareness, appreciation of each part's internal agenda, and for extending compassion and empathy to that part (like a centered, present parent might give to a distressed child). Schwartz calls this inner core "self." Hal and Sidra Stone call it the "Aware Ego." The focused attentive relationship given to a distressed personality part (whether it is located within someone else or with yourself) results in that part becoming less extreme in the moment and sometimes for the long run. This actually happens within people as they and you observe it. People are often unaware that they have such a conscious, nonjudgmental, even compassionate entity inside their personality. This is good news. A therapist's initial role is to help people access this entity and experience the use of it from within. The power of this internal entity, called "self" in IFS terminology, to make transforming relationships inside the person has changed the strategy and tactics of psychotherapy. It has increased the effectiveness of treatmenting people with serious difficulties, such as eating problems, addictions, suicidal behavior, and PTSD, and it has changed the clinician–patient relationships in which psychoactive medications are prescribed (F. Anderson, 2013, personal communication). There is accumulating evidence that this approach may be more effective and efficient than the traditional strategies used alone such as cognitive-behavioral, psychodynamic, mindfulness, dialectic behavioral therapy (DBT), medication, biofeedback, etc. More evidence-based comparative studies are under way (Shadick et al., 2013). Clinical validation is already abundant.

Each division of personality is willing to be interviewed directly by a trusted, curious, nonjudgmental person (IFS calls this *direct access*; it is the usual tactic in Voice Dialogue). Each has a unique narrative to share about what it believes is most important, its emotions, at what age it got formed within that person, and a version of the person's history—never before heard by the person in whom the part resides. Usually most parts are out of sight doing their jobs within people, but sometimes they get super-activated because feelings of vulnerability are being triggered by reality circumstances. A painful illness is one such circumstance. A loss of a loved one is another. Both vulnerable parts and their protectors get activated in these circumstances.

Observations of the existence of parts have been so ubiquitous as to be considered the normal state of the mind by increasing numbers of scientists and the public. Rather than viewed as a unitary or monolithic "I" with sub-divisions like instincts (the id), the conscience (the superego), and the executive controller and defender (the ego), it proves to be more useful to view the personality is as a community of full personalities plus an awareness function which can integrate the system. The awareness function is much like the compassionate leader of a family or a nonjudgmental orchestra conductor who respects all the players.

Furthermore, the personality parts are observed to interact as a system; some protect the vulnerable, and others are like children in a family. They contain different versions of a person's explicit and implicit emotions, beliefs, and behavioral tendencies. As you may recall from the section on Emotional Regulation, placing a word on an emotion has been proven to regulate it, not make it stronger. That regulation appears to be even more long lasting when the person labels the emotions held by *many* of their personality parts, not only the one dominant part showing at that moment—or if you think monolithically, the *only one*. A fuller exploration of the personalities within us is a type of "being with" our personhood, and appears to foster a process of transformation. The full understanding of, and conscious relationship to, parts or selves within a person is reported to help that person's brain, body, and relationships. For example, Hal and Sidra Stone have observed that when a person is heavily identified with their "pusher" (what we used to call "type A personality"), they overdo whatever they are invested in so continuously that they are at risk for developing bodily illness via immune mechanisms, including coronary inflammation, diabetes, chronic fatigue syndrome, and the collagen diseases. Shadick et al. (2013) conducted a random controlled trail at Harvard's Brigham and Women's Hospital that indicated that working with personality parts of people with chronic rheumatoid arthritis increased, for the first time, their joint mobility and decreased joint pain.

Here is a metaphor that helps some people. The personality parts are like folders in your mind's computer; they are not all visible at one point in time, and sometimes they pop up onto your desktop. They can be opened partially or explored fully. There are 10–15 major ones within everyone—unique to that person and also somewhat similar in function. Richard C. Schwartz identifies two general types of personality parts. One type *protects* people from intense emotions coming from their vulnerable emotion-filled parts left over from childhood—the scared, lonely, ashamed, or abused inner children. Examples of common *protector parts* are pleaser, care taker, pusher, perfectionist, know everything, blamer, inner critic, unrelenting responsibility, running away, substance using. Examples of young emotion-filled *vulnerable parts* are parts carrying implicit memories of childhood experiences that resulted in too much emotion for a child to handle, such as parental absences at an age when it felt like forever; the unrelated babysitter; angry, fighting parents; loss; moves; medical procedures that overwhelm the coping capacities of the child and are not well soothed by well-meaning parents and clinicians.

Some childhood personality parts also carry joy, creativity, and desire to explore the world, and also sexuality and sensuality. Sometimes they are "happy campers" within the person's inner system and contribute readily to the person's relationships. Sometimes they have been locked away by protector parts, including the inner critic, in the interest of maintaining love and connection in a person's family culture at that time.

Spawned from years of observation and clinical experience, the hypothesis of mind multiplicity is a heuristic, like all models, and its value is determined by how well it explains, predicts, and informs strategy, and by the results of research testing.

RELATIONSHIPS IN HEALTH CARE AND PERSONALITY PARTS

Protective parts serve the person in whom they reside (you) and appear to be out of tune with the needs of others (such as your patient or your spouse). Here is the inner dynamic. As the locked-up emotional memory gets closer to consciousness and more emotion is experienced coming from inside, the protector's behavior gets activated. Whatever the person's protectors are will begin to dominate their behavior—such as perfection, working, pleasing, withdrawing, eating, etc. As you will see later, it is the conscious mental use of the aware core-self that releases us from being caught in a dynamic that is internally locked in time from our past ways of coping.

There are dozens of examples of this internal dynamic in health care within both patients and clinicians. There are patients who after signing consent for surgery decide to cancel. Legal consents are often signed when a rational personality part of the patient is dominating their personality, or when a compliant part is dominating even before evidence-based information is assimilated. Later, different personality parts often emerge, for example—an extreme autonomous part invested in taking more time to decide is protecting a vulnerable childhood part that is carrying an unprocessed memory of aloneness, fear, or pain experienced from previous health care. This pairing of different protectors that emerge at different points in time and contradict each other is common in health care. This multiplicity paradigm has shifted the strategy of relationship building in health coaching and has begun to be researched for efficacy (Wennberg, 2010; Livingstone and Gaffney, 2013).

CLINICIAN EMOTIONAL SELF-CARE AND PERSONALITY PARTS

Although clinician self-care has been discussed as a separate topic earlier in this chapter, now that we are discussing the personality parts concept there is more to say about the implications that parts work has for clinician self-care.

Clinicians have their own protector parts paired up to protect their vulnerability. For example, often a paternal scolder part and a know-everything part pair up to protect the clinician against the vulnerability feelings that accompany a clinical "failure." This dynamic often blocks clinicians from facilitating patients to assimilate evidence-based information. For the protective parts to soften, the clinician would need a method to soothe the underlying vulnerable part's emotions. Understanding about parts and relating to their own personality parts enables clinicians to emotionally care for themselves.

For example, if you notice that excess *pleasing* of others is getting activated within you (you're up working very late because you've said yes to too many people), you will be able to shift your behavior if you "go inside" and become curious and aware that this extreme pleasing behavior is only coming from a part of your personality, not from all of you, and that it is attempting to cover some emerging vulnerable part with which you are *not yet* in touch. For example, perhaps it is covering an intense fear of not being included in the group you aspire to. Pleasing and striving for perfection may have been your life-long way to protect yourself from that painful fear of imagined exclusion. As you will read in Chapter 8 on tactics, the first step of self-care in this situation is to take some time (1–2 minutes) to focus inward, to become aware of, and get curious about, what is happening inside, to extend caring to parts that you may notice, and ask them to show you their agenda. Notice that we are not recommending that you bury what you notice or meditate it away. Going **toward** what you notice with caring softens your inner system and in-the-moment allows you to stop working and trying to please and to get some sleep—at least for that episode. To mentally revisit (the next day for about 15 minutes) the activated pleaser part and be open to notice and breathe into the underlying vulnerable part's emotion that it was protecting you (from the one carrying fear in this example) proves to be very helpful and needs to become a self-directed and ongoing self-care practice if a more permanent shift in your inner dynamic is to take place. In fact the fear may be unnecessarily intense from an earlier experience for which you received too little relational caring at the time. You could learn to re-parent yourself in the present and heal the old experience. This shifts things inside your psychology.

Another example involves your inner critic part. The inner critic is a part commonly experienced by clinicians, especially when they have other parts that expect them to be, for example, all-knowing or perfect at fulfilling responsibilities. The inner critic appears from the inside and may overdo it and say some very critical things. If the clinician believes them, he/she will feel quite down. The inner critic can generate guilt and painful shame from the inside and may prompt the clinician to find relief from the pain by blaming and shaming colleagues and patients. Stone and Stone (1993) wrote a wonderfully readable book, *Embracing Your Inner Critic*. Learning that nobody can do enough to beat their inner critic, it is best to realize that the inner critic's job is to enforce the rules of the protector parts, such as the voice of responsibility. The protector parts soften when a clinician can be with his or her particular brand of vulnerable feelings. When the protector parts soften, so does the inner critic. We all have our brand of inner critic.

Understanding about parts and relating to their own parts has provided the newest tool for clinicians to emotionally care for themselves. For example, as a clinician, what helps me right away is an awareness (1) that a marked increase in perfectionism in my professional work would be coming from a personality part, and (2) that it is just a part (Schwartz) or self (Stone) within me and is not all of me, that is, it is *not me*. Also, my inner critic part is going to back up my perfectionist part and scold me on the inside if I do not follow his rules. Therefore, it also helps me to realize that my critic too, is only a part. Parts team up—one is the perfection seeker and the other is the enforcer, the inner critic. The pair have the agenda to protect me from feeling, for example, extra intense anxiety about failing that somehow has been activated within me. My knowing this inner situation is a good start. A routine for clinicians to conduct a self-directed internal process has been developed by us and appears in the list of tactical competencies in Chapter 8. An earlier version for health coaching has been published (Livingstone and Gaffney, 2013). Interestingly, the single most powerful self-care method in the workshops with rowing programs was the athlete's realization in-the-moment that the feelings and thoughts that pop up before and during a competition are coming from parts, not all of them, and that the part can be asked to soften back until later in the day. This aspect of the IFS model works for them.

Regarding clinician emotional self-care when working with LGBTQ patients, Jennifer Potter, Associate Professor of Medicine at Harvard Medical School-affiliated Beth Israel Deaconess Medical Center, wrote an important review that addresses how external and internal bias impacts direct patient care, for example, clinicians making insensitive remarks and jokes (Potter, 2015). She illuminates helpful strategies and clinician self-care tactics informed by the IFS model and by Diane Goodman's work (Goodman, 2011), for clinicians to address their tendencies toward making insensitive remarks/jokes and other factors that derail their care of people who have LGBTQ issues.

IMPACT OF PERSONALITY PARTS ON INTIMATE RELATIONSHIPS

The Stones demonstrated with couple relationships that working with parts of the personality (the selves) reduced patterns of bonding between the selves in each partner that were resulting in painful arguments that had a self-perpetuating energy—with anger, sadness, anxiety, and loss of connection (Stone and Stone, 2000). Schwartz (2008) and Herbine-Blank et al. (2015) describe a vast experience that relationship connection can be maintained or regained by a couple when each partner works with their own personality parts on the inside and speaks on their behalf but not from them, thus not dumping emotion on the partner who would become emotionally triggered. This means that misunderstood partnering dynamics might better be understood and remedied through a multiplicity lens. Partnering dynamics impact clinicians and patient relationships, especially during a decision crisis, and clinicians inadvertently get pulled into the marital dynamics of their patient.

Role of implicit memory

Verbal and action behaviors generated by intense affects do not appear to be softened significantly by suppression, avoidance, cognitive manipulation, or breath work alone. Cozolino (2010) asserts that they are softened by brief interventions that are informed by the specific concepts of *implicit memory reconsolidation*.

Ecker et al. (2012) and other workers believe that implicit memory reconsolidation tactics are a significant advance over the previous methods of behavior change. The previous methods they include are all those methods that primarily use cognitive behavioral approaches (CBT) and empathic/active listening (e.g., Progeria, Imago, and Motivational Interviewing). They classify these models of behavior change and psychotherapy as "counteractive" methods, whereas those methods that embed *implicit memory reconsolidation* (IMR) are "transformational" methods.

Ecker also argues that the approach of reactivating implicit emotional memory while in a relationship "unlocks" the previous consolidated emotions and cognitions associated with past events. At the moment when the old situation is open for reorganization, an opportunity to bring in a new set of feelings and thoughts is available. Furthermore they specifically mention that the Internal Family Systems approach, along with some others, is one of those methods compatible with IMR. The Psychology of the Selves and Aware Ego (Stone and Stone, 1993) also needs to be included in their list. IMR describes a hypothesis about mechanisms and core tactics. We recommend more research when neural measurement tools improve. Both Internal Family Systems (IFS) psychotherapy and Voice Dialogue (VD) make use of Implicit Memory Reconsolidation and conduct it diligently with many personality parts, not only with the one showing at any given moment.

IFS and VD are multiplicity-based and attachment-based transformational strategies and tactics. At least one specific mechanism at work in both could be described as IMR. Research, however, needs to be done to assess what aspects of any of these methods are the most effective transformational forces. For example, in IFS work one potent transformational force may turn out to be the attuned interviewing of many different parts of the personality even without invoking specific cognitive or emotion-based tactics of IMR, such as the identification of disconfirming knowledge and pointing out reality that is fundamentally incompatible with the emotional learning that was buried.

Those who are most familiar with IFS strategy and tactic would say that what is being described as IMR has been a feature of IFS since its beginning, and they would add that there is much more to IFS than the behavioral processes of IMR. IFS in addition provides an opportunity for *each* personality part to undergo transformation of its own unique set of implicit emotional and cognitive memories and within the context of a relational attachment both from within the patient's core self and from the therapist's core self. This is a double and often synchronized experience. This could be described as bringing about *transformation on the systemic level*, that is, on the interacting system of personality parts within the patient. The same is basically true for the other multiplicity method, Voice Dialogue. VD emphasizes awareness and energy consciousness, whereas IFS is more of a relational model. They are both interactive, relational systems-based models.

Working with each personality as separate whole personalities is definitely not the operational mode of the monolithic approaches that may use memory reconsolidation with whatever personality happens to be dominant in the interview at that moment in time. The monolithic approaches that may use IMR are said by Cozolino to include Accelerated Experiential Dynamic Psychotherapy (Fosha, 2012);

Coherence Therapy (formerly Depth Oriented Brief Therapy; Ecker and Hulley, 2011); EMDR (unless used with a personality part during IFS therapy; Shapiro, 2002); Emotion-Focused Therapy (Greenberg, 2010); Gestalt Therapy (Zinker, 1978); Hakomi (Fisher, 2011); and Neuro Linguistic Programming (Vaknin, 2010).

IFS clinicians believe that the IFS process of facilitating reconsolidation ("unburdening") of many personality parts is a significant advancement of the use of implicit emotional memory reconsolidation (IMR) over monolithic approaches that may incorporate IMR into their strategy and tactics (RC Schwartz, personal communication). For example, when clinicians view personality as a monolith structure, they will use the IMR strategy with the "person" with whom they are talking. In other words, from a multiplicity perspective they have worked only with the emotions and beliefs of the presenting part dominant at that moment, leaving out the implicit memories carried by many other personality parts.

Since no comparative outcome research has been done, we don't know if the outcomes from using IMF in a monolithic paradigm are significant. If they are, we wonder what is going on in the sessions guided by the monolithic paradigm, especially if a lot of emotion is accessed. Is the clinician taking most of the responsibility for the patient's emotional regulation, or is the patient observed to be taking increasing responsibility for it, much like an IFS session? We hypothesize that for transformation to occur it is important for the therapist and patient to work with a vulnerable part. The advantage of working in an attachment-based IFS frame is that the clinician possesses a framework to track where he or she is going and can time the IMR interventions.

When the clinician uses IMR with *several* personality parts—a standard process in IFS without it being called IMR—the change that occurs is reported to be significant (Sowell, 2013). What has yet to be done is a blind outcome study comparing a monolithic frame with a multiplicity frame that includes recordings of the actual encounters to check fidelity and to discover common features and differences. This type of research would be quite illuminating.

Medical decision making: A process involving emotions and relationship, not only reasoning about facts

The heart has its reasons of which reason knows nothing.

Blaise Pascal, 1640

Decision making often may be a combination of intuition and rules of thumb, perceptual visualization, emotions held in the body, and reasoning based on data. It is influenced differently by different emotions, cognitions, their intensity, and valence. These emotions and beliefs seem to be organized into clusters of personality that can be interviewed separately.

Lowenstein and Lerner (2003), the latter a social psychologist and director of the Decision Science Lab at Harvard's Kennedy School, wrote about the role of affect in decision making in 2003. In 2001 they had already reported that fear and anger have opposite effects upon risk perception during decision making. One take-away from this study is that it makes clinical good sense to process both a patient's anger and their fear on the front end of their decision making process. Lerner's latest publication is *Emotion and Decision Making* (Lerner et al., 2015). They write,

> A revolution in the science of emotion has emerged in recent decades, with the potential to create a paradigm shift in decision theories. The research reveals that emotions constitute potent, pervasive, predictable, sometimes harmful and sometimes beneficial drivers of decision making. Across different domains, important regularities appear in the mechanisms through which emotions influence judgments and choices. We organize and analyze what has been learned from the past 35 years of work on emotion and decision making. In so doing, we propose the emotion-imbued choice model (EIC), which accounts for inputs from traditional rational choice theory and from newer emotion research, synthesizing scientific models.

However, they do not account for the well-substantiated shift in paradigm of personality organization from monolithic to multiplicity. Embracing this observation changes everything, and the authors are considering making this shift (personal communication, 2015).

The author's survey of research since 1970 indicates "one overarching conclusion: emotions powerfully, predictably, and pervasively influence decision making." They define the types of emotion: emotions arising from the judgment or choice at hand (i.e., *integral emotion*), a type of emotion that strongly and routinely shapes decision making (Damasio, 1994; Greene and Haidt, 2002). Internal emotions can be a beneficial guide, and they also can bias a decision. An example of bias was given by Gigerenzer in 2002 (and 2007 by personal communication) as feeling afraid to fly and deciding to drive instead, despite that the risk of death by driving is much higher than the base rates for death by flying the equivalent mileage. Also, they report that researchers have found that *incidental emotions* (defined as emotions carried over from one situation to another) can affect decisions that are and should remain unrelated to that emotion.

They also concluded that evidence reveals that the effects of emotions on a decision occur via changes in (1) content of thought, (2) depth of thought, and (3) content of implicit goals. Interestingly, the latter conclusion supports the need to revisit the work of this group through the lens of the multiplicity paradigm because the thoughts and goals of each personality part possess all three of the above characteristics and seem, by clinical observation, to have a pivotal impact on how an emotion affects someone's decision process. The difference between making decisions while feeling angry compared with feeling fear were also mentioned.

The Emotion-Imbued Choice (EIC) model of Lerner, however, continues to treat the personality as a monolithic entity (as only one "I") rather than as a multiple entity. This monolithic viewpoint, perhaps a by-product of the isolation of research work, is maintained despite what other researchers and clinicians have been observing for many years, that *each of the different personality parts within one person* carries different emotions with different intensities, that each part is linked to particular belief systems within each personality part, and that this setup influences decision making process. Which personality within the decision making research subject was their researcher examining? Which interviewing tactics facilitate a person's decision making process?

What is the decision making process for clinicians? It has been studied vigorously. Carey, in *Learning to See Data,* recently explained that "scientists working in a little known branch of psychology called perceptual learning have shown it is possible to fast-forward a person's gut instincts both in physical fields like flying an airplane and more academic ones, like deciphering advanced chemical notation—The beauty of such learning is there's no thinking involved" (Carey, 2015). This work on "perceptual learning" is informed by the founder of perceptual learning, Eleanor Gibson (Adolph and Kretch, 2012), and by Gerd Gigerenzer's work (see Chapter 3). Comparative controlled research at University of Virginia shows that learning is much sharper and learning scores are four times faster when using a perceptual module for learning gall bladder surgery via video demonstration (Guerlain et al. 2004). John Greally (Golden et al., 2013), director of Albert Einstein College of Medicine Center for Epigenomics, says regarding biological data, "We need some way to capture the gestalt, to develop an instinct for what's important." This applies to evidence-based data statistics, patient interviewing process, and decision making.

Gerd Gigerenzer believes that clinicians and perhaps patients make medical decisions best by an intuition heuristic called Fast and Frugal Rules of Thumb. A psychologist at the Max Planck Institute of Human Development (Berlin), Gigerenzer wrote *Gut Feelings: The Intelligence of the Unconscious* (2007). When he and I talked in 2008, he went beyond Gladwell's *Blink* to posit that medical decisions by clinicians and perhaps also by patients could be made by conscious and unconscious rules of thumb—by a simple Fast and Frugal Decision Tree. Here is how he thinks about it. There have been two approaches in the past to medical decision making.

In the first approach, called clinical-decision theory, doctors and patients choose between alternative treatments by examining all the possible consequences and then calculating the *expected utility* of each choice. There is a mathematical formula. He sees this method as being characteristic of those methods in which the physician provides the alternatives and consequences and probabilities, and the patient is responsible for assessing the potential benefits and harms. Although health administrators think of this as a type of shared decision making, it does not agree with our understanding of the word *shared*, which to us means processing emotions and values within a relationship. Gigerenzer observes that compared to using intuition, many doctors and most patients do not favor using the expected utility approach proposed by economic consultants. No researched proof exists that expected utility methods are best.

The second approach, Gigerenzer notes, was to encourage the use of statistical aids for physicians to make treatment decisions that presumably would be superior to using their intuitions alone. These statistical decision aids are more widely adopted by doctors than expected utility calculations, but a majority of physicians don't understand these complex decision aids and end up abandoning them. He believes that most physicians are "left with their own clinical intuition biased by protective treatment to lower liability." He thinks that most physicians already use simple rules of thumb to add to their intuition, "but for fear of lawsuits do not always admit it and use them covertly." He believes that the solution for medicine is to develop a science of rules of thumb decision making, to help them be conscious, to discuss these simple rules openly, to "connect them with the available evidence, and to train medical students to use them in a discipline an informed way."

According to Gigerenzer, when it comes to professionals making medical decisions, "simplicity is a solution to uncertainty," and "intuitive judgments are usually based on one good reason." He cites the University of Michigan decisions study about patients entering the ER with acute chest pain. The research discovered that not only did doctors send most of the patients to the ICU (two million patients in the United States per year, at great expense), but they sent those who should not have been in the ICU as often as those who should have been there. The doctors' decisions were no better than chance.

The second study revealed that the doctors were looking at the medical record history of hypertension and diabetes, rather than at the nature of the patient's presenting symptoms and those clues in the electrocardiogram that were more powerful predictors. What they decided to do is the most interesting part. The hospital tried to solve the problem with a complex strategy called the heart disease predictive instrument (Green and Yates, 1995). The instrument was a chart of 50 probabilities and a long formula to compute the probability that a patient should be admitted to the coronary care unit. Their decisions improved, and the overcrowding decreased in the ICU. *The clinical team* concluded that the calculations rather than the physicians' intuitions were responsible for the improvement. *The well-trained researchers* were not so sure. They stopped the use of the complex predictive instrument. The improvement in disposition performance, however, did not drop. Their further analysis showed that exposure to the chart improved the clinicians' **intuitions** permanently without further access to the calculating tools. The researchers discovered that all that seemed to matter were the right cues that the physicians had memorized. To us, this is more support that decision making even within doctors is not primarily data crunching.

In the above study, the doctors were still working with their intuitions, but now they knew what to look for. Dr. Green, together with David Mayer, developed a *rule of thumb for coronary care allocations*, which corresponded to the natural thinking of physicians but was empirically informed. The research indicated that physicians tend to avoid the more complicated method of the heavy calculations and probability scores when they conflict with their intuitions—thus proving that under conditions of high uncertainty, simple methods tend to be more accurate. Gigerenzer had already created the Fast and Frugal Decision Tree, which asks only a few yes-or-no questions and allows for a decision after each one; for example, in the tree developed by Green and Mehr (1997), if there was a certain anomaly in the electrocardiogram (the ST segment), the patient was sent to the coronary care unit based on that cue. More information was not required. If that cue is not present, a second cue is considered—*chief complaint is chest pain*; the third cue is any one additional factor. If yes, then the patient was sent to the coronary care unit; if no, the patient was sent to standard nursing bed. Although the triage cues may have changed since then, the *decision process* is the point here. Regarding their own decision making, he believes that doctors and nurses can be trained to side-step litigation risk and "to focus on what is important and ignore the rest." Although not considered by these workers, we suspect that emotions that are triggered within clinicians and/or within patients will trump or distort the Fast and Frugal Framework, and that the emotions and associated thinking will first need to be processed within clinicians who are skilled to navigate the psychological territory with focused brevity. More research will tell us, and this research needs to be completed before organized medicine chooses a decision method for clinicians and spends money on implementing it.

PSYCHOTHERAPY EXPERIENCE WITH MEDICAL PATIENTS IN DECISION CRISIS

Psychotherapies guided by the multiplicity models of Hal and Sidra Stone (Voice Dialogue) and Richard Schwartz (Internal Family Systems), have proven to be new and powerful approaches to medical decision conflicts as they appear in the therapist's office. When the therapist and patient together make separate relationships with each of the personality parts involved in the conflict, and vulnerability is given a relational attachment, a decision emerges. There is internal psychological and physical space for the downsides of the decision as the patient choses the upsides of the decision. The decision is made in self-awareness. The polarization of opposites (ambivalence), stress (which impacts a patient's response to anesthesia), and postdecision remorse are vastly reduced.

There is a national push in the United States to improve medical decision making. An Institute of Medicine report in 2011 on overall US health spending concluded that about 30 percent, or $750 billion/year, reflects overtreatment, excessive costs, and other problems (IOM and NAE, 2011). A national spotlight was directed toward improving two relationship-based tasks believed to be related to these costs: facilitating patients to (1) change health behaviors and (2) make quality treatment decisions. Enhancing clinical power regarding these two tasks is important for many reasons besides reducing cost, including to improve outcomes and patient satisfaction, to reduce suffering, and to prevent clinician burnout.

ADVANCES IN NURSING

Nursing has always been heavily focused on healing and patient care while also paying attention to disease. Recently, nursing researchers developed a list of 24 evidence-based practice competencies for registered nurses and advanced practice registered nurses to use in real-world clinical settings (see Appendix). These are of value and can be elaborated as research unfolds.

Cropley described what is called the Relationship-Based Care (RBC) model in nursing and has evaluated its positive impact on patient satisfaction, length of stay, and readmission rates (Cropley, 2012). Carabetta in 2013 described use of RBC in primary care around experiences with anesthesia (Carabetta et al., 2013). Also, an implementation of RBC was outlined by Winsett and Hauck (2011). The descriptions of RBC, like models of the past, are at the level of external descriptions that promote verbal relationships between clinicians and patients. Although the deeper intrapersonal tactics to implement and conduct such relationships were not specified, RBC is an important focus on the power of direct relationships between patients and clinicians to improve health care outcomes.

Holistic and integral nursing continue to be practiced and taught, and we expect they will be increasingly informed by scientific advances in clinical psychology and neurobiology and the updates in this book.

The ARN (attending registered nurse) is just one of the many new roles for nurses in a changing health care system. These new roles are empowering nurses to play a greater role in improving patient care. They could receive training in health coaching. The January 2015 monthly newsletter from Robert Wood Johnson Foundation reported the following:

> Nurses are helping improve access and quality, and lower costs through care coordination, prevention, a fuller role in providing primary care, and more. Today, a venerable Boston hospital is testing out another innovation, but this time it's in the field of nursing. When a patient arrives at Massachusetts General Hospital (MGH) now, he or she is assigned an attending registered nurse (ARN) for the duration of the hospital stay and after discharge. The ARN builds a relationship with the patient and his or her caregivers, and ensures that all members of the patient's health care team follow a shared care plan. Unlike other RNs, ARNs are designed to promote continuity of care, ideally with a five-day, eight-hour work schedule.
>
> "The role is designed to be a constant throughout the patient experience," says Jeffrey Adams, PhD, RN, director of the Center for Innovations in Care Delivery at MGH and a Robert Wood Johnson Foundation Executive Nurse Fellow (2014–2017). "The person the patient sees every day is available ahead of admissions and post-discharge. This is different than anything we've seen before. We evaluate this work closely and we know ARNs have significantly contributed to improved quality and patient satisfaction."

CONCLUSIONS ABOUT ADVANCES IN RELATIONSHIP PSYCHOLOGY

The advances point toward two clinical tasks that have not been separately explored by previous workers that could be added to the psychological content of PCC. They have become more salient as research and clinical work have unfolded. Both Clinician Emotional Self-Care and Information Transfer are now viewed as major determinants of patient outcome in addition to the tasks of health behavior change, shared decision making, diagnosis, treatment, and prevention. Starting in Chapter 6, you will see that these two tasks are among the elements selected for integration into the new model and into the list of clinical competencies for physicians and nurses.

We have used the same general time placement (after the early 1990s) for these relatively new topics of Clinician Self-Care and Information Transfer as we have for the neuroscience discoveries using fMRI (that also started after the early 1990s).

The seven advances included in this chapter are either based on controlled comparative trials on patient care and professional education or based on hypotheses from accumulated clinical experience that appear to be universal, that is, used successfully by a diverse group of clinicians across cultures. I have tried to be clear about which advances are based on control trials, which on retrospective studies, and which on accumulated clinical observation. Another organizing factor is whether a finding also correlates with one of the advances in neurobiology or seems worthy of neuroscience research. Most clinicians and psychologists familiar with these advances are not bothered by the "soft-science" status of evidential linkage to neurobiological findings. Instead, they seem to feel reassured by the experimental and clinical evidence so far. We encourage you to keep a distinction between psychologically-based data and neurophysiological data. Sometimes the studies of experimental psychologists are being called neuroscience. These workers are getting as close to the boundary of neuroscience as they are able under the present limitations of work with human subjects, yet often they are not tracking neural level activity in real time. As yet, there are too few tools to do that. The theoretical and strategic advances are supported ("from top-down") by prior abstract theories (for example, attachment theory and theory of the unconscious) and "from bottom-up" by concrete laboratory findings with humans, findings from outcome studies in health care, and from observation of psychotherapeutic interventions with medical patients. An example of one such observation is that compassion and empathy are ingredients of relationships that foster affect regulation in the other person. Of importance is that many of the same observations about relationships and personality dynamics have turned out to be ubiquitous across all arenas of human relationship (for example, in theater and literature, legal negotiation, business management, athletic competition, and patient care).

But, logicians caution psychologists and neuroscientists to be aware that the language of the mind (that is, sentences about thoughts and emotions) are only "linguistic substantives" (a word or phrase that is meant to function only syntactically as a noun). They counsel that because these words have an independent existence and logic in syntax, it doesn't make logical sense to search for neural events that directly stand for these nouns. It is a trick that language plays upon us. We believe that hypothesis development in clinical psychological research would benefit from more questioning as to whether it is inherently possible to locate exact neural correlates of particular thoughts and feelings.

Included in this chapter are extensions of knowledge in the field of relationship science. Many programs, however, still focus mostly on psychopathological conditions or the traditional health psychology models mentioned in Chapter 3. Our faculty experience discovered sparse teaching of contemporary contributions made by psychology and psychiatry about "normal" relationships and about interviewing patients for the sake of their medical care. In psychology/psychiatry there has been a paradigm shift in understanding and in clinical relationship strategy resulting from three hypotheses: *attachment theory* (Bowlby, Ainsworth), *implicit memory reconsolidation* (as applied by Cozolino, Fosha, Schore, Siegel, Badenoch), and *multiplicity of personality* (as applied in the IFS and Voice Dialogue models of psychotherapy).

These are mutually enhancing hypotheses at different levels and inform powerful new intervention strategies in patient care, psychotherapy, and sports psychology. The paradigm used in the IFS Model of psychotherapy makes effective use of mindfulness and the breath to facilitate healing relationships with parts of the personality (Schwartz, 1995). The practice of mindfulness has reached the mainstream in health and clinical work. RC Schwartz included it and went significantly beyond it. Updated hypotheses are heuristics (see Glossary), that is, aids to *explain and predict* what was formerly not possible. For example, the multiplicity of personality hypothesis embraced by Richard Schwartz and Hal and Sidra Stone, that everyone's mind consists of distinct and discernable personalities, predicts the sudden change of mind by patients who previously had consented to a certain treatment or who had agreed to take prescribed medications.

Bonnie Bradenoch (2008) and Daniel Siegel started to integrate Interpersonal Neurobiology (IPNB) into psychotherapy—an important step that linked understandings gained from both brain biology and modern psychotherapy to strategies that could be applied to relationships in health care. Fosha (2012) focused on emotions.

There is also another finding relevant to learning patient interviewing. Neuropsychologists like Spratling, working in London, wrote about feedback models of perceptual learning (Spratlin et al., 2006). The medical school at UCLA has adopted perceptual modules as part of its standard curriculum to train skills like reading EKGs, identifying skin rashes, and interpreting tissue samples from biopsies (Carey, 2015). Those workers say that stimulating intuition via visualizations and body awareness is relevant for any field making subtle distinctions. We think that patient interviewing is the quintessence of subtle distinction combined with evidence-based reasoning. It makes sense to use intuitive functions in addition to reasoning for medical decision making by both patients and their clinicians. This idea fits with what Gigerenzer said about gut feelings and rules of thumb (Chapter 3 and this chapter). It also jibes with our experience that visualization of a framework is helpful to those who are learning interviewing. This idea and evidence from the advances provides a necessary counter-balance to the growing notion that everything has to be reasoned and based upon facts.

5

Present advances in neuroscience (starting with the early 1990s): Possible neural substrates of mind functions

This quote bears repeating:

It ain't what you don't know that gets you into trouble. It's what you know for sure that just ain't so.

Mark Twain

Rather than organize this chapter according to anatomical or functional neural regions, such as cortical, limbic (amygdala and hippocampus), brainstem (vagal), and cellular level work, we chose to organize this chapter by neuroscientific topics that appear to be directly and indirectly pertinent to the four relational domains of patient-centered care on which we are focused: decision making, health behavior change, information transfer, and clinician emotional self-care. The advances listed below touch on several topics in neuroscience: neural connections between learning and recall and emotions, and between labeling emotions and self-regulation; mirror neurons, brain plasticity, and interpersonal relationships; the neural substrates of empathy and those between empathy and self-regulation; implicit memory and subcortical activity; vagal tone and attachment relationships; and neural phenomenon in decision making.

The anatomical designations made in the neuroscience advances list and discussion below are subject to revision as neuroscience measurement tools improve and as studies are found that we may have missed. The neurophysiological processes may or may not be fairly similar in all regions of the CNS, even though those regions have overlapping functions that are not yet fully understood. The systems, reduplications and redundancies are built for adaptation and survival. Whatever future research may unfold about these processes and the spontaneous and reduplicated involvement of various regions in the CNS/PNS, it seems unlikely that it would totally invalidate clinical strategies and tactics that are currently informed by observations simultaneously corroborated by cellular neuroscience, experimental neuropsychology, human development, relational psychology, and psychotherapy.

NINE ADVANCES IN NEUROSCIENCE

1. **Learning and Memory: Emotional arousal, learning, and memory are interconnected.** (A hypothesis supported by discovery of interconnections between neural circuits within and between anatomical and functionally different regions: **amygdala, hippocampus, cortex.**)

2. **Affect Regulation and Connections of the OMPFC, Amygdala, Cortex: Labeling emotions with words and creating narratives are connected with affect regulation functions of the nervous system.** (A hypothesis supported by discovery of interconnections between anatomically and functionally different regions: **orbitomedial prefrontal cortex [OMPFC], amygdala, anterior cingulate, and prefrontal cortex.**)

3. **Mirror Neurons and Plasticity: Relationship is a brain-to-brain connection: Mirror neurons and neural plasticity are found to be a substrate for intersubjectivity.** (A hypothesis supported by discovery of cellular-synaptic circuitry interconnections and interconnections in regional anatomy: **fronto-parietal [cognitive control and decision making] and Broca's area [motor/speech].**)

4. **Neural Correlates of Relational Attachment: Interconnectedness is not only a feature of one brain but exists across brains, and that separation/rejection in childhood correlates with persistent neural changes. There appear to be brain circuits and biomarkers associated with relational affiliation, separation, and rejection. Circulating oxytocin appears to be a biomarker of shared states in parenting and romantic partners. Early childhood emotional abandonment and separation experiences correlate later in childhood with dysfunctional responses to social rejection. The neural correlates are increased activity in the left middle temporal gyrus (MTG) (a key region for processing, storage, and retrieval of highly arousing personal emotional experience) and persistent functional changes in the anterior cingulate cortex (ACC) and dorsolateral prefrontal cortex (dlPFC).** (A hypothesis supported by several RCTs of human subjects—adults and children—using current fMRI and physiological measurement tools.)

5. **Role of Prefrontal Cortex: The prefrontal cortex governs both empathy and emotional regulation.** (A hypothesis supported by discovery of neural circuitry and interconnected regional processing of **prefrontal cortex and OMPFC.**)

6. **Plasticity and Activation of Subcortical Memory: Emotionally charged subcortically stored implicit memory can be highly**

reactivated by current experience. The memories are not indelible but are subject to neural plastic processes known as "memory reconsolidation." (A hypothesis supported by discovery of cellular-synaptic interconnections, regional processing and storage, and interconnections between regions: subcortical limbic, perhaps right-brain function.)

7. **Vagal Circuitry and Relationships: The building of vagal circuitry and networks of descending control are fostered by attachment relationships and operate bidirectionally.** (A hypothesis supported by discovery of CNS–PNS interconnections and physiology that have balancing functions concerning emotions, that is, a social engagement cardiovagal tone [VVC, ventral vagal] and a fight–flight viscerosensory tone [DVC, dorsal vagal], each being a pathway to chest and gut, respectively, from the brain stem [10th cranial nerve].)

8. **Neural Substrates in Decision Making: There are common neural substrates for decision making for both complex, emotion-filled issues and simple ethical matters. Reason and emotion appear to intersect (functionally) in the ventromedial prefrontal cortexes and also in the amygdala.** (A hypothesis supported by comparative brain imaging studies of human beings as yet only in laboratory settings.)

9. **Neural Substrates of Emotional Awareness and Mindfulness: Emotional awareness is associated with activation in the anterior insular cortex (AIC) and the ACC. Both PET and fMRI studies indicate that the AIC is associated not just with subjective feelings from the body but with subjective feelings from the brain's activities related to stages of consciousness. Significant signal decreases were observed in midline cortical structures associated with interoception (including bilateral anterior insula, left ventral ACC, right medial prefrontal cortex, and bilateral precuneus). Signal increase was observed in the right posterior cingulate cortex.** (A hypothesis supported by repeated observations via current but crude tools of human brain observation associated with human behavior.)

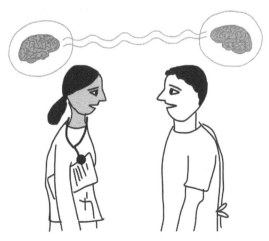

NEURAL ENGAGEMENT

GOING DEEPER INTO EACH ADVANCE

1. Learning and Memory

How emotional arousal impacts learning and memory is important regarding the process of information transfer. *The ability to learn new information and memory* is not only a cognitive function; it is highly influenced by the level of emotional arousal. At modest levels of arousal, amygdala activation stimulates and supports (by enhancing neuroplasticity) hippocampal-mediated learning and explicit memory. There is a balance between the amygdala (and OMPFC) and the hippocampus (and dlPFC). At modest levels of arousal, amygdala activation stimulates and supports (by enhancing neuroplasticity) hippocampal mediated learning and explicit memory (Kim and Diamond, 2002; Williams et al., 2000).

At high levels of emotional arousal, the amygdala (visceral–emotional processing and fear-based learning) stimulates hypothalamic–pituitary–adrenal (HPA) activation, which interrupts hippocampal-mediated (declarative-conscious processing) learning and explicit memory formation. At the University of Washington, Jeansok Kim and David Diamond overviewed the interactions between stress, memory, and hippocampal function (*the stressed hippocampus, synaptic plasticity, and lost memories*; Kim and Diamond, 2002). These and other researchers are working on identifying and defining the mechanisms of how emotions impact learning and memory.

This highlights the importance for clinicians to have the skills to provide direct care to help patients regulate and process emotions so they can tolerate stress and are able to take in information and/or learn from the present experience with the clinician. This is motivation for mitigating patients' stress through the use of clinical interviewing before providing information and when providing information to do it in the context of a connected relationship which modulates affect. Compromised cognitive functioning hampers both the process of information transfer and decision making. Also, as we will discover later, emotions play an additional and different role in shared decision making process.

Elizabeth Karuza and her team in the Department of Brain and Cognitive Sciences at University of Rochester encouraged research that concurrently observes fMRI recording during learning. We agree with their focus on understanding the process, *Invited Review Combining fMRI and Behavioral Measures to Examine the Process of Human Learning*. Their review of the literature reveals that many fMRI studies of learning either (1) focus on outcome rather than process or (2) are built on the untested assumption that learning unfolds uniformly over time. They discuss here various challenges faced by the field (Karuza et al., 2014). Again, because of gaps in research mentioned in the review, we encourage adding the variables of emotion and a concurrent human attuned relationship into such studies. These added dimensions increase expenses, which few studies can afford, and require that a researcher in experimental psychology who is sufficiently experienced in interpersonal dynamics design it well. We discuss these research issues further in Chapter 14.

2. Affect Regulation and Connections of OMPFC, Amygdala, Cortex

Labeling affects with words has been shown to downregulate activation of the OMPFC, the amygdala, and the anterior cingulate (Rushworth and Behrens, 2008). This downregulation is experienced by the person as increased tolerance of emotion (a partially validated physiological hypothesis). Amygdala-right frontal activation is inversely correlated in a homeostatic balance mediated by the OMPFC (Leiberman et al., 2007).

Labeling of emotions correlates with decreased amygdala response and an increase in right prefrontal activation (lateral and medial), which correlates with increased affect tolerance and regulation (Hariri et al., 2002; Johnstone et al., 2007). *Journaling* (creating narrative) about emotional issues was found to correlate with increases in prefrontal activation which downregulated the HPA (and increased hepatitis-B antibody levels, lower heart rates, and skin conductance levels, Dolcos and McCarthy, 2006).

Mathew Lieberman and team in 2011 at UCLA conducted four studies examining the effect of affect labeling on self-reported emotional experience. In study number one, self-reported distress was lower during affect labeling, compared with passive watching, of negative emotional pictures. Studies two and three added reappraisal and distraction conditions as pictures. Affect labeling showed similar effects on self-reported distress as both of these intentional emotion regulation strategies. Thus, affect labeling seemed to them as an incidental emotion regulation process. Study four employed positive emotional pictures, and here, affect labeling was associated with diminished self-reported pleasure relative to passive watching. This suggests that affect labeling tends to dampen affective responses in general, rather than specifically alleviating negative affect (Lieberman et al., 2011).

In 2014, the University of California and Pittsburg's Carnegie Mellon Center for the Neural Basis of Cognition collaborated on the study by Burklund et al. (2014). Although diminished limbic responses (amygdala) and self-reported distress had been shown to correlate with both intentional and incidental efforts to regulate emotions, there was no research about underlying mechanisms of each type of regulation strategy, intentional and incidental. The authors posited that affect labeling may be one of those examples of affect modulation occurring at the limbic level but not requiring a conscious and intentional attempt to reduce and reappraise. They devised an experiment using 39 healthy older adults that separated affect labeling and the processes of intentional reappraisal and emotion reduction.

When affect labeling and reappraisal of belief were directly compared by fMRI, it showed that both activate common areas in several prefrontal regulatory regions, with affect labeling producing the stronger responses. Affect labeling and reappraisal were also associated with similar decreases in amygdala activity. Finally, both affect labeling and reappraisal were associated with correlated reductions in self-reported distress. The researchers believe these results pointed to common neurocognitive mechanisms involved in affect labeling and reappraisal, supporting the idea that *intentional* and *incidental* emotion regulation may utilize overlapping neural processes (Burklund et al., 2014).

This finding, in our opinion, confirms widespread clinical experience that affect labeling seems to have an emotion regulating affect that is strong and may be distinct from the actual intention to calm down. We believe it supports the value of helping patients and ourselves to put words on emotions—as distinct from their thoughts—for their own internal sake, because it is healthy for our brain and it fosters communication that has a lower risk of triggering emotional reactions in the listener. In each of Lieberman's studies in 2011, participant predictions about the effects of affect labeling suggest that unlike reappraisal and distraction, people do not believe that affect labeling is an effective strategy to regulate their emotions. These authors report that even after having the experience of affect labels leading to lower distress, participants in their study still predicted that affect labeling would increase distress in the future. Although our and others' clinical experience early in a patient's emotional-learning process tends to confirm this finding, the patient's belief that affect labeling will make matters worse decreases markedly when they realize that their belief is coming from only one particular part of their personality system, not all of them. Often, it is coming from an internalization of Western culture and family rules, which conflate giving voice to emotions with getting out of emotional control. The function of personality parts will be discussed at length later in this chapter and throughout the rest of the book. The point is that most people, after attention is given to their inner reservations about doing so, are then able to embrace an intention to label their affects routinely.

The clinical relevance of studies like those at University of California (Burklund et al., 2014) might be increased by using audiovisual stimuli instead of pictures and by including the relational dimension by studying pairs of people. Again, this increases the expense of the study and requires the researchers to be clinically training in interpersonal work.

Creating narratives about stressful experiences also impacts emotions and body physiology. This is very pertinent to medical care experiences. There is support for the hypothesis that the mental processing of emotions and their accompanying thoughts and the underlying processes in the CNS impacts bodily health. The hypothesis was that creating narratives in writing or telling another person helps regulate emotion and also boosts the immune system. A psychological trauma specialist, Bessel van der Kolk (2014), says in his recent book that the first systematic test of the power of language to relieve the impact of trauma was done in 1986 by James Pennebaker at the University of Texas, Austin (Pennebaker, 1995 and 2004).

Pennebaker asked each student in his psychology class to identify a personal experience that they'd found very stressful. He divided the class of 200 into three groups. For four consecutive days while alone, one group was asked to write about current events in their lives; the second was asked to write about the details of the traumatic personal experience; and the third, to recall the facts and also their emotions and their thoughts about the stressful experience. He had accumulated data for all the 200 students on the frequency of visits and types of illness reported to student health. The third group—which had written about both the facts, thoughts, and the emotions related to their trauma experience— clearly benefited the most from their writing. In the following month compared to the month before the study, they had a 50% drop in doctor visits compared with the other two groups.

van der Kolk (2014) states, "Those reporting a traumatic sexual experience in childhood had been hospitalized an average of 1.7 days in the previous year— almost twice the rate of the others." Regarding research design, it is not clear how the three cohorts were equalized or not for this possible bias.

A summary of 15 studies between 1965 and 1980 by Mumford et al. (1981) found that individuals in talk psychotherapy showed a 13–20 percent decrease in medical utilization compared to controls. In an attempt to replicate his ear- lier study, Pennebaker (1995), at Ohio State University College of Medicine, compared two groups of students who wrote either about a personal trauma or a superficial topic. Again, those who wrote about their personal traumas had fewer visits to the student health center. Their improved health, by testimonial, correlated with improved immune function, as measured by the action of natu- ral killer cells (T lymphocytes) and other immune markers in the blood. This effect was most obvious directly after the study and could be detected six weeks later.

Numerous research studies have since replicated these findings. Writing experiments from around the world with grade-school students, nursing-home residents, medical students, maximum-security prisoners, arthritis sufferers, new mothers, and rape victims consistently show that writing about upsetting events improves physical and mental health. Here is the mind and brain impact- ing the body. The exact route by which this occurs has yet to be worked out. Working it out, as it usually does, may inform further developments in clini- cal strategy. This is why we must do that. We do not, however, have to wait for answers about neuroscientific and physiological mechanisms to apply what has been validated by replicated clinical studies.

The search for neural substrates for emotions continues. In 2013, Kassam and five workers at Carnegie Mellon University Department of Social and Decision Science published "Identifying Emotions on the Basis of Neural Activation" (Kassam et al., 2013). Method actors were asked to self-induce nine emotional states (anger, disgust, envy, fear, happiness, lust, pride, sadness, and shame) while in an fMRI scanner. Using a Gaussian Naïve Bayes pooled variance classifier, they could accurately identify specific emotions experienced by an individual— well over chance accuracy. These sophisticated researchers explained that rather than search for contiguous neural structures associated with specific emotions, they applied multivoxel pattern analysis techniques to identify distributed pat- terns of activity associated with specific emotions. This allowed for the possibility that neural responses to emotional stimulation may occur in many brain areas simultaneously and that each emotion has a "neural signature." It is relevant for any fMRI work on the Internal Family Systems (IFS) Model to "locate" the signa- ture of personality parts or self energy, if one exists.

3. Mirror Neurons and Plasticity

The *mirror neuronal system* functions as the neural substrate of *intersubjectivity* in relationship. It bridges the gap between people, from brain to brain, and is the neural substrate for empathic attunement (Wolf et al., 2001; Cozolino, 2010). That neurons join in a functional cluster in response to experience is supported by Hebb's work and rule (Hebb, 1949). A clarification by Hebb is discussed further on.

Rizzolatti and Arbib (1998), working at the Institute of Human Physiology at the University of Parma (Italy), identified indirect evidence of a mirror neuron system (similar to findings in primates) in the human brain. Transcranial magnetic stimulation and positron emission tomography (PET) experiments suggested that a mirror system for gesture recognition exists in human and includes Broca's area. It is an observation-execution matching system which provides a bridge between actor/sender and observer/receiver. This has been confirmed by many other workers. In 2002 Nishitani and Hari at the Brain Research Unit in Helsinki explained in *Viewing Lip Forms: Cortical Dynamics* that "viewing other persons' actions automatically activated brain areas belonging to the mirror-neuron system (MNS) assumed to link action execution and observation." Using magnetoencephalographic cortical dynamics, they followed subjects who observed still pictures of lip forms, imitated them, and made similar forms in a self-paced manner. They said, "In all conditions and in both hemispheres, cortical activation progressed in 20–70 ms steps from the occipital cortex to the superior temporal region (where the strongest activation took place), the inferior parietal lobe, and the inferior frontal lobe (Broca's area), and finally, 50–140 ms later, to the primary motor cortex. The signals of Broca's area and motor cortex were significantly stronger during imitation than other conditions. These results demonstrate that still pictures, only implying emotion, activate the human MNS in a well-defined temporal order" (Nishitani and Hari, 2002).

The discovery of mirror neurons was a major breakthrough in locating the neural substrate for a number of human behaviors, for example, *On Being Moved: From Mirror Neurons to Empathy*, edited by Stein Braten (2007). Braten is also author of *The Intersubjective Mirror in Infant Learning and Evolution of Speech* (Braten, 2009), a volume that illustrates how recent findings about primary intersubjectivity and mirror neurons provide a new understanding of children's nature, dialogue, and language. Contributors to this volume respond to such questions as why an 11-month-old infant responds to and reciprocates care. These volumes shifted the paradigm in child development from viewing the development of the capacity for relationships and thinking as evolving through stages over many years (as did Freud and Piaget) to one of observing with an open mind the early forms of relational reciprocity and intersubjectivity during infancy. Rather than by discrete stages, development seems to be more of a layering and integration of elements one upon the other without loss of the prior abilities. Rather than a stage model, it is an interactive confining system in which both earlier and later abilities can be used adaptively.

Gallese et al. (2007) posited that the mirror neuron system, "together with other mirroring neural clusters outside the motor domain," constitute the functional neural mechanisms of intersubjectivity. They concluded that by means of our embodied simulation of the experience of others, we are intentionally attuned to others and provided with a sense of familiarity. Not only do mirror neurons of primates mimic other's actions, but they also go beyond the mere storage; they create complex information about the details and options of actions. The regions proven in primates to be involved are identical with Brocca's area in humans. While at the present no studies entailing recording of single neurons could be done on humans, all the indirect neurophysiological evidence indicates that an adapted and sensitized mirror neuron system is the neural substrate support for relational attunement in human experiences.

These are ideas replicated by many workers in the United States, Italy, Finland, and Norway who, since 2002, have published hundreds of papers and books that report the projects that measure and create models about the brains of humans and primates and correlates of social behavior, like empathy. Noninvasive scanning has extended the findings in primates to human brains. Rizzolatti and Arbib (1998) and Fadiga et al. (2009) wrote on the role of Broca's area in encoding sequential human actions. Badino and Fadiga (Fadiga et al., 2009) published on the computational validation of the motor contribution to speech perception. Molnar-Szakacs et al. (2006) at UCLA wrote "Observing Complex Action Sequences: The Role of the Fronto-Parietal Mirror Neuron System," and Ramachandran (2011), working in San Diego, published *The Tell-Tale Brain: A Neuroscientist's Quest for What Makes Us Human.*

4. Neural Correlates of Relational Attachment

There appear to be brain circuits and biomarkers associated with relational affiliation, separation, and rejection. They operate bidirectionally. Circulating oxytocin appears to be a biomarker of shared states in parenting and romantic partners. Early childhood separation experiences correlate later in childhood with dysfunctional responses to social rejection. The neural correlates are increased activity in the left MTG (a key region for processing, storage, and retrieval of highly arousing personal emotional experience) and persistent functional changes in the dorsal anterior cingulate cortex (dACC) and dorsal lateral prefrontal cortex (dlPFC).

The bidirectional nature of the nervous system was given a boost in 2005 when cell biologist Bruce Lipton, whose theories are controversial, posited that cellular DNA may be influenced and controlled from outside the cell, even by the nature of conscious thoughts coming from the brain (Lipton, 2005).

Feldman et al. (2011) showed that when mothers and their infants engage in strong visual and emotional face-to-face interactions, their heart rhythms become virtually identical to each other during such interactions. Weisman et al. (2012) showed that soon after fathers received a dose of oxytocin during their interactions, there was a significant increase in their infants' oxytocin levels although the infants did not receive oxytocin and were not in the same room when the parent received it. Ilanit Gordon and others working at Yale Child Study Center reviewed the research on this emerging topic in 2014 (Gordon et al., 2014).

In December 2014, a well-designed neural and behavioral comparative, controlled study of 25 children in foster care who experienced significant, repeated, early separation from parents before age 2 (Early Life Stress: ELS), appeared in the child psychiatry literature (Ruttle et al., 2014). The control group was 26 children raised by their biological parents and matched with the experimental group by history, demographics, and neurologic characteristics. For example, the number of current close friends did not differ between the experimental cohort and control group, and impacts of major diagnosis such as fetal alcohol syndrome were controlled. The authors, collaborating between the United States, UK, and Germany, interviewed current families, evaluated the children, and studied their fMRI and behavioral responses to a well-standardized, fMRI-adapted, social-exclusion paradigm (*Cyberostracism*, Williams et al., 2000). Between-cohort comparisons in neural data showed that children with ELS exhibited significant reduced brain activation in the bilateral dACC extending into the superior frontal gyrus, including the left MTG. Complete lists of whole brain fMRI and psychophysiological interaction (PPI) results were provided. Behavioral data show that children with ELS, by comparison, felt significantly more excluded and had more distress by interview and questionnaire. Authors concluded that the data suggest dysfunctional neural processing of social rejection in children with ELS "despite best-case conditional in stable and caring family environments." It is unknown how long term these affects are or what interventions might mitigate them. We would like to see the above study replicated. Perhaps we may have a research situation to compare the impact of different interventions, such as an IFS-informed treatment of child and caregiver compared to a treatment within a monolithic assumption, that is, that works only with the emotions, thoughts, and memories of the personality part that is dominant in the treatment room.

Affective resonance (what we call "connection") is perhaps what the researchers meant by "warmth" when Judith Morgan conducted her study reported in 2014 at the University of Pittsburgh (Morgan et al., 2014). The participants were 120 boys and their mothers from a longitudinal project on vulnerability in low-income families. Families were recruited when the children were ages 7–17 months. Maternal warmth was observed during mother–child interactions at 18 and 24 months and again at 10 and 11 years. Because the brain's reward circuitry is associated with depressive illness (low striatal and high mPEC activation) and other disorders, and is activated by positive affect from a loved one, a longitudinal study was planned to understand how maternal depression impacts children's brain development in those regions associated with reward functioning. Without going into the design of this well-controlled complex study using valid measurement tools and well-done fMRI, they concluded that the experience of warmth and affection from mothers may be a protective factor for reward function and brain development in boys exposed to maternal depression, possibly by engaging the brain's vulnerable neural reward systems through affiliation. Their findings are a step toward understanding how warm parent–child relationships create a healthy context for brain development. This has implications for the clinician–patient relationship.

5. Role of Prefrontal Cortex

When many workers use the word *empathy* they are probably not distinguishing—as do we, Schwartz, Siegel, and others—between compassion (a felt sense of the other person's affective experience) and empathy (an extension of compassion to verbalizing or just sensing a cognitive understanding of the other's experience).

Empathic behavior, without this distinction above, is believed to be linked to functions of the prefrontal cortex. Damage to this area in childhood often results in deficits in learning social roles and taking the perspective of others, which is needed to be empathic. The prefrontal cortex plays a part in forming ideas about the intentions, beliefs, and perspective of other people (Goel and Dolan, 2003; Stuss and Knight, 2002). Damage to any area of the prefrontal cortex may prove to impair aspects of empathic behavior, said Peter Eslinger (1998) from Penn State University, Department of Neurology (Eslinger et al., 2004). Eslinger and colleagues reviewed ten cases of early prefrontal cortex damage from clinical literature. They said conservatively that "there is preliminary evidence to support distinctive developmental differences in integration of cognitive, social-emotional and moral development after dorsolateral, mesial, and orbital-polar prefrontal lesions" (Eslinger, 1998). He defines empathy as referring to "the cognitive and emotional process that bind people together in various kinds of relationships that permit sharing of experiences as well as understanding of others." Empathic changes are particularly evident after focal prefrontal cortex damage and closed-head injury in adults, and early frontal lobe damage is associated with poor empathic and social development.

Low glucose metabolism is a significant finding in both the dorsal and orbital sections of the frontal brain in many murderers. Perhaps this is also implied evidence of a brain substrate of the capacity to be empathic. Damage to the OMPFC in Phineas Gage resulted in a significant change in his ability to control emotions, make decisions, and adhere to conventions of social relationships (Damasio, 1994).

Many studies confirm that empathy for pain is associated with activation of the dACC and the anterior insula (AI), but it has been unclear if the same is true for other affects. Using fMRI in 2014, Morellii, Rameson, and Lieberman (Morellii et al., 2012) at University of California researched the neural components of empathy for pain, anxiety, and happiness. They also included whether daily prosocial behavior could be predicted. They moved beyond earlier limitations in the linkage between psychological models of empathy and the neural basis. Studying 32 participants they assessed the empathy responses to more than one affect, namely pain, anxiety, and happiness, and also sampled their real-world helping behaviors over two weeks. The result demonstrated that empathy for positive and negative emotions selectively activated brain regions for negative and positive affects and that what they called the "mirror system" was more active during empathy for context-independent events like pain. The cognitive system was more active for events like anxiety and happiness, which are more dependent on the context. Also, they found that the septal region was the only region activated across empathy for all the affects. They concluded that limbic regions are involved in affective congruence, which support an emotional state in the observer that is complimentary with the other; and that there are two pathways to sharing emotions, which are differently engaged depending on the amount of context that is provided to understand the other's experience (includes a cognitive operation). The septal area seems to facilitate an *other-focused*, caregiving state of mind. Empathy, they believe, may be induced by simply observing another's experience. They go on to say that at other times, it seems necessary to take the other person's perspective in order to connect with their emotions and that the neural components of empathy, regardless of the affect, heighten the focus on others.

For us, there are many further questions to research. One of our usual suggestions about relationships is pertinent here, that is, to use live emotionally upset people rather than still photographs in order to include the "brain-to-brain dimension" and to replicate the same protocols. It also makes good sense to us to study the recipient of the empathy, that is, to study pairs of people. We strongly recommend that fMRI research take this direction when the experience studying individuals has been further replicated.

Regarding clinical work, these findings may reflect the distinction some clinicians (Schwartz) make between feeling compassion (emotional resonance) and empathy (a more cognitive perspective-taking in addition to compassion) toward another person and whether it matters regarding the other person's experience.

Empathy by health care clinicians seems to require both cognitive flexibility and affect regulation (to put one's own needs on a back burner), and an ability for perspective about the needs of others. The neutral systems of affect regulation and ability to relate with empathy are tied together functionally. In clinical psychology, the linkage between these two functions (affect self-regulation and capacity for empathy) has been known for some time. To know exactly which regions of the brain are involved (probably several at different levels of function) will not alter the finding that the ability to be empathic and to regulate affects are associated neurophysiologically and anatomically with the prefrontal cortex, the *same* brain region. This correlates with longstanding clinical and naturalistic observations that link these two psychological functions and were gained independently of what brain science were discovering. This finding supports the recommendation that clinicians who work with patients learn how to regulate their own emotions before and while trying to relate to their patients.

6. Plasticity and Activation of Subcortical Memory

We do understand that the mind–brain–body is one interconnected dynamic system. The research in the domain of *memory reconsolidation* sometimes seems to go over the boundary from cellular and systemic neurophysiology and functional histological and gross anatomy into the category of experimental psychology of human behavior and strategies of psychotherapy—while invoking untracked brain events. Workers in memory reconsolidation do this less than workers in many other fields. We hope that some day measurement instruments of human brain functioning will be sufficient to link the two domains in increasing ways. Multiplicity-based psychotherapy utilizes the process of memory reconsolidation for each personality discovered within one patient's systems. This has proven to be a powerful facilitator of change, presumably on a neural level (van der Kolk, 2014).

While honoring testable hypotheses that help us integrate, we have erred on the side of continuing to separate the findings in the field of memory reconsolidation that are related to CNS/PNS neurophysiology and functional anatomy from those which are primarily derived from observations and research in human psychology.

We believe that the concept of memory reconsolidation will increasingly straddle both fields and that information may flow in both directions, as it does more fully with other organs than with the brain at present. The brain, however, unlike other organs, also produces language. Language expressions are *substantives* (see Glossary) that by definition do not require a *substance* to justify their existence or to understand them. We have to be careful not to get into a misdirected search for "reasons," a *substance* (like a neural network) behind the language of thought and of feelings, *substantives*. It is probably not a one-to-one correlation. It is only language. And, there is a human nervous system that registers emotional activation and produces language.

Tanaka et al. (2008) said, "When neurons fire together—within a few milliseconds of each other—they strengthen their existing synapses and form new ones; this is how they 'wire' together." Here is one mechanism of how mental activity might change neural functions.

7. Vagal Circuitry and Relationships

Neuroscientists in the past thought that the vagal tone was largely a stable characteristic. Fredrickson's data show that this part of our brain-to-heart connection, the vagal tone, is plastic and amenable to change (Fredrickson, 2013). Our ventral vagal tone can be increased by our engaging and caring social habits. Ventral vagal tone is central to interpersonal contact; it is responsive to facial expressivity, comforting touch, and the frequency of the human voice. As we expand our capacity for person-to-person connection, empathy, and harmony, we increase our ventral vagal tone. In short, the more we are affectively attuned to others, the healthier we seem to become. This mutual influence also explains how a lack of positive social contact diminishes an individual's vitality. Our heart's capacity for friendship, just like our muscles, obeys the biological law of "use it or lose it." If we don't regularly exercise our ability to be in relational contact, we will eventually lack some of the basic biological capacity to do so, and the opposite is true.

Vagal tone and relationships status seem to impact each other in both directions. This may correlate with and explain what people experience in a comforting relationship when hyper-aroused. But, just as important is the impact on vagal tone of the relational-boosting effects of interventions that adjust ventral- and dorsal-mediated vagal tone such as breath work and mindfulness practices (increases ventral tone and decreases dorsal tone). These viewpoints were asserted in the early 2000s by Porges (2011) in his Polyvagal Theory and later reiterated by van der Kolk (2014).

The work of Linda Rinaman at University of Pittsburgh (Rinaman et al., 2011) emphasized the importance of visceral–sensory pathways from the brainstem (caudal) including noradrenergic pathways, in stress responses, and affective/emotional states.

Lisa Diamond and colleagues in Utah demonstrated in male subjects that vagal tone was negatively associated with attachment anxiety in relationships and positively associated with perceived security in current attachment relationships. Men with high perceived security in current relationships showed more effective recovery from laboratory-induced anger. Vagal tone mediated this association. This has implications for medical decision making, which we will cover later. The actual presence of the person to whom they were romantically attached had no moderating effect; it was the inner perception of the relationship that mattered (Diamond and Hicks, 2005).

Diamond et al. (2011) studied 68 cohabiting couples for 21 days. They demonstrated an association between cardiac vagal tone (indexed by respiratory sinus arrhythmia, RSA) and daily relational interactions with positive affect. They did not speculate the direction of cause and effect. Our experience is that these body-mind dynamics are usually bidirectional and are impacted bidirectionally by interventions, for example, as seen in the impact of breath work on affect regulation and relational attunement and also the impact of relational connection on breathing and presumably RSA.

Barbara Fredrickson reported from the University of North Carolina that her research team conducted a longitudinal study on the effects of people cultivating warmer interpersonal connections in daily life. They designed a 6-week program that trained participants to develop more warmth and tenderness toward themselves and others. The researchers discovered that by the end of the program the participants not only felt more lively and socially connected, they also altered by measurement a key part of their cardiovascular system—their vagal tone (especially the ventral complex, VVC). She states that recent research has discovered that minute variations in our heart rate reveal the strength of this brain-heart connection and, as such, provide an index of our vagal tone. The vagal tone can be either dorsal or ventral. The dorsal reflects passivity and a shutting down that occur when there has been cumulative neglect and a lack of relational contact. The ventral reflects pleasurable social engagement that comes from such activities as nursing, eye-to-eye contact, soothing touch, kissing, pleasant voice tones, bodily cues of acceptance, and relaxation. They assert that the higher our VVC (Porges' "smart" division of the vagal nerve), the better we are able to regulate the internal systems that keep us healthy, such as our cardiovascular and immune responses (Fredrickson, 2013).

We wish to emphasize again that vagal dynamics appear to be bidirectional, that is, vagal tone and balance impacts the quality of clinician–patient relationships, and the quality of clinician–patient relationship, including attention to breathing, impacts vagal tone.

8. Neural Substrates in Decision Making

Antonio Damasio, MD, UCLA Professor of Neuroscience, Neurology, and Psychology said, "Correlations suggest an interaction of the systems underlying the normal processes of emotion, feeling, reason, and decision making" (Damasio, 1994). He was referring to the ventromedial sector of the prefrontal lobe and his and other's clinical experience with brain-damaged people who had both impaired reasoning/decision making *and* impaired emotion/feeling, in otherwise intact neurological profiles. He hypothesized that emotions and feeling may provide a bridge between rational and nonrational brain processes and that reasoning does not culminate in decision making without intactness of brain structures involved in processing emotions.

In 2003, Heekeren and his team in Berlin (Heekeren et al., 2004) used fMRI to study regional neural activation during different types of decision making, ethical in particular. Because previous research had already demonstrated during complex emotional-filled (often violent) moral decision making a consistent involvement of the ventromedial prefrontal cortex (vmPFC), left posterior superior temporal sulcus, and the posterior cingulate cortex, they decided to study simple ethical decision making not containing issues of bodily harm. They found that simple ethical decisions compared to semantic decisions resulted in activation of the left posterior superior temporal sulcus (pSTS), middle temporal gyrus, bilateral temporal poles, left lateral prefrontal cortex (PFC), and bilateral vmPFC. They concluded that the pSTS and vmPFC are a common neural substrate of decision making about both complex emotion-filled issues and simple ethical matters.

Few clinicians would disagree that medical decision making is filled with the processing of emotions and is also affected by the ability to learn and remember evidence-based information. Neuroscientific research substantiates that acute stress impacts learning and memory. Psychological research also indicates that stress shuts down accuracy and recall of information provided during a patient's stressed state. This is what some neuroscientists have to say about the neural factors. In 2010 Tallie Baram and her group at University of California, Irvine, working with rats and mice discovered that short-term stress (even for several hours) can impair brain-cell communication in critical areas (at the dendritic spines) used for learning and memory within the hippocampus (Ivy et al., 2010). They found that acute stress activated corticotropin-releasing hormones (CRH) (not cortisol) that disrupted the process by which the brain collects and stores memories. By blocking CRH, it seems reversible; "The dendridic spines grow back," Chen et al. (2010).

Once this is replicated in primates, it would be important to measure learning and memory of new health information with and without stress—external and internal—then measure before and after the administration of CRH blockers, then compare this drug effect, if any, with the impact of two different clinical strategies of stress reduction, for example, brief mindfulness meditation vs. brief relationally attuned implicit memory work on personality parts. Such comparative studies, if well controlled, are expensive, yet they would solidify the scientific underpinnings of using multiplicity methods to process emotions with patients simultaneously with their cognitions. Mather and Lighthall (2012) have already studied human decision making under stress conditions. They indicate that stress (for example, time pressure to make a decision imposed from the outside) affects more than memory and the hippocampus. They posit that "Stress affects other regions involved in cognitive and emotional processing, including the prefrontal cortex, striatum, and insula. New research examining the impact of stress on decision processes reveals two consistent findings. First, acute stress enhances selection of previously rewarding outcomes but impairs avoidance of previously negative outcomes, possibly due to stress-induced changes in dopamine in reward-processing brain regions. Second, stress amplifies gender differences in strategies used during risky decisions, as males take more risk and females take less risk under stress. These gender differences in behavior are associated with differences in activity in the insula and dorsal striatum, brain regions involved in computing risk and preparing to take action." We think that pressure covertly felt (physiologically measured) but not overtly verbalized by the clinician would induce "pressure stress" in the patient that would impact his or her medical decision making. This has not yet been studied, to our knowledge.

9. Neural Substrates of Emotional Awareness, Mindfulness

Neural correlates of mindfulness have been demonstrated at the University of Capetown (Deliperi, 2011). During mindfulness meditation, significant signal decreases were observed in midline cortical structures associated with interoception (including bilateral anterior insula, left ventral anterior cingulate cortex, right medial prefrontal cortex, and bilateral precuneus). Signal increase was observed in the right posterior cingulate cortex, middle prefrontal cortex, and right anterior insula appear to thicken with the practice of mindfulness meditation (Lazar et al., 2007). Increased activation of paralimbic cortical structures may possibly correlate with increased abilities to regulate affect (Tredway and Lazar, 2009). All these findings suggest that mindfulness meditation may change brain function and programming.

Although these are major discoveries in pure neuroscience, for example, the role of von Economo neurons (spindle neurons) as neural correlates of consciousness (Craig, 2009), we believe that these kind of findings are not yet able to inform how to process emotions and relationships in patient care. If measurements on how the brain is activated by emotions and relationships turn out to inform clinical work in ways that would otherwise not be possible, it will be a major clinical advance for patient care.

DISCUSSION

Some of the nine advances mentioned above seem to parallel the advances in relationship psychology and are relevant to relationship-based aspects of Patient-Centered Care. Although we are aware that neuroscience—particularly the interpersonal realm—has a long distance to go before research about neural substrates of human personality becomes robust, we want to update you in a field in which you may have growing interest. We have done two things: (1) in Chapter 3 we have outlined past basic knowledge in neuroscience relevant to relationship psychology, and (2) we have presented here in Chapter 5 a few pertinent advances in neuroscience enabled by the research use of fMRI since the early 1990s.

As clinicians, you may be reassured to learn about the findings that may eventually be linked to the clinical strategies and tactics you are asked to learn. For example, when facilitating patients to put names on their *feelings/emotions* as distinguished from their *thoughts*, it might be reassuring to know both that clinically it has been proven to help regulate affects and that in cognitive and affective neuroscience there are research findings that correlate with the clinical observations.

If you look closely, however, at some of the ideas being called "neuroscience," you will discover that they are not evidence based at the level of observable neural synaptic system activity. They have been loosely correlated with increases in physiological activity by fMRI in certain regions of the brain. Some people call it "soft science." The rest of the theorizing sometimes sounds like speculation and tends to conflate with findings from experimental behavioral psychological. That seems to be the current status. This is understandable in an evolving field, and yet it is important to keep reminding ourselves that there are gaps in neuroscience research that make it hard to translate findings into clinically useful hypotheses. For example, in the use of EEG neurofeedback, the baselines that correlate mind events with neural events have not been fully established so that it is premature to begin examining pairs of people in relationship (personal communications 2014 with Kenneth Kaplan, MD, about neurofeedback and with Jennifer Leaner, PhD, at the Decision Science Lab). When these individual baselines are better established, simultaneous psychic and neural events while two people are relating will be possible to study. We believe this type of information will fill gaps in the neuroscience dimension of clinician–patient relationships.

Jon Lieff said that much of the knowledge in neuroscience has been discovered within the past several years. Lieff, a specialist at Harvard Medical School on the interface between neuroscience and medicine, published *The Limits of Current Neuroscience* (Lieff, 2013). He says that "conclusions that many of 500,000 neuroscientists have espoused are unproven and speculative viewpoints and that results from fMRI are being over interpreted." For example, he cautioned that most fMRI studies in the design of experiments make an incorrect assumption concerning the control group. The incorrect assumption is that the cohort performing a task activates a specific part of the brain which is *a simple addition* to the control group's brain activity. Another problem he sites is that there is "no known center of subjective experience, no understanding of what it might be, and little evidence that imaging devices actually are related to subjective experience. With a few notable exceptions, the relationship between neural circuits and behavior has yet to be established." Furthermore, he believes there is no evidence that fMRI measures neuronal activity as currently used. Astrocytes, not neurons, are believed to be the cells that determine blood flow by "having feet on each vessel and opening and closing them to provide local neurons with blood." This is a relatively slow process compared to neuronal signaling that occurs in milliseconds.

As noted earlier, we find that some of the neuroscience advances discovered appear to contain a conflated mixture of neuroscience and experimental human psychology. This is a prevalent conflation in this field partly because there are limited measurement tools to observe specific functions and regions of the human brain. Another contribution to the conflation is that professionals trained in experimental psychology tend to label their work as "neuroscience." Yet, their data is primarily from observation of human psychological behavior rather than from direct observation of the nervous system on the cellular, physiological, or anatomical levels. With neuroimaging, fMRI, it is possible now to observe human behavior and neuroimaging concurrently. The neuroimaging, however, is relatively crude compared to the observational tools evolved in psychology over the years. Calling the research "neuroscience" is often more of a hope for the future than it is a present reality. This is understandable because researchers find themselves studying what they can observe directly, that is, mostly human cognitions and behaviors and a limited amount of direct but still fairly crude data on brain dynamics.

Ecker et al.'s interesting book *Unlocking the Emotional Brain* (Ecker, 2012), when referring to the tenacity of implicit memory, says, "Research showed that extinction training forms a separate learning in a physically separate memory system from that of the target learning." In our view, saying "physically separate" is an example of the overinterpretation to which Lieff refers. From our perspective, when we see a "hot spot" of blood flow in a brain scan, we remind ourselves that the rest of the brain is still on-line and that neuronal circuits are firing and changing much faster than changes we are viewing. The authors try to support the notion of a so-called physically separate memory system with references to work at the NYU Department of Psychology. Phelps, in a lab, conducted behavioral studies on extinction learning in humans. They did not support a "physically" separate system. Testing eleven right-handed human subjects using mild shocks to their wrists in a conditioning paradigm with psychophysiological measurements, they concluded: "The fMRI results support animal models suggesting that the amygdala may play an important role in extinction learning as well as acquisition and that vmPFS may be particularly involved in the retention of extinction learning. The present results provide a demonstration that the mechanisms of extinction learning may be preserved across species." They are also quoted as saying, "Behavioral studies of extinction suggest that it is not a process of 'unlearning.'" That is as far as the cautious research team apparently went. We support this caution since it is known that there are functional overlaps in the brain.

Another example of a gap in neuroscience research is the omission of relational forces in most studies. It would be more expensive to study pairs of people relating, partly because for the research to be clinically valid, the researchers would also need to be experienced in the specific relational skills illustrated in this book. That would require more interdisciplinary collaboration than currently exists on most research teams. The existence of mirror neurons and new understandings about brain plasticity open up hypothesizing about how relationships impact both brains, brain-to-brain, in real time. Failures to account for the neural impact of being in a brain-to-brain:body-to-body relationship with another person is a serious limitation in design of many studies. We seem to be more aware of it with our animal pets than with each other. Talking and cognitions seem to be overrated. For example, being in a relationship may shift the way the brain processes and recruits regional capacities, including after severe psychological trauma and physical brain trauma. Although the fMRI indicates blood flow, not the much faster neural activity, we could at least study the impact of relating on what we can measure. It is unclear whether it makes sense yet to conduct comparative studies in and not in relational space on a number of dimensions such as extinction studies, learning and recalling new information under stress, emotional regulation studies, and using relationship work alone to work within the personality to heal severe trauma experiences. The newer fMRI using water molecule diffusion techniques might get at the changes in a neuron's cell membranes and be a more accurate or timely indicator of neuronal activity than the current fMRI.

The impact of being in a relationship does not show up in the peer-reviewed literature, yet we think it is relevant to include it. For example, Mark Bouton, Professor in Behavioral Psychology at University of Vermont, conducted a selective review and integration of the behavioral literature on Pavlovian extinction. According to the results he reviewed, extinction does not involve destruction of the original learning. Instead, new learning appears to be the main behavioral factor that causes the loss of responding to a stimulus. Although original learning (is it emotional learning or not?) seems to survive extinction, we do not know from this particular research design whether the same neural patterns are followed during the conditions of relationship-less learning (solo in a booth) compared to relationship-related learning (in a diad). For example, clinical experience indicates that the introduction of an attuned relationship makes a significant difference in what is heard, understood, and how well a set of reactivated implicit memories are extinguished. Lerner's Harvard Decision Science Lab, for example, was designed to study individuals isolated in booths where they are hooked up to physiological measurement tools. Interpersonal biological research has implications for informing the treatment of PTSD in veterans and trauma reactivity in children.

There is another example in *Unlocking the Emotional Brain* (Ecker et al., 2012) where caution is needed not to overinterpret evidence regarding a transformational process they call "implicit memory reconsolidation." This term for them describes the mental process that allows people to transform the grip that past experience has on them—that is to change the psychic core of what drives emotions and behaviors that people wish to change. It needs saying that both of us for years have used the features of IFS therapy that embrace the tactics of implicit memory reconsolidation—without any idea of what might be happening on the neural level. This has been powerfully transformative for patients worldwide. What Ecker et al. say, however (quoted from their table on page 21), is that memory reactivation and memory mismatch is a "requirement" for inducing reconsolidation. Just to be clear, the evidence is from animal and human laboratory studies in which the subjects were not in a relationship with another person. Also, the authors frequently use the term "synapse unlocking." Caution is needed when hearing such metaphors. The authors call it the "brain's requirement" without anyone being able yet to access brain activity data on that level of specificity. At this point, it would be helpful to re-emphasize that many of these statements are hypotheses based primarily on *psychological behavioral and cognitive data* while making inferences about brain functions. The ideas are not yet based on separate neuroscientific evidence. This is what many mean by "soft neuroscience."

For us, this work is within the legitimate realm of experimental psychology and is valuable. It is helpful to stay realistic, however, about the status of our knowledge in neuroscience as this informs us of what is not "known about what" and what more needs to be discovered.

The knowledge gained since 1995 and even in the past 3 years about the CNS/ PNS is impressive. Yet, it is at gross regional levels based on blood flow seen in the fMRI in humans and at cellular levels in animals. And, specific neural events have not yet been tied by research to specific human behaviors. What is known are mostly untested hypotheses from a number of sources: repetitive observation of deficits in function resulting from specific damage to the brain, from fMRI studies in humans, and from work with animals including primates on a cellular level. This a status statement not criticism.

Some workers ask why it matters clinically that we directly measure brain dynamics since we can validate data from human behavior for clinical use. Although we all realize that we are investigating one interconnected system, specific data on the neural side helps in the development of testable hypotheses on the psychological side and vice versa. For example, if we were to discover on a neural level that the "unlocking" and alteration of synaptic circuits proven to be carrying emotionally charged implicit memories requires that those circuits be reactivated in present time, we would test what personal experiences count as a reactivation on the neural level (measured independently) and under what conditions clinically for change in the circuitry occur. Could the clinical conditions for activation and change (by neural measurement) be from *experiencing video presentations* designed for the task? Or would a change on a neural level (measured independently) require facilitation *within a relationship* that is empathically attuned and exploratory? For example, researchers could use observations made during interventions that strongly include memory reconsolidation, namely, eye movement desensitization and reprocessing (EMDR) or IFS Personality Systems Parts work, to discover which elements (if any) in both these interventions correlate with independently measured changes in the neural system.

So far, we can say that the emerging findings about the functional anatomy and physiology of the CNS, although some distance from being able to test specific hypotheses in humans, seem generally consistent with psychological observations in the domains of implicit memory, affect regulation, relationship bonding, and the impact of emotions on learning and recall. Depending on how far beyond the first publication date you are using this book, you may be able to adjust and add to our neuroscience information.

It may help you to carry a visual image of the interconnected unity of the entire nervous and circulatory system that was embedded in my mind from *Bodies, the Exhibition* (Premier Exhibitions) created in China. This exhibit, although ethically controversial, showed human dissections of both systems together on the skeletal framework with all the soft tissue removed. It looked amazing—like an interdigitated treelike network of anatomical relationships between nerves and blood vessels reaching into every corner of the body. I was reminded that scientists create compartments for the sake of study, and yet functionally the body and mind are an amazing interacting, overlapping, and reduplicating constellation of shifting networks.

BASICS OF UPDATED FUNCTIONAL NEUROSCIENCE

(As recently described by personal communications with Augusto, 2013, and Anderson, 2013.)

- **Neural networks:** neurons interconnect to form networks; "neurons that fire together, wire together" (Tanaka, 2008), neurons interconnect to perform various functions; association areas bridge and direct multiple networks; there is neural integration, i.e., coordination and balance of separate areas; there are vertical and horizontal networks.
  Neurons fire when we have experiences. Firing grows and strengthens new synapses (neuroplasticity) and new nerve cells (neurogenesis).
- **Vertical networks top down:** omfc > right hemisphere > amygdala > brainstem olpfc > Lft hemisphere > hippocampus.
- **Vertical networks bottom up:** (visceral) (brainstem) > (limbic—amygdala, hippocampus) > (Ant. Cortex, cingulate, insula) > (Prefrontal cortex).
- **Horizontal networks:** (right–left) (dominant functions).
- **Right-brain functions:** unconscious, experience represented through imagery and feelings; intuitive, focused on present, direct connections to body, site of relationship attunements and memory of expectations. Right frontal lobe > limbic system locus of emotions > brainstem locus of ANS.
- **Left-brain functions:** conscious, experience represented verbally, focused on logic and detail, analysis of past/planning for future; little direct bodily awareness; connects to hippocampus, psychological managers and inner critics are associated with activity here.
- **Defined implicit memory:** Involves brainstem, amygdala, and right hemisphere.
  Starts in first 18 months of life, generalizes experience, tenacious, unconscious; involves perception, emotion, and the body.
- **Defined explicit memory:** Starts at about age 2; is conscious and requires the hippocampus; involves focused attention (dlPFC); is factual, linear, brings past into awareness, helps create sense of time and a narrative.

ENABLING ADVANCES IN TECHNOLOGY

Functional magnetic resonance imaging (fMRI) is a technique for measuring brain activity. It works by detecting the changes in blood oxygenation and flow that occur in response to neural activity—when a brain area is more active, it consumes more oxygen, and to meet this increased demand, blood flow increases to the active area. fMRI can be used to produce activation maps showing which parts of the brain are involved in a particular mental process. Hemoglobin makes MRI sensitive to brain activity. Oxygen is delivered to neurons by hemoglobin in capillary red blood cells. As neuronal activity increases, there is an increase in demand for oxygen. The local response is an increase in blood flow to regions of increased neural activity. Hemoglobin is diamagnetic when oxygenated but paramagnetic when deoxygenated. Diamagnetic atoms all have paired electrons. Paramagnetic atoms have at least one unpaired electron. This difference in magnetic properties leads to small differences in the MR signal of blood, depending on the degree of oxygenation. There is a momentary decrease in blood oxygenation immediately after neural activity increases. This "initial dip" is followed by a period where the blood flow increases—not just to the level which meets oxygen demand but overcompensating for the increased demand. This means the blood oxygenation actually increases following neural activation. The blood flow peaks after around 6 seconds and then returns to baseline. Since blood oxygenation varies according to the levels of neural activity these differences can be used to detect brain activity. Zald and Rauch (2006) reviewed methodological issues in neuroimaging, and Gerber and Peterson (2008) discussed them again.

Neurofeedback is a high-tech adaptation of EEG, giving information to the brain about the brain. It confirms the hypothesis that some brain circuits are plastic. The neurofeedback therapist and the patient together can see the brain's activity in real time and train the brain to self-regulate. Hirshberg at Warren Alpert Medical School, Brown University (Hirshberg et al., 2005), and Gapen and van der Kolk in Brookline, Massachusetts (www.traumacenter.org), reported that neurofeedback enabled patients to be with their emotions with more calmness and to use psychotherapy more easily. Efficacy research has been planned and is needed. In a recent personal communication to us from Scott Rauch, MD, Psychiatrist in Chief at McLean Hospital and a researcher using fMRI, he said: At present, other than ruling out general medical causes of psychiatric disease, there is not proven value for imaging (fMRI) in clinical psychiatry.

CLOSING COMMENTS

Cognitive–Affective neuroscience is a huge field, and to review it cannot be the focus of this book. The take-away here is that there are enough findings to confirm that there are neuronal observables that have already been found to correlate with common observations in child development and adult relationship behaviors such as relational attunement, social and informational learning, affect regulation, decision making, empathy, and compassion. Examples of these hypothetical neural "substrates" are suggested by plastic neuronal networks, attachment schemas, physiological dynamics, and bidirectional regulatory mechanisms.

This is the best science we have ever had. There is much work to be done to replicate existing research and deepen validation. These neurobiological findings motivate hypothesis building and research about psychological models of patient care. How well any psychological model will prove to correlate with emerging findings in neurobiology remains to be seen. We can imagine that as neuroscience findings emerge over the next 20 years, the clinical models of relational interviewing in medicine and nursing will get fine-tuned. Most needed is for neuroscience researchers to study pairs of people in a relationship. The Decision Science Lab at Harvard's Kennedy School has the potential to do this, but the baseline studies have not yet been done and they are not able yet to use fMRI to study relationships. It will take a cross-disciplinary team to do so. Now, mainstream professional education in nursing and doctoring has opportunities to catch up with the psychology of relationships in patient care and doctoring provides limited opportunities that may support it.

Building New Theoretical Hypotheses, Strategies, and Tactics for Clinicians

PART 3

Building New Theoretical Hypotheses, Strategies, and Tactics for Clinicians

6

Integration of past with present advances (selections of elements to include in a new model)

We shall not cease from exploration
And the end of all our exploring
Will be to arrive where we started
And know the place for the first time.

T.S. Eliot

INTRODUCTION

We have arrived at the exciting and challenging place of integration. As you know, research by its very nature is continuous. Yet, periodically, the time is right for accumulated knowledge to be integrated and applied to patient care. This is one of the first times in the evolution of the science of relationship that we are able to shine new light on places where we have been before. And, because of pressures coming from evolving health care policy to influence patients' health behaviors while controlling costs, it is imperative that we do not wait to create a new model for the relational side of patient care that is grounded as much as possible in existing science.

Also, we want to say at this point that the newly defined field of Interpersonal Neurobiology (IPNB) and Cognitive–Affective Neuroscience (CAN) are crucibles of integration for the future, especially when they embrace the Internal Family Systems (IFS) Model of personality organization.

Ultimately what makes it possible to integrate the scientific components of clinician–patient relationship is that they are aspects of one intertwined biological process, and that the clinical tasks of say, behavior change and information transfer, have at their core the same fundamental strategies and tactics involving the patient's emotions, cognitions, and memories—and require the same core competencies in clinicians. For example, the processes of working with decision conflict are quite specific, yet they require a simultaneous process of information transfer. Without both, patients cannot make medical decisions that are informed and are a conscious choice. The process of behavior change requires that certain conflictual lifestyle decisions be made by the patient. Although not high-risk treatment decisions, they are decisions involving opposite sets of emotions and beliefs carried within their personalities. For behavior change to be enduring, the clinicians must also help process decision making and must have skills to offer more information as the patient is ready to assimilate it. Conducting interviews is like conducting a symphony orchestra with sections of instruments representing personality. In the past nurses and doctors could be overheard to say, "Nurses cannot tackle medical decision making because it requires specialized knowledge about disease and treatment statistics and requires training in the formal Shared Decision Making® protocol." Consequently, it remained separated from most curricula on behavior change. And, information transfer, thought to be only a cognitive communication-science process, had also remained separated. Various "courses" were given on apparently different topics when in fact they required common understandings and clinician competencies.

The previous three chapters paved the way to use past and present findings to craft relational theory, strategy, and tactics that empower clinicians to facilitate behavior change, decision making, diagnosis, treatment, and prevention. Behavior change models and the Shared Decision Making protocol, despite their quasiscientific status, have been officially considered clinical tasks within Patient-Centered Care (PCC) for several years. Two additional relationship-based tasks need inclusion, as discussed in Chapters 4 and 5. These two tasks are Clinician Emotional Self-Care and Information Transfer. This makes **four** relationship-based tasks (behavior change, shared decision making, information transfer, and clinician emotional self-care) in addition to the **three** disease-based tasks (diagnosis, treatment, and prevention). By using these seven overlapping items, perhaps a clinician with a patient would always be able to answer the orienting questions, "What am I doing now and where am I headed?" The nurses that both of us trained in interviewing found that this orientation helped them discover, with a sense of relief, when it was time to end a patient encounter.

Both Clinician Emotional Self-Care and Information Transfer have been underresearched topics. Although the prior models (Chapter 3) separately addressed the clinical tasks of behavior change and decision making, none focused specifically on the clinician's inner process of emotional self-care during their encounters with patients. Our analyses of recorded clinical interviews by many clinicians and with a diverse group of patients showed that this item had a pervasive influence on patient engagement, ability to change, and make decisions right for them, and on the clinician's well-being (Livingstone and Gaffney, 2013). Oncology and palliative medicine seem to be the only arenas where clinical self-care has been studied and programs have been developed (Sanchez-Reilly et al., 2013). It is possible now to add significantly to their scientific understanding and to the importance of this domain. Their work is discussed below.

About relationships

How many times have each of us heard that something called "the relationship" is important in patient care? Acknowledging this idea makes sense despite not knowing exactly what is meant by the word *relationship*. The case for the importance of developing a relationship was based for many years upon it being the humane thing to do. Hippocrates talked about it, later so did Sir William Osler, and Francis Peabody said that finding out "who the patient is" was important. But it represented a goal or an idea without ways to walk the talk and to teach competency. Then the importance of *relational* aspects became a key to patient satisfaction and risk management. When it became clearer that treatment outcome of bodily illness was determined by qualities of clinical relationship and that even teenage-onset of type II diabetes was influenced by whether the family physician had processed a recent loss of a parent with the teenager, the quality and content of clinical relationships received more focus. Without dismissing the importance of cognitive processes, most of the psychotherapies and health psychology models, such as Self-Determination Theory and Motivational Interviewing (MI), and holistic nursing, placed the relationship of patient and clinician at the hub of symptom relief, healing, and behavior change in general medicine. It was implied by the word *shared* in Shared Decision Making and by the words *patient centered*. Still to this day, the science is ill-defined, and we hear faculty and practitioners say, "Skills of making effective relationships with patients cannot be taught—it is talent." Growing evidence indicates rather that it is science, and that it includes the science of self-care of reactive emotions and burnout that block the personal sensitivity of which almost every clinician has a larger supply than he or she is using.

The exploration of existing models and advances made in psychology and neuroscience in the past decade has brought us back to where we began—focused on the relationship, emotions, and personality. But, we now "know this place for the first time" *with scientific grounding*. Besides making use of new tools for studying brain activity, relational science is becoming a bigger trend in research. This viewpoint may in part reflect our interest and experience-based bias.

What we mean by relationship includes a state of the clinician's psychology and neural activity that the patient experiences as presence, resonance, attunement, and a sense of safety while being seen and accepted by the clinician for having competencies, protections, and vulnerabilities. To become a feature of clinician–patient relationships, clinicians must conduct their own emotional self-care so they can be emotionally and cognitively available from their core in order to extend genuine compassion, curiosity, and empathy to their activated parts (pleasers, inner critics, pushers, shamers, etc.), and then to focus on and self-regulate what is underneath them, for example fears of failing and frustration. He needs to reestablish caring and curiosity about his patient's vulnerable emotions which are underneath the part that is protecting and to have an alternative set of tactics. This will be demonstrated in video and discussion. For example, the clinician can ask his patient to recall his earlier emotions (probably confused and scared) and *ask him to notice if* this may be blocking his taking in the information (as compared to being paternalistic by impatiently repeating the information). When the clinician and patient can join together to look at what is going on between them, this establishes some perspective and lowers the negative energy in the dynamic. It often helps both people become aware of their vulnerable emotions—in this case a clinician, who has a part who is fearful of failure and is frustrated, and a patient, who has a part who is confused and fearful; rather than a clinician who is critical and a patient who is zoned out or becoming rebellious. This is a strategic goal to repair relational bonding patterns and establishes a workable atmosphere. The clinician can then slow things down to enhance the patient's awareness of how he is responding to the diagnosis and treatment plan. In diabetes it is often feelings of loss, with whatever meanings and memories (realistic and unrealistic) are activated by the diagnosis and the new health-management responsibilities, that need to be processed within the patient (that is, that need to be brought into awareness in relationship with a clinician, reality checked, and regulated from both inside and out). This example has given you the idea of how the personality parts play a pivotal role in clinician–patient relationships and what to do about it.

Some people feel comfortably familiar with the personality parts hypothesis, and others become skeptical and find it disturbing, at least at first. Again, all we ask is that you get curious about thinking this way and obtain some mentoring about your questions. The writings of Hal and Sidra Stone (for example, *Embracing Your Inner Critic*) and Richard Schwartz and others (for example, *Introduction to Internal Family Systems, The Mosaic Mind*, and also *There Is a Part of Me*—by Jon Schwartz and Bill Brennan, 2013) that provides a nontechnical avenue into the topic. For understanding the use of the personality parts hypothesis in health care, you can read our chapter on health coaching (Livingstone and Gaffney, 2013), Sowell on changing the course of chronic illness (2013) and her randomized controlled trial with rheumatoid arthritis patients (Shadick et al., 2013).

About information transfer and Information Interweave™

Information Interweave™ is a term we coined to refer to the relational process of the broader public health concept called information transfer. In concert with modern communication theory, information is always shaped to fit the patient's cognitive capacities, and if DVD or printed materials are used as supplements, there is content for most everyone that matches their learning styles. For interweave to take place, the psychological readiness of the patient gets to determine when, how much, and what information is provided. The term *interweave* means that information is interwoven at a time and at points within a process of relational exploration of emotion, beliefs, and memories of the patient. Interweave is information provided via a relational conduit. Checking as to whether information supplied is information heard—both facts and implications are one part of the interweave process. Slowing the process down and lowering quantity goals is often needed. Readiness is defined as checking with those parts of the patient's personality that are activated by the nature of the new or restated information. These parts may come hard up against implicit old beliefs or activated by a perceived threat to relational ties or to income-earning employment. For example, meds or radiation treatments or surgeries may directly affect sexual functions or be viewed as impacting desirability. Patients respond to information in hidden and significant ways. It is the clinician's job to enhance awareness for both patient and herself about these forces. The patient's emotions and beliefs need to be articulated and reassessed by them. The provision of information is interwoven into this exploratory open relational process. It takes less time than you imagine. Some data suggest that psychoactive medication compliance and even the medication's physiological effectiveness beyond placebo effect are enhanced by writing prescriptions within an interwoven process (F. Anderson, 2013, personal communication).

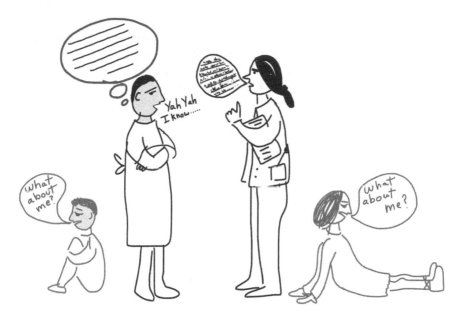

NEGLECT OF EMOTIONS CLOSES INFORMATION TRANSFER

That information transfer involves *more than a cognitive matter* or just a matter of sweeping emotion away so cognition can dominate is supported by the fact that there are interconnections between brain regions that process emotions generated in relationships and those that process learning and memory. What "more than a cognitive matter" looks and sounds like needs to be addressed by any clinical model that medical and nursing students are expected to learn.

It is interesting how the conflict over measles vaccination in the winter of 2014 magnified the need for clinicians to gain the relational skills to work with parent's beliefs and emotions rather than repeatedly presenting the same or new evidence-based facts. The opting-out of having children vaccinated was said by the media and medical establishment to be caused by an information gap. Yet, the observation was that providing more information to opting-out parents did not alter their reticence but actually increased it. The experience at UNICEF showed that African mothers and fathers, despite plentiful information from health workers about infant diarrhea, began to boil water used in infant formulas only when they were prompted by people indigenous to their culture. Parental behavior change seems unlikely without exploring and respecting parent's belief systems and their emotions, including through people indigenous to their local culture. The medical community questioned whether "opting-out parents were fully informed by the research data." From the perspective of this book, however, the question would be put differently. The issue is whether the parents are informed both from the outside (evidence-based information well transferred) and from the inside about their own beliefs and emotions that are not sufficiently conscious for them to check. The latter type of information is gained by talking with a clinician with skills in personality exploration. The stricter requirements for parents to opt out of vaccination by having to obtain a signature from the child's pediatrician, nurse practitioner, or physician assistant creates a powerful public health opportunity provided that the child's clinician can provide credible information while nonjudgmentally exploring the parents' beliefs and helping them to regulate their emotions. At the moment, too few clinicians are being trained in those interviewing skills.

We have included the cognitive dimensions of communication models from the field of health communication and marketing that promote shaping information to fit the patient's education and needs for clarity and control of quantity. The disadvantage of all these models, however, has been that they omit the role of relationship bonding and polarization between sets of emotions, beliefs, and memories in the process of communication of new information. We do not view these models as stand-alone approaches. Advances indicate that the process of transferring evidence-based information (Chapter 4, section "Information transfer") to patients involves two dynamics: *the state of the patient's readiness* (including degree of emotional arousal, beliefs, and nature of attachment to clinician) and *the state of the clinician's mentality* (including their freedom from judgment and coercive agendas). Both domains can now be addressed by the strategies and tactics of contemporary relationship psychology.

Although these topics and clinician training about Information Interweave are discussed in depth in later chapters, there are a couple of principles we want to offer here. In addition to teaching clinicians how to shape and pace the material to match their patients' cognition, research shows that the patient's emotional system needs to be *prepared* by the clinician. Reflecting back on beliefs, emotions, affect labeling, and the clinician's nonjudgmental emotional disposition are of central importance in this preparatory process. In a first interview the clinician does not know enough about the patient's knowledge of their diagnosis, their history (personal and family), their present life responsibilities and stressors, and their current emotions to front-load them with facts about their illness. In many cases, demonstrated by our recordings, front-loading facts pushes patients into denial, glazing over, and/or rebellious behaviors. Clinicians who are untrained in this domain often react to rebellious patient behaviors by giving even more facts and doing it with a tone of voice that inadvertently shames the patient. This clinician behavior is the foundation for ongoing polarization (sometimes subtle) between clinician and patient.

In subsequent chapters we indicate criteria of patient readiness and demonstrate Information Interweave in audiovisual form. None of the past models of health behavior change (see Chapter 3) were sufficiently informed by contemporary understanding of personality organization or relationship dynamics to be useful as a guide to help patients to assimilate and remember the information they may hear or read.

Also, none of them seems to illustrate specific interviewing tactics. For example, "roll with resistance" or "be empathic" are strategic concepts, not tactics, and they don't (as observed in current medical school programs) carry most learners to the point of skill competency. In the past, how could a clinician help their patients when there was so little theory linked to strategy and tactics of what needed to happen relationally in order for patients to assimilate new information.

About our process of integration

Although this young field has been in a state of fragmentation and has been embracing models thinly grounded in existing science, we want to include elements from prior models that are partly in concert with new advances, for example, some of the elements from narrative medicine, mindfulness practices, and integral/holistic nursing, MI, and Shared Decision Making. For a field still in its early adolescence it is important that the scientific bar for inclusion not be placed too high yet that we remain aware of the scientific status of what we do include. Too few randomized controlled trials (RCTs) exist on this topic due to the egregious expense of such projects, gaps in understanding by gatekeepers in funding agencies, and a scarcity of measurement tools. In addition to comparative RCTs, as evidence of efficacy we have included case reporting, pilot studies, and prospective trials comparing one method with care-as-usual. Also, heavily weighted for inclusion are sets of strategies and tactics that are widely used and claimed to be effective by large numbers of pertinently trained clinicians across diverse cultures, for example, elements of Psychology of the Selves and IFS Model. Another boost to qualification is the amount of independent discovery associated with a method, for example a hypothesis independently discovered both in psychology and in neuroscience is weighted heavily for inclusion. Combinations of many of the above inclusion criteria strengthen the rationale for inclusion.

Our criteria for inclusion of theory, strategies, and tactics from past models and advances since 1990 are as follows: (1) whether the theory/hypothesis is at least partly compatible with some established theory and observation, (2) whether at least one fidelity-checked, controlled research study has validated the hypothesis, and/or (3) whether the strategies and tactics linked to the hypothesis are in regular clinical use with widespread and documented reports of efficacy.

We have selected psychological elements from the past (Chapter 3) and from the advances since 1990 (Chapter 4) that we think could be included in an updated model. Then we have selected elements supported by both behavioral psychology and neuroscience from Chapters 3, 4, and 5—that is, with triple support. In Chapter 7, we formulate the resulting theory and strategies, and in Chapter 8 we list and discuss tactical competencies for clinicians to learn. The reason why selections are chosen from Chapters 3 and 4, despite not yet having been researched by neuroscience for lack of adequate measurement tools, is that they are sufficiently validated by behavioral research or wide experience. Some of the elements selected are present in several models and some are model specific.

SELECTION OF ELEMENTS FOR INCLUSION IN A NEW MODEL

Selections supported by Chapters 3 and 4: Psychology past and present

Despite the fact that many important concepts from traditional psychotherapies, holistic nursing, and past health psychology models (such as MI and Self-Determination Theory [SDT]) have been one-dimensional, or narrowly cognitive, or abstract without much tactic, or concrete without much theory, they have been included in the updated model by placing them within a contemporary context of theory, strategy, or tactic.

ABOUT EMPATHY AND COMPASSION

Several past models emphasized the importance for clinicians to have empathy for patients. This has been included in the updated model, but the concept has been broadened and the strategy and tactics are specified. Empathy is treated as a subtopic of the larger concept of attuned relationships, which includes both right- and left-brain aspects of empathy (emotional and cognitive), compassion (extending caring), and reciprocity. Empathy, seen this way, is included as one of several features of attuned relationships (attachment theory)—the platform upon which most clinical tasks rest. As you will see, attuned relationships have the advantage also of helping people regulate emotions. Current usage, as you have already read, defines empathy as having two components: (1) cognitive understanding of the person's ideas (not agreement), and (2) resonance with the person's emotions (standing briefly in the shoes of the other not so intensely as to become the other person). Compassion is a crucial feeling for clinicians to extend toward patients and sometimes toward themselves to regulate their own emotions; parents and teachers extend compassion toward children. It is different from empathy. It is an extension of warmth and appreciation (not so intensely as to become the other person). In prior models it is omitted or conflated with empathy, which is also vaguely defined. Compassion also can be extended by the mindful clinician toward personality parts that "reside" within them, for example, to their vulnerable inner childhood part that carries the extreme responses to illness and loss and who can be soothed by being given inner focused attention. This is a powerful tactic in clinician self-care that is discussed later.

ABOUT BEHAVIOR CHANGE AND DECISION MAKING

Both behavior change and decision making are emotional and cognitive. With this in mind, here are the ideas featured by prior models and our rationale for included them or not. Supporting the patient's competency and enhancing internal and external sources of motivation, relational connectedness, autonomy, and reflective capacities are aspects contained in SDT (Chapter 3, section "Self-determination theory"). Although it is not always clear what the proponents meant operationally, in general these ideas qualify for representation in the updated model. So does the statement embraced by SDT, "The most enduring and robust motivation to changing behavior is an internal psychological matter in a dynamic relationship with external variables." This notion needs to be reconfirmed, yet it is not new and has long been an aspect of traditional and contemporary psychotherapies and holistic nursing. (Recent telephone communications with the proponents have indicated that they had not fully operationalized their ideas.) The ingredients of this "internal psychological matter" that are associated with behavior change and the "dynamics" with external variables are more operationally defined by this book so that strategy and interviewing tactics can be taught.

ABOUT MOTIVATIONAL INTERVIEWING

The importance of the relational aspects of interviewing inherent in Motivational Interviewing (Chapter 3, section "Motivational interviewing") is in harmony with a contemporary approach. The ideas in MI that the clinical relationship is important and that ambivalence is a factor in behavior change are included in this work. What will not be adopted is MI's definition of ambivalence. The development of MI antedated the science that clarified that ambivalence includes conflict between internal personality parts that carry different agendas, emotions, and beliefs and that it is also influenced by relationship dynamics within their clinician and loved ones. These interacting forces can be tracked and accounted for. There also are other barriers to change, for example, failed information transfer, especially when both clinician and patient are unaware that accurate information has not been heard or assimilated by the patient. Also, we do not adopt the vagueness of MI tactical instructions, for example, "Give advice, express empathy, and decrease the desirability of the status quo." How and why these tasks are to be accomplished during an interview by clinicians seem to be missing. MI, in its day, did not elaborate sufficiently the interviewing tactics for applying their strategies in the context of maintaining an attuned interpersonal relationship. In our view, this is no small matter. Those medical and nursing students and experienced practitioners (faculty) we have directly observed trying to use the eight strategies and five principles of MI often use the protocol to manage the patient's behaviors and feelings, especially when the clinician seems to feel frustrated. Sometimes this is quite subtle, yet patients' personality parts have radar for such subtle forces. Often the empathic statements sound OK but do not ring true to the vulnerable parts of the patient. These features of interviewing are antithetical to enduring change and stable decisions. We have tried to remedy this situation and enhance those who use MI by embedding new strategies and tactics within the updated model and by creating video demonstrations.

ABOUT THE STAGE THEORY OF CHANGE

The Transtheoretical Model (Chapter 3, section "Transtheoretical model and stages of change") is not being brought forward since other dimensions of change are now understood to take precedence over the concept of *stages*. The latter continues to be controversial (West, 2005). Self-efficacy (Chapter 3, section "Self-efficacy theory") as an outcome of reflective cognition and modeling, although important in its day and not to be ignored, is not positioned in the updated model as the primary force in behavior change.

ABOUT THE HEALTH BELIEF AND PRECAUTION ADOPTION MODELS

Perceived susceptibility, benefits of diagnostics, and severity of illness are the focus of the Health Belief Model (Chapter 3, section "Health belief model"). It was created in the 1950s by TB public health professionals and modified in 2004 by Strecher. This touches upon a cognitive concept that subsequent studies have confirmed and is worth including as one aspect of medical decision making. The Precaution Adoption Process Model (Chapter 3, section "Precaution adoption process model") is another stage model that does not match well enough with current findings. That people's conscious (and unconscious) intentions (Theory of Planned Behavior, Chapter 3, section "Theory of planned behavior") would be a determinant in behavior seems to be a well-known (but not major) factor and can be found within the update.

ABOUT SHARED DECISION MAKING

It is helpful to distinguish between shared decision making as an idea and the protocol Informed Shared Decision Making (ISDM) as promoted by the group in Ottawa, the Foundation for Informed Medical Decision Making (FIMDM), and taught by others. It seems likely that the Institute of Medicine (IOM) embraced the idea of shared decision making but not any specific protocol. The finer details need to be reformulated in light of recent scientific advances, and the use of a stand-alone questionnaire to discover the patient's "values" needs to be research validated.

Hereafter, our using the term *shared decision-making* refers only to the generic use of the term. A stipulation for the development of shared decision-making has been written into the Affordable Care Act (2010) as section 3506.

It was helpful, indeed, when the workers in SDM in Ottawa discovered that the *values* of the patient play an important role in medical decision making, not just the *sharing* of evidence-based information between clinician and patient. Without fully realizing it, they were including the psychological realm of the internal life of the patient—not just their values but also their emotions. From our viewpoint, several dimensions have been omitted from the mainstream concept and SDM. Gigerenzer's findings on the conscious use of intuition supported that much had been omitted (Chapter 4, section "Medical decision making: A process involving emotions and relationship, not only reasoning about facts"). Both SDM by the Ottawa group and the mainstream generic concepts of shared decision-making seemed far from complete. The advances presented in this textbook expand the concept to include many pivotal factors in the science of decision process.

In a way, Gigerenza and I are saying that the human mind is organized to take care of the person, and we clinicians need to provide a more aware context that welcomes the safety of this organization for the person. The concept "shared" has been in metamorphosis for several years. We are now able to expand the concept to a new level, which includes pivotal factors in the science of decision process, namely, awareness of emotional influences (Lerner et al., 2015), the reality of conflicting agendas within the patient's personality (Sowell, 2013); improved knowledge of the process of information transfer (Livingstone and Gaffney, 2013), and use of a self-directed protocol to help clinicians process their own emotions and the thinking, which are activated by aspects of their patient's illness and behaviors (Livingstone and Gaffney, 2013; Schwartz, 2013).

Exactly how interviewing clinicians go about helping values and emotions to be aspects of the patient's process is a pivotal part of the update. As you know, the Ottawa group used a cognitively based questionnaire. It is not only the patient's values that matter; it is also their emotions, relational ties, and memories. The goal is not for the clinician to identify them. Evidence supports that the goal is to enhance the patient's self-awareness so that their emotions, beliefs, memories, etc., are included within the left- and right-brain functional dynamics of their processing. For this to happen, the clinician has to be "present," meaning, in relationship to both their left- and right-brain processing. Otherwise their right-brain functions dominate the process with the patient.

When my journalist friend explained that even though she had all the information, she still had to make a decision, she was referring to her sense of this cognitive-conscious and emotion-conscious process. The clinician does not have to "manage" all the content of the patient's process but needs to facilitate both a left- and right-brain process and be supportively present for it.

In conclusion, shared decision making, as we have come to understand it, is included in the new model but is expanded to become a cohesive, dynamic process going on within the patient, within the clinician, and between them. Current understanding of personality makes it possible for an interviewer to learn tactics to work with all three dimensions while using evidence-based information and conscious rules of thumb (see Gigerenzer, Chapter 4, section "Medical decision making: A process involving emotions and relationship, not only reasoning about facts").

Also, it makes sense to include printed and electronic Patient Decision Aids (PDAs), provided that they are tailored to fit the timed process of Information Interweave. Until more research is conducted on the updated versions of shared decision making proposed here, including how PDAs are used in an interpersonal context, it seems premature to create international standards for the development of PDAs as has been done with IPDAS (see Appendix).

An advance we have included by Gigerenzer (Chapter 4, section "Medical decision making: A process involving emotions and relationship, not only reasoning about facts") promotes a more humanly realistic process than "expected utility calculations" or "statistical analysis." It is the conscious use of rules of thumb matched with intuition. He calls it *Fast and Frugal Rules of Thumb* (Gigerenzer, 2007). It is more scientifically grounded than is clinical intuition left vague and unconscious—something we do not recommend. I include, however, the perceptual module (Guerlain et al., 2004) for acquiring interviewing skills during training and resonating with patients during an interview. Applied to interviewing, this means that the clinician, in addition to using reasoning with evidence-based information, is open to using their body-based (gut) feelings and visualizations of the spheres being tracked and of the personality parts within the patient (like their vulnerable childhood part) as supplementary guides for choice of direction, that is, both left- and right-brain functions. Diagrams and line drawings help to jump start such visualizations.

It is a positive sign that Fallowfield (2002) found that doctors asked for more of the active mentoring about medical interviewing that was used in his training program. Our work during the past 10 years confirms this receptivity for more rigorous training in this domain. As discussed in Chapter 4, fear incitement and persuasion have no place in a contemporary model of patient care. There are abundant clinical examples and theoretical understandings of how fear and persuasion-based techniques activate opposing protective systems within patient's personalities and ultimately block the goals of both patients and their clinicians. These techniques may be viewed as effective in a marketing and business context where escalating vulnerability activates buying, but it does not belong in health care where escalating vulnerability activates resistance and denial.

ABOUT HOLISTIC AND INTEGRAL NURSING

Over the years holistic nursing (Chapter 3, section "Holistic and integral nursing model") has accumulated many interpersonal concepts that we include, despite that the ideas seem thin in tactical details and seem unlinked to a comprehensive and testable theory. The updated model helps to integrate many ideas of holistic nursing, upgrades many of its strategies, and elaborates it into interviewing tactics. Some of the strategies of holistic nursing we will not include, such as the Santiago Theory of Cognition and their definition of empathy. And, the update adds a specific system of clinician emotional self-care from moment-to-moment that goes beyond mindfulness meditation—so that nurses have additional self-directed routes to be the holistic clinicians they aspire to be.

ABOUT THE NEUROSCIENCE OF PSYCHOTHERAPY

Embraced by our updated model is Cozolino's summation of the common principle he thinks applies to all traditional forms of psychotherapy: "Intellectual understanding of a psychological problem in the absence of increased integration with emotion, sensation, and behavior does not result in change" (Chapter 4, section "Role of implicit memory"). Some forms of traditional psychodynamic psychotherapy, however, promoted the labeling of affects because it helped with interpersonal communication and it seemed to reduce the intensity of the emotion. Doing it cognitively without interpersonal resonance was always thought to be ineffective. It was not known then that the placing of a symbol (a feeling word) on the emotion actually changed how that person's brain is processing it. There is now every reason to include this affect-labeling strategy in the updated model as long it is used within an attuned relational context.

ABOUT MINDFULNESS

Mindfulness (Chapter 4, section "Role of implicit memory") is taken forward into the new model and is a crucial aspect. In the 1990s, Jon Kabat-Zinn's continuing seminal work proved its usefulness in medical settings (Kabat-Zinn, 2007). The helpful impact of mindfulness practices is now supported by behavioral and neuroscience research on the brain and vagal system. Our health care model has extended beyond mindfulness alone into specific additional strategies and tactics that make full use of the mindful state. Different from Epstein's viewpoint in 1999 that "mindfulness cannot be explicitly taught," we and others have evolved tactics to access mindfulness both for in-the-moment and longer-term use, and to use it as a platform to do specific personality work. There is abundant clinical evidence of its value even without the discovery of neural correlates (Deliperi, 2011; Rowers Mind-Body Routine—RMBR™, Livingstone and Clark, 2015, unpublished). It is a process that is woven into our update for clinicians to use with their patients and with themselves for emotional self-care when with patients. The tactics are discussed in this chapter and demonstrated in subsequent chapters. The question that needs asking is what more can be done with what is noticed when clinicians are in a mindfulness state. First, we propose an openness and curiosity toward inner reactions that clinicians notice in themselves when witnessing specific patient presentations or behaviors. These reactions come from personality parts (see "Multiplicity," this chapter). Second, we are proposing a specific self-directed routine that clinicians can use regularly with these same activated personality parts. The combined strategy of mindfulness that is incorporated into the inner personality work proposed in this text has been found to lower the risk of unwarranted verbal and action behaviors toward patients (Livingstone and Gaffney, 2013).

ABOUT ATTACHMENT THEORY

Attachment theory (Chapter 3, section "Attachment theory of relational development") (supported by years of observation of parent–child relationships) is one of the core hypotheses for the update as are the interpersonal interview strategies it informs. There are years of abundant evidence of value from worldwide observation of parents and developing children and of adults with unsatisfactory childhood attachments. This theory and intersubjectivity were topics included in Chapter 3, section "Attachment theory in human development", and Chapter 5, sections 3 and 4. We put the theory to work in the updated model by formulating strategy and interviewing tactics based on some of the findings in interpersonal neurobiology.

ABOUT TRADITIONAL NEUROANATOMY AND NEUROBIOLOGY

Traditional functional neurobiology (Chapter 3, section "Traditional anatomical and functional neurobiology"), although quite crude, laid groundwork for multi-directional interconnections in the CNS and PNS. Establishing the functional and anatomical linkage between brain, body, and mind has been an uphill climb since the philosophy of Rene Descartes promoted their separation in Western culture.

Jumping ahead to the advances, the updated model brings the brain and the body's participation in emotion into clinical use. Badenoch (2008) represents a major effort to integrate neurobiology and psychotherapy, yet much of it could also be applied to clinician–patient relationships in health care. The recent text about trauma, *The Body Keeps the Score*, by our physician colleague Bessel van der Kolk (2014), presents the growing evidence for the role of the body in mental matters that the psychological sciences have long ignored. As you will see later in the model building, the observation of nonverbal behaviors and also asking patients to notice what they are experiencing in their bodies during an interview are important clinician tactics for exploring the emotions and beliefs of health care patients. Nonverbal reactions are a trailhead leading to implicit thoughts and emotions.

Selections supported by Chapters 3, 4, and 5: Psychology and neuroscience, past and present

The findings in neuroscience used to support the hypotheses below show that activity in the CNS measured by relatively crude current tools does correlate with many relational and psychological phenomena. As we have said before it is reassuring to discover that the interpersonal psychological events that have been observed for years are not constructed out of "pure ether"—existing solely in the minds of those involved and without corresponding neurophysiological events taking place. We have plenty of correlating evidence of neural events in animals and now in humans, although not very specific yet.

It is not possible to conclude that the regions of the CNS mentioned below and in Chapter 5 in the supportive research are specific or exclusive regions where specific psychological functions take place or that the effects might be unidirectional. A good bet is that they are bidirectional effects operating according to systems theory and that even though certain regions show up in an fMRI that correlate with an emotion or a behavior, that does *not* mean that the rest of the brain is off-line. Remember also that neurons fire in the range of 10–200 Hz, and blood flow responses seen in fMRI are slower phenomenon, lagging 1–2 seconds behind.

I think, however, that it is not necessary to wait for more neural evidence before applying those psychological and neural strategies—like neurofeedback— that are proving to be clinically effective, provided we are willing to reshape them as research unfolds. We need to remind ourselves that the psychological strategies, although further along in verification, are also works in progress. Here, we are integrating evolving knowledge—such as it is—and drawing attention to possible areas for future research. Bonnie Badenoch (2008) in Portland, Oregon, informed by the work of Schore (2003), Siegel (2011, 2013), and others, has been integrating psychotherapy and contemporary neurobiology.

As you review the seven psychological and nine neural advances and review the prior models and methods in Chapters 3, 4, and 5, perhaps you would agree that the evidence currently available leads to the following hypotheses:

- The process of affect labeling in interviews is necessary for emotional regulation and building of relational connection and is supported by current knowledge of neural connections and by long-standing clinical psychological experience (Chapter 3, sections "Motivational interviewing", "Holistic and integral nursing model", "Attachment theory of relational development"; Chapter 4, section "Emotion regulation"; Chapter 5, section 2). Emotional regulation is fostered by building an attuned relationship with the patient. Within this context empathy and affect labeling sensitive to the patient's self-awareness can occur.

- The regulation of emotions and an attuned relationship with a clinician are necessary ingredients for the cognitive assimilation of information by patients. This is supported by current knowledge that emotional arousal, learning, and memory are interconnected in the amygdala, hippocampus, and cortex. This is also supported by observations and clinical case reports that patients and parents who are experiencing intense emotions are at risk for distorting what is said and failing to recall what they think they heard (Chapter 3, section "Information transfer models"; Chapter 4, sections "Information transfer", "Medical decision making: A process involving emotions and relationship, not only reasoning about facts"; Chapter 5, section 1).

- Interpersonal relationships are both psychological and neural brain-to-brain interactions, and the brain's regions involved in regulating distress from social exclusion appears to be specifically and functionally altered by interruptions of attachment relationships in early childhood. This is supported by studies using biological markers of heart rhythms, circulating oxytocin, and vagal circuitry; by comparative, controlled behavioral and fMRI studies of children; and by psychologically based observations that affective relational connection (in childhood and adulthood) can lead to increasing attunement, affective resonance, and reciprocity (Chapter 3, section "Attachment theory of relational development"; Chapter 4, section "Relationship platform"; Chapter 5, sections 4, 7).

- An interpersonal relationship based on attachment theory and its strategies supports patients to change behaviors that are driven by intense affects and beliefs. This hypothesis is supported by current knowledge of neural plasticity (well-substantiated) and subcortical implicit memory reconsolidation (weak neuroscience evidence as yet)—both well-substantiated in clinical work in cognitive and motor rehabilitation and in those psychotherapies that stimulate new functions and retrieve and reconsolidate implicit memory (Chapter 3, section "Attachment theory of relational development"; Chapter 4, section "Role of implicit memory"; Chapter 5, section 6).

- The hypothesis of personality multiplicity unifies other theories, integrates the various pathways of relational attachment, and explains and predicts behaviors of patients and clinicians. It orients the clinician to be aware that he or she needs to be willing to make a relationship with several distinctly different and sometimes opposing personalities within the same patient that are activated by the stress of their situation. This is a hypothesis and heuristic now supported by 20 years of experience worldwide by thousands of highly trained clinicians and researchers and by observations of everyday life by writers, actors, negotiators, and others (Chapter 4, section "Shift in view of paradigm of mind organization"; Chapter 5, sections 6, 7).

- The development of attachment-based relationships requires clinicians to possess the interviewing skills that affectively connect to the patient, to understand they are relating to personality part within their patient, to resonate with emotions (their own and the patient's), and to feel genuine compassion and empathy. This is supported by current knowledge that activity in the prefrontal cortex (OMPFC and septal region) correlates with both emotional regulation and interpersonal empathic behavior, and by a vast clinical experience showing that the ability to regulate one's own emotions enables genuine empathy to be felt toward others and received by others (Chapter 3, section "Attachment theory of relational development"; Chapter 4, sections "Emotion regulation", 4; Chapter 5, section 5).
- Without a relationship on the level of attunement, upon which depend intersubjectivity, affect regulation, empathy, and implicit memory reconsolidation, it would be difficult to facilitate behavior change and medical decision making and the assimilation of new information required to support each. This is supported by current knowledge of (1) the existence of mirror neurons, neural plasticity (supported by fronto-parietal regions and Broca's area); (2) the connection between the OMPFC, amygdala, anterior cingulate, and prefrontal cortex; (3) the biomarkers of relational interconnectedness such as heart rate, oxytocin, and vagal control; and (4) the role of the prefrontal cortex in both emotional regulation and empathy. And, it is supported in the psychological domain by clinical research indicating that a relational platform enhances the facilitation of decision making, behavior change, and the transformation of blocking beliefs and emotions (Chapter 3, sections "Seven selected behavior change models", "Shared decision making", "information transfer models"; Chapter 4, section "Medical decision making: A process involving emotions and relationship, not only reasoning about facts"; Chapter 5, sections 3–8).

In order to **affectively connect and resonate** with the emotions of the patient and to maintain that state it is necessary for the clinician (1) to acquire a method for **emotional self-care**; (2) to know a theory of personality that helps to explain, organize., and predict what he or she is observing; and (3) to acquire the **skills to track three dimensions** (within patient, within himself, between them), **and** (4) **to explore different (sometimes polarized) aspects of the patient's personality**. These four requirements are supported by the nonspecific finding in neuroscience—that **activation of the anterior insular cortex and anterior cingulate cortex** is correlated with all the different subjective feeling states reported by humans. They are also supported psychologically by the observation that feeling states along with their associated beliefs, memories, and body sensations (1) are stored in both explicit and implicit memory and (2) are organized as multifaceted feeling and belief states in distinct programs of the personality, each of which, like an autonomous person, can form a distinct relationship with an interviewer (the "direct access" interviewing of personality parts) (Chapter 4, section "Shift in view of paradigm of mind organization"; Chapter 5, sections 6, 7, 10).

7

Formulations of theoretical hypotheses and strategies of relational patient care

FORMULATION OF UPDATED THEORETICAL HYPOTHESES

Clinical relationships are governed by the following testable hypotheses:

1. That both intrapersonal and interpersonal psychological and neurobiological factors operate in health care relationships, and they are determining forces in behavior change, decision making, information transfer, and clinical outcome.
2. That activation of these forces within the clinician's personality system (mind and brain) may interfere with their successful facilitation of behavior change, decision making, and assimilate of evidence-based information, and that these forces within the clinician's personality system are reduced by self-directed methods used in-the-moment.
3. That the psychological and neurobiological forces within patients can be altered by clinicians who develop a direct, attuned interpersonal relationships with the personality forces within their patients and who include their emotions, beliefs, body sensations, and thinking.
4. That the clinical process governing the transfer and assimilation of evidence-based information by patients involves relating to the different emotions and beliefs within the personality of the patient. It is a new theory of health communication called Information Interweave™.
5. That it is useful to guide health care interventions by the assumption that human personality is organized into distinct full subpersonalities or personality parts, some that have the role to protect or shield that person from vulnerable emotions and others that carry those vulnerable emotions, and that each personality part has a different set of emotions, belief systems, values, preferences, memories, and body sensations.

6. That when the interviewing clinician develops awareness of several active personality parts within the patient in a medical encounter, it facilitates a safe and open relationship that promotes change, decisions, and improves outcome.

FORMULATION OF UPDATED STRATEGIES

Strategies are conceptual operations to reach goals informed by theory. They are expressed at different levels of abstraction but are always less behaviorally concrete than statements about tactics.

Strategies supporting decision making, behavior change, and assimilation of information (information interweave) are as follows:

1. First take care of your own reactive emotions, bodily sensations, beliefs, memories, and agendas before and during your interaction with patients and their relatives. This permits maintaining self-awareness and nonjudgmental curiosity, compassion, and empathy toward all aspects of your patient and their history, that can occur even in the context of cognitive disagreement.
2. Build and maintain attuned relationship with your patient's leading/presenting personality part (this is usually a part with a protective role) in order to facilitate Information Interweave.
3. Wait for vulnerable parts of the patient to show through, and acknowledge and mirror them as well as the presenting part. Your calm, attuned mirroring relationship with your patient's presenting personality parts generates the psychological safety your patient's system needs for connection to you and to be able to show or express vulnerable emotions.
4. Facilitate emotion and affect regulation only within the context of maintaining an attuned relationship.
5. Facilitate the patient to discover implicit emotional memories that relate to their past health care or other experiences. Support the awareness of discrepancies with the present and help downregulate those emotions and beliefs by mirroring, affect labeling, and breath work.
6. Facilitate your patient to discover from within themselves what medical information needs to be repeated or explained for the first time. Assimilation is both a cognitive and emotion-based process, and patients need time and assistance to process the meanings and emotions that are activated within different parts of them by each piece of information.
7. Facilitate the patient who faces a medical decision or behavior change to become aware of the different, sometimes polarized opposite, personality parts that may have different agendas and sets of emotions, beliefs, body sensations, and relational needs.
8. Facilitate your own awareness of possible dynamics between your personality (and its parts) and those of your patient or their loved ones (and their parts).

A SUMMARY OF UPDATED STRATEGIES IN SHARED MEDICAL DECISION MAKING

Our current scientific understanding of medical decision making is that the process consists of facilitating the patient to become conscious of the following elements and then allowing space and time for integrated intuition to enter their system. From this process a decision emerges. It is *decision emergence*, more than decision making. The latter tends to activate mainly cognition about facts for a process that we now know requires combining left-brain (cognition) with right-brain (emotions, relationships, body, and integration of intuition) processes.

Strategic elements (clinician's goals) that support medical decisions that are likely to be enduring and that diminish backlash (decision remorse, poor healing, nonadherence, and litigation) are as follows:

1. Develop a *simultaneous* aware sense in the patient of several main personality parts that have been activated.
2. Facilitate the patient to gain awareness of the thoughts, beliefs, emotions, and agenda of each of the above.
3. Support each personality part of the patient to assimilate (hear, take in, react to, recall) all the relevant factual evidence-based information—using Information Interweave.
4. Facilitate the patient to gain simultaneous awareness of polarized (conflicting) personality parts and to tolerate the tension between them as opposites.
5. Facilitate the patient to tolerate consciousness of all parts activated by the decision process while also allowing intuition to play some role.
6. Gain awareness of the influence of the beliefs, thinking, and emotions of those people with whom the patient has an important relationship (loved ones, other clinicians).

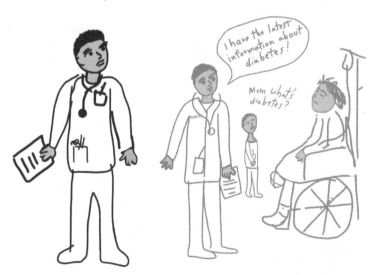

MEMORIES MATTER TO CLINICIANS

DISCUSSION

Embracing the theoretical hypothesis of full-personality multiplicity has advantages for clinicians when facilitating emotional self-care before and during encounters, and building an attuned relationship with their patients. The latter, although depending heavily upon clinician self-care, is not found to develop between clinicians and patients unless the clinician continually mirrors voice tone, body language, and verbalizations of the patient. These specific tactics are discussed in Chapter 8. The finding is that this works best when clinicians notice and get in tune with the dominant personality part of their patient who is present. The goal is reciprocal resonance. This can be understood as mind-to-mind and brain-to-brain resonance. Lack of attunement will be indicated by the patient's body and facial language.

If you wish to mirror back your patient's words, thoughts, and feeling-tone (even when you are confused or disagree), you will need to be in a relational mode within yourself. Understanding that your patient's personality is a multiplicity of distinct parts is an advantage. It allows you to understand that there are other aspects of your patient not showing through at that moment and that they could. For example, if your patient is covering over their unconscious fears by presenting with flat affect and a palpable reserve, you cannot expect your patient to respond to humor or an inquiry about emotion. Although your patient might contain such a personality part somewhere inside of them, at that moment it is being covered over. It is important that that clinician does not perceive the entire patient as having a certain character, such as "flat and reserved." It is not true and also closes off the possibility of noticing and flowing with the shifts that commonly occur during interviews. This understanding gives the clinician a tactic to perform what Motivational Interviewing perhaps meant by "Roll with Resistance" although the MI model does not include tactics.

The advances indicate that the determining factors of the successful facilitation of behavior change and decisions are as follows: (1) the quality of the clinician's ongoing emotional self-care of activated parts and ability to remain curious and nonjudgmental; (2) the ability to track three spheres: within himself, within the patient, and dynamics between them; (3) the clinician's ability to help patients to notice and explore polarized sets of beliefs and emotions; and (4) the clinician's ability to use Information Interweave.

Factors that determine the success of transfer of the evidence-based information correlate with successful emotion regulation within the patient, which includes affect labeling, interpersonal compassion and empathy, and all those clinician behaviors that support *emotion regulation*. These behaviors by clinicians have been found to correlate with activation of the *same regions of the brain* in the patient. This is another way of stating a hypothesis that emotional regulation is associated with relational empathy, affect labeling, and the attunement of attachment. Future research may indicate that mirror neurons and plastic aspects of brain function are activated by attachment relationships and that these neural activations, in turn, correlate with the regulation of emotion and assimilation of information—both of which are required to make decisions and change behaviors. This would prove that attachment relationships not only feel good but are crucial to medical care for a number of connected reasons.

Plentiful anecdotal clinical observations show that decisions and behavior changes based upon a process informed by multiplicity theory and strategy appear to be enduring and without remorse. Everyday observation and language by the lay public support the concept that personality parts determine behavior (see Chapter 4, Steinbeck, Hargitay, Nellan). Theoreticians about mind organization and neuroscience support it (see Chapter 4, Damasio, Minsky, Rowen). Some physicians in medical schools support it (see Chapter 4, Potter, Shadick, Warrier), and thousands of psychotherapists worldwide who work with medical patients support it.

The current high level of support for this hypothesis about personality parts, as we see it, warrants conducting random controlled trials to test comparative efficacy and outcomes of (1) using this theory and its strategies as a guide to patient care and (2) using the tactics as a new approach to medical decision making, behavior change, and clinician emotional self-care. Research design is discussed in Chapter 14.

8

Tactical competencies and frameworks

Every word, facial expression, gesture, or action on the part of a parent [and a clinician] gives the child [vulnerable patient] some message about self-worth.

Virginia Satir
American author and social worker

INTRODUCTION

Chapter 7 outlined updated theory and strategies. This chapter describes the tactical competencies we find to be common interviewing components *within all the strategies*. For example, we have talked about making an attuned relationship with the patient's presenting personality part. We now describe how to notice the presenting part, what becoming "attuned" during an interview entails, and what working with behavior-determining inner experiences looks and sounds like. No matter how elusive it may seem at first, these competencies are possible to acquire. After the competencies and framework are learned, they can be made your own. Not only is this degree of detail necessary for effective learning and training, it is also necessary for research. When conducting comparative clinical research in this field, there can be little validity in such research unless reliable intervention adherence scales for assessing interviews are developed.

The videos demonstrate the competencies of one clinician while, without being formulaic, she remains within the framework of theory, strategy, and tactics of this updated approach to facilitate behavior change, shared decision making, and information transfer. You will be able to use her behaviors as a model as you evolve your own ways of being and saying things. To us, the competencies described below also seem to rest upon a fundamental caring for patients and yourself.

A word about what we mean by the term *soften* or *soften back*. These are the words clinicians use to help a patient's personality part (and their own) to become background in their mind instead of foreground. It is a visualization in space. We ask a personality part to soften back or step back; we don't ignore it or *push it back out of awareness*. This would promote the old way of "managing" feelings and pushing emotions and thoughts out of mind and reburying them. That is antithetical to your relationship goals with your patients. Inside yourself the goal is to welcome all parts as partners and be able to make use of them without having them become extreme and dominant. Awareness of parts opens the possibility of a conscious choice of behavior. Perhaps it will help you to think of yourself as a parent or teacher who, after listening to a child's story and emotions, asks her to stand beside you rather than leaving her and/or sending her to her room.

As you have read, an aspect of learning this subject involves *visualization* and *gut feeling*, in addition to reasoning. Learning by perception-visualization is one of the newest approaches to learning specific data processing skills in surgical medical training (Chapter 4). Health profession schools might benefit from adding this dimension to learning interviewing, if this works for the learning style of that student. Some adults use bodily sensation rather than visualization as their primary mode of inner learning. Inner visualizations of what you are tracking and the personality parts of your patient, and being able to tap into your gut feelings, supplement and apparently sharpen your reasoning over data. As you create space for inborn and semiconscious capacities as a guide to obtaining truths about patients, you become a more efficient and accurate learner—much like the examples of the microsurgeons and pilots learning to use instruments. To do this requires a willingness to move beyond your reasoning brain and a receptivity to experiencing your patient's beliefs, emotions, and nonverbal manifestations, leaving space for this, without having to explain and sort all of it through reasoning functions alone. This is the "data" that comes from being *with* the patient, which is not gained from electronic records, laboratory results, and weighing statistics and is akin to the well-known implicit dimension of decision making. It is not either/or. It is both. This function is operating within the clinician during the audiovisual interview demonstrations while she is also using her reasoning and procedural frameworks. We have offered you diagrams and frameworks to support your use of visualization.

TWO FRAMEWORKS TO VISUALIZE

There are seven tasks and three spheres of relationship to keep in mind. At first, learning to use these will involve conscious cognition. Then via visualization and your bodily senses, they will become more automatic aspects of your inner road map while you interview.

The seven tasks

The past models and the advances taken as a whole prompt the addition of two more relationship-based tasks to those suggested by the Institute of Medicine (IOM), i.e., behavior change, and shared decision making. They are **transferring new information** from clinician to patient, and psychologically based **care-taking by clinicians** of their inner emotional responses to the illnesses and behaviors of patients and to memories of their own past health care experiences. This puts four relationship-based tasks in the spotlight for improvement and as topics for training physicians and nurses along with the three usually mentioned tasks of diagnosis, treatment, and prevention. This makes seven tasks in clinical care. Disease-based tasks: (1) diagnostic evaluation, (2) treatment planning and delivery, and (3) prevention; Relationship-based tasks: (4) communicating evidenced-based information, (5) health behavior change, (6) medical decision making, and (7) clinician emotional self-care.

All seven tasks overlap and also have credibility as separate entities, have similar core elements, and are mutually supportive during any one encounter with a patient. For example, information transfer may be interspersed when you are primarily working with your patient's intrapersonal conflict about a decision or a behavior change or when you are conducting an examination for diagnostic purposes. You can bring in diagnostic and treatment data into other tasks as it becomes pertinent to the patient's readiness to receive it. Although your emotional self-care may be operating throughout your encounter, there are some moments when increased focus on your internal system may be necessary.

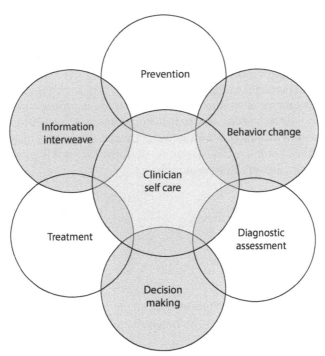

SEVEN TASKS OF PATIENT CENTERED CARE

Three spheres of the relationship triad

Three relationship spheres for clinicians to visualize and be aware of at all times in their encounters with patients are: (a) within the patient's personality, (b) within the clinician's personality, and (c) the bonding pattern dynamic between them. We call this the *Relational Triad*. All of these domains are continually impacted by the vulnerable emotions within both patients and their clinicians that are associated (presently and historically) with illness, health, death, and treatments. The nature of each domain in the triad has been explored psychologically by many thousands of clinicians who work with patients as therapists, health coaches, and holistic nurses (Herbine-Blank, Dossey, Sweezy, Livingstone and Gaffney, Schwartz). The processes within each domain, as you have seen in Chapters 3 through 6, vary as to their current scientific status. The scientific status for use of the interactive triad itself is relatively new in health care. For example, although psychologically we have studied pairs of patients and clinicians for several years, we could not find any brain imaging research to date that has studied simultaneously the neural activations in patients while in various types of dynamic relationship with clinicians or with loved ones when health behavior change or decision making are issues. In the past 10 years, much more understanding in this interactive domain is available from clinical psychology than ever before (Stone and Stone, 2000; Livingstone and Gaffney, 2013; Herbine-Blank, 2013). From a systems perspective, there are spheres of influences on several dimensions. They are within the patient's personality parts, body, and brain biology; within the clinician's personality, body, and brain biology; between them as interpersonal parts dynamics; and between the patient and loved ones who carry family and cultural expectations. Relationship dynamics of personality parts operate between patient and loved ones and between clinician and patient. To track these spheres of interaction may seem like a daunting task for the average clinician, who also needs also to focus on diagnostic-evaluation, treatment, and prevention. With practice, awareness of the relational triad makes the other tasks easier. They become an integrated set of skills. The total is greater and more effective than the sum of the separate spheres.

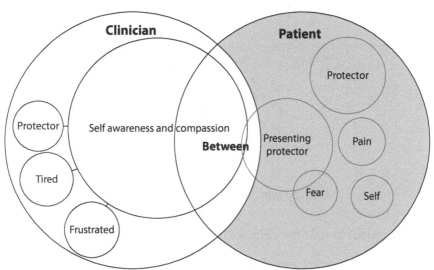

THE RELATIONSHIP TRIAD: INSIDE CLINICIAN, INSIDE PATIENT, BETWEEN THEM

Notice in the diagram above that the internal setup within the clinician is different from that of most patients. The clinician strives for a large core of awareness of his or her own parts so they will remain softened back and he can remain present and focused on the patient's ways of coping with the visit. The patient is expected to be using an automatic protector part to shield the vulnerable emotions inherent in the situation. The part that is automatically being used, for example, a "know it all," although it protects the patient from too much emotion, may pose difficulty for the clinician who is unaware that when he respects and relates to this protector part, it will soften, allowing vulnerability to appear gradually.

There appears to be support from many directions for inclusion of the following tactics in any updated model for clinicians to employ in patient care: (1) establishing an interpersonal relationship by safely exploring thinking and beliefs, by noticing body sensations as clues to emotions, and by utilizing methods that foster attachment (mirroring, affect labeling, respecting personality parts, and reconsolidating implicit emotional memories as needed), (2) using mindfulness and breathing and going beyond it to work with parts, and (3) using the type of clinician emotional self-care that enables the clinician to extend curiosity, compassion, and genuine empathy to the different personality parts noticed within themselves during their interventions with patients.

CORE TACTICS IN INTERVIEWING: COMMON TACTICAL COMPONENTS THAT IMPLEMENT ALL THE STRATEGIES

Tactical competencies

1. Using Steps I and II of clinician emotional self-care
2. Paying attention, being quiet, and waiting
3. Mirroring and validating
4. Helping patient to locate and/or identify and become aware of bodily sensations
5. Helping patient find words for emotions, distinguishing between emotions, thoughts, and body sensations
6. Extending empathy—both components
7. Noticing, exploring, and enhancing awareness of the set of emotions, thoughts, and body sensations carried by each personality part, especially the presenting part
8. Enhancing awareness of each personality part that is involved in a polarization (a pair of opposites) and prompting the patient to tolerate having them both in awareness simultaneously during their process of change and decision.
9. Interweaving information when patient is ready and shaping it to fit the interview process
10. Asking for feedback (emotions, thoughts) from patients of what they heard and its impact; check on influences from family and other clinicians

Tactical competency descriptions

TACTICAL COMPETENCY 1: USING STEPS I AND II OF CLINICIAN EMOTIONAL SELF-CARE

> Definition of a totally mindful clinician: "Someone who you don't know very well."

There are two steps: Step I (30–60 seconds) is used before and during your encounter with patients. Step II (10–15 minutes) is used later in a quiet place to revisit and continue processing the emotions, thoughts, or body sensations that came up earlier. The more you make use of these tactics, the easier and more "organic" it becomes.

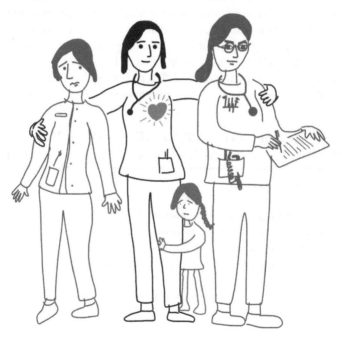

SELF-CARE PREVENTS BURN-OUT

Step I (Self-care in-the-moment: 30–60 seconds): Before starting with the patient, the clinician spends time focusing inward and noticing whatever thoughts, emotions, or body sensations he or she is having and then breathes into them, whatever they are, until there is more self-awareness and curiosity. The clinician reminds him- or herself that what is being noticed is coming from personality parts, **not all of him- or herself**. We call these parts *pop-ups*, which consist of thoughts, emotions, and body sensation, such as "I'm late already," neck tension, feeling worried, "I don't know about this disease," or "You have to rush." They come through into consciousness when activated by the situation—sometimes we are aware of *only one aspect of a pop-up*—often the body sensation—and can start with that.

The other aspects we could discover are the emotions, the thinking, and any imagery that are linked to the body sensation. The key tactic is to go *toward* these pop-ups and notice them and get curious about them, as compared to the usual and intuitive habit of trying to push them out of your mind. This business of getting curious and going toward is a nonjudgmental and relational approach. It can feel good and does not make it worse. This tactic invariably softens the emotions and body sensations of the pop-up. If placing a label on the emotion of the pop-up is possible, this is also done, for example (clinician to self), "So there is some fear going on right now." "So, I am sensing a need to rush in my shoulders." "I am aware of the thought 'I don't know enough about ____ (disease), and the feeling it gives me is ____.'" The clinician then does the following: (a) breathes into what is being noticed, (b) makes an inner intention for later in the day to revisit the pop-up to learn more, (c) then asks the pop-up to soften back so that the clinician can focus on the reality task. Step 1 takes about 60 seconds, a long time to give the psyche. And, it can be repeated even during the patient encounter for the same pop-up or additional ones. Step II is used later in the day and is essential not to forget. It will take about 15 minutes of being alone and focusing inward.

Step II (Ongoing self-care; 15 minutes, 4–5 times per week): Revisit the earlier pop-up, whatever aspect can be recalled. Notice it. Notice any specific sensation in your body. Go toward whatever you notice and breathe into it. Notice if more emotions, thoughts, or images come through. Go toward them (not away from them). See if they cluster into different aspects. Recognize that these are pop-ups and are coming from personality parts, even if it is not exactly clear what they are. Just focus on whatever you notice and extend your curiosity toward it. Ask whatever else is coming through that is judging or concerned to ease back. Check what you feel toward what you are noticing. If it is judgment, fear, or skepticism, ask what it would need to give you space to just be with this **one** part, **to learn more about it**, yet not letting it take over. Refocus on the pop-up you wish to work with that came up when with your patient, and invite it to share anything it wants you to know about it. Just notice and stay tuned. Explore the memories, emotions, beliefs, history. Ask the part its agenda—what it does for you or what it thinks might happen if it did not exist within you. This process is just like an interview with a young person and the building of a relationship—not fixing or judging. This process alone of being *with* a pop-up lowers the chance that the pop-up will reappear as an intrusion during your work. If you spend time with your inner pop-ups, when they come up during your work, you can then immediately recognize them and ask them again to wait until later. This is how inner trust develops. The more you practice this process, the better the results. Just as you do workouts for your body, this is a mind workout to add to your daily routine.

This tactic can be visualized as building an internal relationship with your inner personalities—the younger versions of yourself. It becomes a useful personal skill for the clinician that enhances his or her patient care in stressful situations and prevents short- and long-term burnout.

Emotional self-care in-the-moment (Step I) is pivotal in order for you to initiate and maintain attuned relationships with your patients. As we have explained, mindfulness has been the only protocol for this tactic until the shift in understanding of mind organization provided a new pathway (Chapter 4, section 5). Steps I and II include mindfulness and go beyond it by using the power of awareness of the personality parts within the clinician's system. Clinicians are at their best when they are attending to and soothing their own internal vulnerable emotions (whatever their source) so that their protector parts (fact-finders, doers, knowers, pushers, and affectless robots) are not doing the entire job of protecting them from emotions that they think are too intense for them. Please be aware that in the interview demonstrations you are observing a very experienced clinician who does not have to use Step I vigorously, since it is almost organic for her to help her activated parts to remain in the background of her mind so she can attend to Tactical Competency 2, below.

More than 4500 psychotherapy practitioners, now guided by the Internal Family Systems Model, practice a form of emotional self-care that clinicians in medicine and nursing can adapt. I have adapted it successfully for athletic coaches and elite athletes. Before a big event, athletes normally experience mental activations (called mind pop-ups), for example, a sick stomach or thoughts such as, "What am I doing here," "I might let everyone down," or "I'm going to be the greatest!" These pop-ups (either negative or positive sounding) stimulate cortisol, block optimal performance and team collaboration. The same is true for clinicians. A pop-up can be an image, emotion, body sensation or thought.

The best goal for the average nurse and physician is to discover the personality parts that are their main protectors during their clinical work and also know something about the vulnerable inner children they shield—because younger versions carry the vulnerability. Your places of vulnerability may be linked to your past experiences with health care, illnesses of relatives, losses, or school experiences with authorities. The common protectors in health clinicians are observed to include the "voices" of responsibility, perfection, pusher, caretakers, "gotta know everything," inner critic, and parts that judge others. Common vulnerable parts in health clinicians are observed to include a fear of failing the patient or superiors, feeling shame, feeling overwhelmed, and running out of time. The inner task is getting to know and be with these emotions, many of which can be extra-strong because they carry the past in addition to the realities of the present. This is self-empathy. The goal is not to get rid of them. When clinicians gain this awareness within, they can regulate their emotions and parts that carry them. They are then able to maintain a state of nonjudgmental, curious, compassionate energy. They have some choice about their verbal and action behaviors toward patients and colleagues, and can give themselves the time to consider the impact of what they might say and do.

TACTICAL COMPETENCY 2: PAYING ATTENTION, BEING QUIET, AND WAITING

What enables you to (1) pay visual and auditory attention to your patient's verbal and nonverbal behaviors and (2) keep in mind that data from the medical record? It is utilizing the emotional inner care of Step I of Competency 1 above, the most important for mastery of all the remaining competencies. Helping your rational mind to be quiet and your parts to soften back comes with practice and is a key component of maintaining active and open external attention. Using what your body may tell you is another source of information about you and your patient. Allow yourself to listen to yourself and the space to listen to your patient. You might visualize the space or the "emotional oxygen" you are providing. Put the oxygen on yourself before trying to help someone else. You patient has innate capacities that you will block if you don't allow some quiet for their feelings, memories, and imagery to emerge inside them. It saves time to let this happen.

The mirroring back of what you are observing helps maintain active attention on your patient, and active attention is necessary in order to mirror well.

TACTICAL COMPETENCY 3: MIRRORING AND VALIDATING

Different patients need to be mirrored in different fashion. In the beginning and often through an interview, the patient is speaking from their *presenting personality part—a protector*. This is where your mirroring starts. Examples of different protector parts you may notice are: *"You tell me—you're the expert," "I read it—know it all,"* minimizers and maximizers, *malcontents*, and *push through and "be done with it."* Mirror back with respect the voice tone and body language of your patient is dominant part.

If your patient speaks slowly and separates their thoughts, you will be able to mirror during the pauses. In small sound bites you can just repeat softly close to their exact words without editing or you can sometimes review larger chunks prefaced by, "So if I'm hearing you correctly, you—." What you want to watch out for is that your tone when you mirror is not carrying judgment or feeling of confusion within you coming from your parts. Confusion needs to be tolerated while mirroring. There will be more that will eventually clarify what you are hearing, and if you wait, you can ask your patient later, "Could you tell me a little more of what you mean by—?"

If your patient speaks quickly, you will want to slow the process down by mirroring back slowly as subtext or gently *interrupting* with something like, "So to be sure I'm getting it, I'm hearing you say—is that right?" If you don't do that, you will feel flooded (just as your patient may feel) and not be able to recall enough to mirror well. Interrupting the pressured speaking with your presence and a nonjudgmental tone helps to slow things down and helps to downregulate the emotional state of the patient, so that the patient is not as flooded. This is the necessary groundwork for anything else on the agenda of the meeting.

During the entire interview, we suggest you stick mostly with their words and phraseology while expanding on it to convey your clinical views. With practice this will become more automatic for you. You can ask your patient if what they are hearing themselves say makes sense to them. This increases their awareness, as does your mirroring back, which means it is heard twice, once when they say it and a second time by your mirror.

Patience and attentive listening are required. This is hard when there is time pressure. The research has found that it saves time to take time to stay in tune. Self-awareness and care of your own parts is your ongoing strategy—by using Step I of clinician self-care. You need to match your patient's energy style for a while and see what happens. Your job is to remain present, to help them notice what is happening inside their thinking and feeling, and help them express this so that they can contain and regulate, not either to bury it or push deeper.

When emotions appear in the patient, the tendency, however, is for clinicians to protect themselves by getting active or ignoring them. Both of these behaviors shut down felt relational connection. Examples of activities we have observed that are designed to protect clinicians (rather than patients) are inquiring more, getting falsely empathic, prematurely making statements that sound reassuring, and in the patient's presence, looking up and presenting more facts. Your calm, attentive presence is more powerful than you realize.

If you mirror and match your patient's style and be with him or her, in one interview a shift is likely to occur as they feel safer. The shift would be toward allowing more vulnerable feelings to be safely shared with you. This gives you and your patient together a powerful ability to facilitate information assimilation, behavior change, and decision making. This is truly a shared and informed process.

Sometimes, despite your best efforts, patients get flooded with emotions. If your patient should enter with a flood of emotions—such as terror-filled anxiety or tearful sadness—you need to acknowledge that they are feeling a lot, mirror it back, help them place a word on it, but do not push them to feel more by going into detail of what it is about or offering sympathy. This would bring up more than they (and you) can regulate—which feels awful. You need to facilitate their safety in being with the emotions and staying with what they notice, asking them to take a few deep breaths as you extend your presence. This is the relationship regulator to which all humans respond.

TACTICAL COMPETENCY 4: HELPING PATIENTS TO LOCATE AND/OR IDENTIFY AND BECOME AWARE OF BODILY SENSATIONS

The feelings that people have are often only available to them from what they can notice in their body. So asking someone to notice what they are aware of in terms of their bodily sensation can help them become more aware of their feelings—help make feelings more explicit. "So, try going to your body to see what you notice." It might be a generalized sense; it might be tension in their shoulders, a sinking in their stomach, heaviness in their chest. Accept whatever they notice. Even if your patient is already expressing an emotion in words, he or she can increase the level of awareness by noticing how their body is responding. When you ask them to breathe into what they notice, this helps downregulate intense emotions of fear and anxiety, and the body sensation provides grounding for their emotion.

TACTICAL COMPETENCY 5: HELPING PATIENTS FIND WORDS FOR EMOTIONS (LABELING AFFECTS) AND DISTINGUISH BETWEEN EMOTIONS/FEELINGS AND THOUGHTS

You can also wonder, along with your patient, what thoughts go with an emotion and what emotion goes with a thought. By doing this you are enhancing the width of their awareness.

Helping you and your patient to make this distinction between thoughts and emotions is for the health of your patient's brain. It facilitates experiencing and regulating emotions that otherwise are neglected because they were expressed as thoughts. This can be done organically by nonjudgmentally reframing what your patient says. For example, when your patient says, "I feel that—," and believes they have verbalized a feeling, you could say, "So when you *think*—, what emotion comes up for you? You can check your body." Emotions are one word and felt in the body. You can invite them to make up a word. Remember, you are helping your patient to find the best word for them to symbolize their felt emotion. You are helping what is implicit and semiconscious to be explicit for the patient and to share that with you verbally. This deepens the attunement. *You* are not supplying the label. You are asking them to name the sensation or feeling from inside of them. Chapter 5 describes the neuroscience supporting this tactic. You can offer a brief list of words people use for emotions. One they settle on their word, you can mirror it and use it for the remainder of the interview. If later on your patient wishes to change their word, go with their adjustment. Stay in tune.

You are helping patients perceive and be with three awarenesses: thoughts, emotions, and body sensations. You can also help them to perceive and differentiate personality parts by accepting and tracking contradictions of thoughts, emotions, and body sensations during your interview. The contradictions are held by different personality parts—each having their own set as a full personality (Chapter 4, section 5). It is normal for people to have a part that feels or thinks one way and another part that feels or thinks another way. **This type of differentiation of parts enables your patient later in your interview to develop a felt awareness of polarities between personality parts, which is crucial for working with ambivalence during behavior change and decision making.** Take care of your inner reactions to their emotions so that you can stay separate and still remain tuned in.

Memories can enter consciousness as images, body-based feelings, and/or thoughts. Invite your patient to stay with whatever they notice, and you stay with them by paying attention, mirroring, and remaining open and accepting. It is not appropriate to go deeply into detail with an emotion or traumatic event, as this is likely to make the patient feel overwhelmed and trigger protective parts, which will shut down their process and trust of you. On the other hand, it is not helpful to avoid their psychological process. It saves time to keep within the framework of purpose for your meeting while acknowledging your patients' inner experiences. You will notice that the demonstration interviews in Chapter 9 keep this balance.

You will notice in several interviews, near the end when clinician and patient are in tune and more emotions are being tolerated, the patient's inner critic emerges and may say things like, "You are making too big a deal out of all this." The clinician needs to connect to that part and help it soften, since it is likely to try closing off, as it is in the habit of doing, the patient's access to their emotions—the access that is needed between interviews to process decisions and behavior change.

TACTICAL COMPETENCY 6: EXTENDING EMPATHY—BOTH COMPONENTS AND COMPASSION

The *feeling dimension of empathy* is a brief standing in the other person's shoes and resonating with their emotion and acknowledging in some way that you "get it." The acknowledgment can be expressed by a body motion such as a head nod or verbally as, "Yes, I see," or you can mirror the patient's words, especially words that label emotions. The *cognitive dimension* is an understanding of the thinking of what your patient is saying, and can be acknowledged by a comment such as, "I follow you." Otherwise, wait for more information and ask the patient to say more about that. This empathic procedure does not imply that you agree or fully understand; it is only that what is being said "makes sense" in the context of the patient's feelings. Mirroring facilitates awareness of explicit and implicit emotions (Chapter 4, section 6) and is a pathway for patients to place words on their emotions and locate where they might experience them in their body. You can extend compassion and both aspects of empathy and hold space and time in the interview for them to *be with* the emotions and thoughts they are experiencing in their body. As you have read in previous chapters, this helps to downregulate and is supported by advances in both clinical psychology and neuroscience.

TACTICAL COMPETENCY 7: TRACKING, EXPLORING, AND ENHANCING AWARENESS OF PERSONALITY PARTS, ESPECIALLY THE PRESENTING PART—WITHOUT "TEACHING" PARTS LANGUAGE

Most everything people say is generated by some part within them. Parts run our lives. They are indispensable. Clinicians can learn to track them during interviews. Either we use them with awareness and have some choice in the matter, or they *are* us and we experience ourselves as being whichever part happens to be most activated at any point in time. Actors willfully access a part for their performance; this is what makes a performance genuine. Patients automatically use a part to cope with their medical visit. As we've stated before, patients will usually be speaking from one part of themselves without awareness that they have more than that one part. Especially in health care, where vulnerability is activated when seeing a clinician, a protective part of the patient is usually operating. It is often a strong one to protect from vulnerable feelings overwhelming their inner system, for example, their talker or fact finder, a tough one, or one that spaces out. This is the normal way humans shield themselves from being overwhelmed by emotion. Health care clinicians can learn to facilitate an alternative pathway in order to accomplish optimal care. We hope that Tactical

Competency 1 helps the clinician not to be blended with a protective part of his or her own. In the diagram "Relationship Triad," notice the "ideal" internal differences between the clinician and patient at the start of an encounter. The clinician is taking care of her protective parts, and the patient is blended with them and behaving from them.

However, the patient's presenting part may pose a difficulty for you to engage with. For example, the presenting personality part may pose as being tough when there is a very scared child underneath who will drive a change of mind after surgery has been booked and a consent form has been signed. Or a presenting part may say (through the patient's mouth) that he knows it all despite it being true that the person needs much more information to make an informed decision.

The above observation means that you need to make your first relationship with the patient's presenting personality part, usually a protector, while knowing that this part is linked to a much more vulnerable part underneath it. **This is an essential awareness for you to have**. This understanding provides a roadmap for you to bypass the initial misstep of aligning yourself fully with this one part of your patient. It does allow you, however, to engage with this part in a genuinely curious and interested way. Engaging with it does not strengthen it. On the contrary, this engagement dynamic between you and your patient is what allows the presenting part eventually to soften and permit the voices of other parts to come through. What we are saying is that the clinician's awareness of more than one part within the patient changes the way the clinician engages with the presenting part (for example, "a pleaser" who agrees with everything, but the behavior will show otherwise). While engaging with this part (listening, mirroring, and being empathic), the clinician is allowing space for other parts to enter and give voice to their different emotions and beliefs (for example, to parts that do **not** agree and want to know more). When this happens in the interview it fosters requests for information coming from more than the presenting part of the patient. This allows the information to be assimilated. Your job as clinician, after helping your own parts to soften back, is to relate to your patients from your nonjudgmental self-awareness, which has the qualities of curiosity, compassion, and calmness. This is your core self relating to your patient's personality parts, whatever they may be, from that place in you that feels safe and in tune with your patient (as seen in the diagram).

In the start of your interview, it is helpful to visualize or get a sense that someone within the patient is talking. What increases your awareness of whom it might be is your sensing it, as you mirror back the thoughts and emotions you are hearing. It is usually a protector part (parts that are super rational, or controlling, or pleasing, or pushing). Also, see if you can visualize a more vulnerable person within them (for example, someone carrying fear or confusion) who is being shielded by their protector. It is not necessary to teach them "parts." It is fine to say "a part of you," as this is common usage, or to say, "one feeling or thought you seem to have is—." But **stay relating to the protector, even if that part carries beliefs that are antithetical to your diagnostic or treatment agenda**. For example, a know-it-all protector is not going to follow your lead, but if you stay seriously interested and appreciative with what the knower knows and how it knows it, and/or how this has been important to the patient's life, a vulnerability will normally start to emerge. Don't shine a spotlight on the vulnerable emotions to go deeper. Just notice it by mirroring and noticing to yourself that there are now two parts in the room with you. As the vulnerable voice gets more frequent, you might comment to your patient that you are "hearing one part of you that—, and on the other hand another part of you that—." This is how you enhance the patient's awareness that they have two distinctly different parts operating. It works best not to start teaching about parts, because that activates cognitive understanding and shifts you and your patient away from the feelings that their brain needs to downregulate. You are normalizing emotions by relational attunement and finding words for them and the body sensations that accompany them.

TACTICAL COMPETENCY 8: TRACKING AND ENHANCING SIMULTANEOUS AWARENESS OF POLARIZED PERSONALITY PARTS

Now that you know how to be aware of several personality parts of your patient and to begin to track polarities and enhance their awareness of the same, you are ready to observe if any two or three personality parts are polarized, or opposites, in conflict, and to help your patient begin to notice the same. That is, there are sets of beliefs, emotions, and agendas that promote opposite behaviors. For example, one part may have the agenda to increase the quality of the person's life by good nutrition with some dieting. The other may be their eater and smoker; that is, have a strong agenda to give the person relief from emotional or physical pain through eating and smoking. This is a deeper understanding of what is called ambivalence. Both parts have the agenda within the person to reduce vulnerable emotions. But, this is unconscious. If these two opposing parts become activated at different times during the week, the behavior of your patient will make shifts—which correspond to each part. One will promote dieting and exercise; the other, the opposite. The behavior of one part, however, activates the behavior of the other. Although this can remain a subtle dynamic, sometime it escalates. Then we may observe a crash dieter opposed by a person who eats to soothe himself, and then probably an inner critic (a third part) that starts to scold on both accounts—all three parts. In this inner escalating conflict, the patient is being pulled first by one set of behaviors and then by the other, and feeling increasing badly about themselves as a result of their inner critic. This is stressful and dangerous for health. It is a kind of open warfare between polarized personality parts. More information, warnings, and appeals to rationality from clinicians have little lasting impact on the polarity situation. Traditional psychotherapies do not fare much better.

When your patient presents with a subtle dynamic of opposing parts, first help them get the sense that there are opposing parts involved in their swings of behavior and get curious. Once you and your patient are in a more conscious relationship with both parts, you can ask your patient to feel and notice **both at the same time and to observe what happens in their feeling and thinking**. Appreciating that both parts are trying to be helpful is important. Doing that takes them to a new place and increases their ability to hold the opposite personality parts or a cycle of parts in their conscious awareness. This reduces the behavioral shifting and de-energizes the conflict. This is what we understand **internal integration** to be. With many patients, three or four 20-minute visits can provide an opening for behavior change and decisions to get made. Health coaching can be ongoing as part of primary care, and it lowers the risk of unexpected action behaviors. Goals beyond that are for psychotherapy.

When polarized behaviors pose serious current risk, as they would with a diabetic person, it is best to stabilize by identifying that there is a cycle of parts within and making a referral to a psychotherapist with training that includes the Internal Family Systems Model. Making a referral is the topic of Chapter 11. You will observe and hear interviews with polarized personalized parts in the video demonstrations in Chapter 9.

TACTICAL COMPETENCY 9: INTERWEAVING INFORMATION WHEN PATIENTS ARE READY AND SHAPING INFORMATION TO FIT INTERVIEW PROCESS

Interweave is a process which includes emotions, not just the provision of facts. It is best to have identified a couple of personality parts which are salient in your patient before you think of supplying more information, unless it is specifically requested. Even then, it is best to know to whom (to which Part) in the patient's system you are supplying the information and best to ask for feedback—"How does this sound to you? What comes up for you when I say that?" You may think communication has occurred, but it may not have. Once both you and your patient know about the existence without judgment of different sets of emotions, beliefs and agendas within them (the patient) that explain their behaviors, their system is more open. Readiness is present when the patient's emotions are in better regulation and the patient is not totally blended with a Part. This is your platform for interweaving evidence-based information. It is best to sense and to wonder out loud what information that they may have already heard needs repeating and what new information needs to be supplied. Be aware to which personality parts the information is most relevant and "speak" to those. You will notice near the end of the demonstration with Joe how the clinician repeats—seamlessly and in-step with the conversation—the three main items to be tracked in diabetes (A1c, **B**lood pressure, and **C**holesterol—the ABCs). This is a good example of Information Interweave™. Our preference is to provide patients with a PDA booklet and/or DVD only after an emotion-processing relationship has been established (usually two visits) and then to go over it together in a third visit and to check what they believe other clinicians have told them. As you listen to your patient talk about their understanding of their disease and options of treatment, you will get an idea of the level and type of language they use. You can then shape the information in the same language. Remember that you will want to ask for feedback about their inner responses of emotions and beliefs to information you provide.

You are not only conveying facts; you're their partner in helping them process and know their internal system so that the facts can be assimilated beyond just hearing them. In decision work, remember, you want to allow for intuitions and rules of thumb (Chapter 4) to be included but not to take over. Also, assist your patient to process, emotionally and cognitively, any conflicting external medical information.

Also keep in mind that opposite personality parts exit between clinicians and patients, not only within each of them. They can push off against each other and get reflected in behaviors. For example, commonly a teaching-professor-knows-best part within you may trigger a rebellious part in your patient. The more extreme your patient's rebellious part gets, the more activated your teacher will become. The attuned relation then is lost. If you do your inside self-care, your dynamic always softens and can be talked about frankly even in "parts" language and an apology made from your side.

TACTICAL COMPETENCY 10: ASKING PERIODICALLY FOR FEEDBACK ABOUT UNDERSTANDING WHAT'S BEING SAID, AND ALSO CHECKING ON INFLUENCES OF FAMILY AND OTHER CLINICIANS

Asking your patients what is now coming up for them at multiple points during your interview is how you help yourself and them to stay in-tune with *their* process and what needs to happen next. Their feedback will be driven probably by one or another of their personality parts you already know, but something different might pop up. Based on what you hear from the feedback, you can supply more information or reemphasize the existence of a polarity, or you can wonder if something else is interfering with their assimilation.

It is always best to ask if anything going on outside of them in relationships with family members or other clinicians needs to be shared. Your patient's side of the dynamics going on with a family member or other clinician over a decision or behavior change can be identified. This awareness and appreciation between patient and clinicians is helpful without trying to do anything specific about it. It is helpful to just know that loved ones and clinicians also have their parts. Sometimes a spouse can be included constructively in a second or third session, yet the patient needs room to take the lead on that decision, and you need to know that you have the skills to work with a pair of people.

VIDEO: We suggest that you now watch the entire set of full video demonstrations. *On the first viewing* the goal is for you to get a general idea, without focusing on note-taking or trying to follow all the annotations in Chapter 9. This first viewing is mostly a right-brain exercise. Although each interview is chosen to highlight a particular clinical task, such as information interweave or behavior change or decision making, *all the videos illustrate the strategies and tactical competencies presented in Chapters 7 and 8.* The clinician is always shaping the strategies and tactics to accomplish a set of clinical tasks. You could review Chapter 2, where many of the suggestions are located about using the videos.

PART 4

Acquiring Interviewing Skills

9

Three interviewing demonstrations, links, and annotations

BEHAVIOR CHANGE (SMOKING): MY FRIEND

Introduction

This is a 67-year-old woman who has been smoking cigarettes since age 10, whose mother died from COPD and who has been told the risk factors by her doctor. She has tried to use nicotine patches, gums, and oral medication. Her primary care physician has referred her to the nurse health coach in the practice to help her stop smoking. At the very beginning of the book you were asked to review only the patient's opening statements and then speculate on your choices of response, strategy, and why. Now that you have read about the updated model, here are the options this clinician chose. Time designations are located on the left side of the page and should correspond to the audio and video track you access via the link.

The text that follows contains an annotated processing of the entire interview that draws your attention to strategy and tactics heard and seen in the video (from a triple perspective—inside the patient, inside the clinician, and the dynamics between them).

This video may be accessed at http://goo.gl/sggT9Q

Annotation

This clinician has gone through Tactical Competency 1, Step II, from Chapter 8, on previous occasions after interviewing patients with the same condition. In this interview demonstration you are observing an experienced clinician who does not use Step I vigorously since it is almost organic for her to help her parts to remain in the background of her mind so she can pay attention, be quiet, and wait, as needed (Tactical Competency 2, TC2 below). If *you* were the clinician in this case, you would use Tactic 1, Step I, to take care of the personality parts that become activated within you so they do not take the lead in your interview, including being with a person who needs to stop smoking, being video recorded, and doing a good job. The timeline is on the left side of the page in seconds. The numbers used throughout the interview (TC1–TC10) refer to the key and corresponding descriptions of tactical competencies explained in Chapter 8.

Key: Tactical competencies used in the interview

TC1: Using Step I of clinician emotional self-care
TC2: Paying attention, being quiet, and waiting
TC3: Mirroring and validating
TC4: Helping patient to locate and/or identify and become aware of bodily sensations
TC5: Helping patient find words for emotions, distinguishing between emotions, thoughts, and body sensations
TC6: Extending empathy—both components
TC7: Noticing, exploring, and enhancing awareness of the set of emotions, thoughts, body sensations carried by each personality part, especially the presenting part
TC8: Enhancing awareness of each personality part that is involved in a polarization (a pair of opposites), and prompting the patient to tolerate having both in awareness simultaneously
TC9: Interweaving information when patient is ready and shaping it to fit the interview process
TC10: Asking periodically for feedback (emotions, thoughts) from patients of what they heard and its impact; also, checking on influences coming from family and other clinicians

C = clinician, M = patient (Mary Lou)

This experienced clinician is able to start with TC2. You would start with TC1, Step I, Self-care.

The interview

0:00–2:54
Note: This is an introduction by Dr. Livingstone about behavior change. The interview starts at time mark 2:55.

2.55
C: **You've indicated to Dr. Eldridge that you'd like to stop smoking.**
M: Nods in agreement.
C: Mirrors the nod and says, **Ya-a.** This is the subtle but intentional start of the attunement (TC3).
C: States that she understands that M hasn't been able to stop—**Is that correct?** (TC3, TC10)
M: **That's correct; it's very difficult.**

3:43

C: Shares that she noticed a bodily reaction (TC3 and TC4).

M: **I want to and sometimes I don't want to really stop; it's part of me, my friend.** Sounds like M has an "intelligent knower" who knows about her ambivalence (TC2). M is conscious of the contradiction within her and is willing to name it in this initial contact focused on quitting.

C: Draws attention to body behaviors attached to wanting to and not able to and goes on to name a conflict. **A little bit of a conflict inside of you—a part of you that does want to stop and another part inside of you that feels that smoking is your friend** (TC7, and beginning of TC8) C mirrors the part that does not want to stop smoking *with acceptance and nonjudgment.*

M: **Absolutely.** The knower part in M is agreeing.

04:22

C: **So what happens with this conflict inside of you?** (TC8) This gentle enhancement of M's awareness that there is a conflict (polarity of parts), naming both sides of it more clearly, and asking what it is like to have two parts in conflict are crucial tactics for beginning what becomes a central feature of the behavior change process. M may sound like she is already aware of what she needs to do, but that is her awareness held by her cognitive/logical part, **not** the emotional part that is activated by her process of moving forward toward a commitment to change her smoking behaviors— an important distinction for clinicians to make.

M: **When happens is—I stop—couple of days—I feel almost a wreck— cause I live alone and it's become my companion—phone would ring and I'd have a cigarette—after dinner, my life is different** [without it]. **The other thing is it's like a reward after working hard—What do I reward myself with now?** (TC8)

C: Notice that as M explains, C is making continuing sounds—**uhuh**—of acknowledgment that M is being heard. There is connected flow—**right**—(TC3).

05:11

C: Acknowledges the importance of the emotional side. **This is really important, because the medical protocol has been focusing on nicotine, but what you're talking about are the rituals and the comforting of the habit itself and without it you feel like you're losing something.** (TC5 and TC6)

M: Nodding head and agreeing—so C continues—(TC3)

05:41 (names focus of the work)

C: **That is important to recognize because that also has to be taken on quite seriously** (TC6) **with a focus, because you can begin to identify, as you have, that you have triggers that make you**

want a cigarette, that you reward yourself with it, and that it is a friend to you. (TC7) This is a naming of the areas for deeper exploration toward the emotions and meanings that C will need to focus on to help M shift *within herself, on her own terms,* if change is going to occur. **Because you live alone—those are three very important factors that need to find substitutes for: rewards—something gets triggered—and having a comfort for yourself.** (TC3 and TC6)

06:09–10

C: (TC2)

(Notice M's sigh as she is nodding her head after the three factors are named—she is able to feel more of whatever this is for her on the inside. The tone is expressing M's connection (not a flood) to these feelings— the essential first step to making a shift.)

M: **But I don't want to eat a lot more—that concerns me.** Now we know more. Living alone contains a lot of underlying emotion and meanings for M, but C is not going toward eliciting more emotion— even though it has been mentioned several times. This is not the place to go deeply into the emotional meanings of that (TC6). *C is balancing stabilization with exploration* in this first interview. If C went too deep with living alone, it might swing M back into smoking even more after she leaves the visit and that would increase her sense of failure.

C: **Right, right—so you want to be careful about what you substitute** (TC3 and TC6). Notice that C acknowledges the eating concern yet does not go deeper into an inquiry at this point about her eating concerns—staying broad regarding awareness of the triggers and behavior around them, so that they *both have an overview first of all the parts activated by smoking cessation.*

C: **Most people** (normalizing it) **are helped with a support group—and something physical that you can look at—an app on your phone—find doing it alone does not work for people. Hotline here, a counseling program—I as a nurse can work with you as a health coach. We are talking about what smoking does for you on the inside, right?** (TC9 and TC6) **I'd like to support you—we can go over how things are working and what isn't working.** C means support for the specific concerns of the parts named, involving living alone, internal triggers, and rituals—all without activating more emotions about it (TC6). This creates space for *all of these parts to be included in their work together* in discovering what does and what does not work.

07:30

M: **That would be good—one of the problems that smoking causes is I have to get away from people who don't want me to smoke— they don't want my grandkids to be around me cause I smell** like smoke—that's more of my reason—my top priority—My health, I'll be fine, but Mother died of COPD—I worry about that. (C: TC2) M is deepening the results of TC5, TC6, and TC7 and beginning to identify (TC8) the values of her polarized parts. Her top priority is seeing her grandkids, but smoking is limited her contact with them. Then there is her health—part of her believes she'll be fine, and another part carries worry about COPD from which her mother died. Each of these will need to be simultaneously embraced and tolerated via the relationship with the clinician. C allows M to shift to the *isolation as being her problem with smoking*. Here is where her pain is. C would *not* have gotten here earlier by telling M about the downsides of COPD or asking M about the downsides of her smoking. Many smokers "worry" about COPD, but deny it because it is the future. Isolation she lives with *daily* and a meaningful sharing of that, that is with some emotion and not just her intellect, was best initiated by M as she became ready.

08:13

C: (TC2)

C: **So, you have an intellectual understanding and gone through an experience with your mother. Am just wondering—as you just mentioned that you took a big—(sigh).** M acknowledges with nodding, C with nodding and yea. M and C are in reciprocal attunement. (C: TC1, is taking care of any emotions about loss of her own mother.) (TC4, TC5 and TC7)

08:32

C: Naming and welcoming, but not going deeper into loss of her mother is an essential tactic (TC1, TC6, TC7, TC8). **I think what you're talking about is the difference between the knowing part of the brain and the feeling part of your brain** (TC9) (acknowledging the presenting part and prompting information interweave). **And as you spend time with this, you maybe realized that although it is your friend, yet it also is isolating you and pulling you away from your family and kids—important for you—negative things.** (TC3, TC8 about polarities) C is including all the feelings that are activated in M as they explore smoking cessation—the focus of their meeting.

M: **New York—used to be—now it is like you're pariah.**

C: (TC2)

C: **Positive things it brings to your life and also negative things it brings to your life. It's complicated.** (TC3, TC6) **Because of that, it's important that you have supports for every step, gradual steps** (TC9).

M: **I would think it would be helpful to have someone who is not personally involved who supported me—not nagging—not helpful.** This response happens organically from an interview in which the patient's parts feel heard and seen. M is initiating a return to a "need for information" that C planted earlier (TC9). Before exploring, however, the support needed by using information, C wants to hear what M's previous experiences have been with support from others (TC7, TC9).

C: **Did you have that experience of someone personally involved and nagging you?** Deepening/exploring both parts of the polarities simultaneously (TC7).

M: **Uh—I did—a girlfriend—they think it's that easy—it's not like I don't want to see them. I'm struggling with it.**

C: (TC2, TC7)

10:47

C: **So, if I'm hearing you correctly, there is something about the nagging and the, "just do it," that makes you feel people don't understand your struggle?** (TC3, TC7)

M: **—would like someone who is not personally involved—**

C: **Not common that people can just do it [stop]. Noticing how aware you are and your reaction—that's a gift and being aware— that could make it harder.** (TC7, TC3, TC6)

M: **That could make it harder for me?**

C: **That makes it harder because you would be feeling everything.** (TC8) Her feelings are not coming from the part that "knows" what she should do.

12:19

C: Starts raising the issue of physiological supports—patches etc. (TC9)

M: **Meds—terrible nightmares.**

C: **Patch or gum or lozenges plus support which we can talk about— combination physician and emotional.** (TC9)

13:32–38

C: **Just wondering how you are feeling about this issue right now?** (TC10) C wants to be sure she is staying in tune with all the parts of M's personality and not getting ahead of her process of change. So, C invites and checks M's thinking and feelings at this point in the exploration of the parts that are activated by cessation.

13:38–39 (Watch M's face and affect.) (TC2)

14:19

M: **Still the idea of never having another cigarette in all my life; I've never stopped—pregnancy—when I stop for a few days I feel like I'm grieving—like somebody died—gotta find something else.**

C: (TC2)

C: **What do you do when you start feeling the grief? What happens?** (TC6, TC8) Notice that C does not go deeper to pull for more feeling; but, she does ask M what she does in reaction to the grieving, to embrace awareness of the behaviors that she engages in to substitute for her feelings.

M: **I get depressed and try to get busy so I don't think. I think exercising more, doing something with my hands—the actions, the lighter—crazy as it is!** M has action as remedies; C gives recognition of the doing rituals in group programs and also suggests that she can learn to be with her emotions and learn to regulate them. (TC6, TC4)

15:50

C: **First is the grief—then depression—then you get busy and then you want the reward. The busy and reward are one set of things, but the grieving and depression are something else.** (TC7 and TC8) **I'm wondering if you've ever considered getting some counseling to help you process those feelings?** (TC9)

M: **Not really** (See, mouth, and body behavior of doubt)

C: **Does that sound OK to you?** (TC10)

16:20

M: **Is that something you really recommend?**

C: (TC2), (trainee TC1)

C: Identifies and supports M's competency in naming *two big factors for her*—and then explains *an alternative pathway for her*, such as getting curious to know them more (TC4, TC8). **Not talking about changing them or doing anything big; but getting curious, gently getting to know more about them a little bit** (M closes her eyes) **so you don't have to jump from it by getting busy and then going for the reward.** (TC3, TC7) C can see M's discomfort, so she is offering right-brain attunement with her tone, eye contact, and facial expressions as she offers left-brain information about the goal and process of counseling. M has already identified a repetitive pattern that happens in response to her feelings and that grief leaves her feeling depressed. **Going for a reward is something that you can work on in support programs. But the first piece** (meaning the grieving and depression) **sounds like something you're aware of but haven't really processed it.** (TC6, TC8)

M: Nods head in agreement.

C: Nods head in acknowledgment (TC3).

C: **My suggestion is to try it and see how it feels to you.** By "it," C is including counseling.

17:15

M: **Start with getting into a support group?** So for M, the "it" that is most comfortable for her at this point is *support group*. It is clear another visit with C and a process with her is indicated before a referral for counseling would hold up. C goes with the part that is available.

C: Explains a *process*: She will write up her notes and share them with her and says again that she realizes that the idea of giving smoking up forever is a setup for failure. Suggests she takes note on what comes up for her as she reviews the notes from the session.

C: Acknowledging again, the loss side of the conflict. **For most people, the idea of giving up smoking forever—etc.—too big—one day at a time, just today! Makes us feel like we are failing if expectations—right?** (TC3, TC6 TC7, TC8)

17:43

M: **You're right—that thought is overwhelming to me—crazy as it is.** This response indicates resonance with C.

C: (TC8, TC9) **No, it is not, this is the way this kind of process works for people—more normal for the process than not.** Normalizing the process of M being with the parts of her process and not letting an inner critic part (saying "crazy as it is") take foreground at this point of the interview.

C and M: Mutual nodding. (Notice the mirroring of nodding that persists all during the interview. This supports the connection) (TC3).

18:10

C: (TC2) (trainee: TC1)

C: **But we are going to have to come to the end of our meeting today.** Sums up the polarities.

(TC8 and TC5) **What I heard, if it's OK if I say it back again?** (M nods yes.) **This is a very complicated and difficult struggle** (TC3, using M's word). **Parts of you that want to give up smoking and parts of you that don't want to because it's your friend** (still using M's words) **and it's something you get a reward from and it's soothing and it pulls you away from people—isolates you in ways that does not feel comfortable. And, you did not respond well to the medication so that's off the books—and you are willing to look at some support for the nicotine addiction which we can talk about—patch etc., and getting into a support group for other people to talk to—ideas about the rituals—and some mental health counseling to actually befriend instead of distraction from the feelings of grief and what feels like depression.** (TC8 and TC5) C is offering some regulation of affect in how she summarizes this meeting to M and includes all the parts that need to be identified before she will be able to change her smoking behavior.

C: **Not saying you are depressed—something you could evaluate.** (TC9) C is not pushing M into accepting something that her body behavior and the interview sequence told C was hard for her to assimilate. **Right?** (TC8, TC5, TC10)

M and C: Mutual nodding and vocal agreeing (TC3).

C: **So—those are three things** (TC10) **to get started with—and then approach for yourself of thinking what's manageable— one day at a time—and work in a reward for yourself each day—manageable?**

M: **Yes—not eating.**

C: **That's what the mental health counseling helps with and also the coaching. You and I—we can meet weekly for the next several weeks.** (TC9)

20:42

M: **Thinking—my reward would be my grandchildren**

C: **Aaawww** (empathic vocal response from C) (TC6) **Yaaa—such an internal insidious process you're trying to change—it helps to have external reminders—cup of tea—pictures of grandchildren? Picture—look at them and take it in—to remind yourself.** (TC9)
(Note: Many of these items are given to patients but not in the context of the attunement exemplified by this relationship that welcomes all the polarized opposites that are identified.)

M: **A trigger for me to stop.**

C: (TC2)

21:32

C: **Wondering if you have any questions or comments.** This maintains attunement, especially with the presenting part, her intelligent knower. (TC6 and TC10)

M: **My mother died from COPD; and the doctor said I have the beginnings of it—will it improve if I stop?** Notice that her protective presenting part allowed more vulnerability to enter at the **end** of the session. M is ready for an information interweave (TC9). C, at this time, does not go into probable fear of dying or into loss of mother, in an attempt to motivate M out of fear. However, C notes them in her mind. These emotions will emerge organically in subsequent visits—perhaps with a therapist or with C if health coaching is M's choice.

C: (TC2; trainee TC1) **Absolutely—will be an improvement and no worsening—something to track with your doctor—documentation and tracking—improvement and no worsening.** (TC9)

22:37

M: **Well, good** (to e-mail her notes).

C: Talk regarding ending the session and an appointment and notes will get sent.

M: **Will notes go to the doctor?**

C: **No** (explains that the notes are for her), **you had so many different parts that came up today**—to see what comes up as she reviews the notes. C is confirming that this is M's internal process and that she is in charge of it. C is still deepening the work with *polarizations* (TC8) and the two of them for meeting next week to process between them. **COPD could be tracked** with your doctor (TC9). **Does that make sense?** (TC10)

M: **I don't think he gets how difficult it is.**

24:14

C: **So he's one of those who doesn't get how hard it is.** (TC3) **I'm here because there is a part of him who knows how difficult it is— and you're picking up on the way he approaches it.** (TC6)

24:26

C: **You know, the most important thing is that you respect how difficult it is.** (TC9) **And that's another thing we'll be working on. Yaaa.** (TC3)

The plan is to meet next week and process the notes and go further—working the polarities and helping M be *with* her feelings as they come up—*increasing her tolerance of* "getting depressed," whatever that is for her, rather than distract herself and getting caught up in the perpetual cycle. Perhaps the counseling referral won't take place and C will work with her in a series of 20-minute health-coaching visits. This remains to be discovered.

Possible takeaway

Behavior change often involves a sense of loss. This is a verbal patient who has not yet integrated the cognitions and the emotions into a cohesive story of opposing parts within her. The patient is caught in a cycle of feelings and behaviors that perpetuate her smoking. Mutual nodding, vocalized noises, and using the patient's own words are crucial to initiating and maintaining relational attunement. This relationship "holds" the space for the patient to *be with* (not blend with) more emotion-laden thoughts in a safe way as they emerge during the course of the interview—to the very end. The clinician starts relating to the patient's presenting personality, which opens the door to her emotional awareness of the many sides to her inner story (the polarized personality parts) and of how complex it is. Behavior change is a process that involves new ways of coping with emotions, competing needs, and healing old wounds. Most important, it is finding pathways of *how* to work at it with other people who understand the complexity. The task of quitting is learning to tolerate through a clinical relationship (of health coaching) what actually is being experienced emotionally as the various parts of the person get activated. This is what a relationship is needed for—to acknowledge the patient's experience of the complexity and to help regulate, in new ways, the emotions that arise. Referring someone to mental health counseling is a gradual process of pacing.

You may have noticed many features of interest to you that we have not mentioned. We encourage you to explore these within the context of multiplicity, your own experiences, and your own style of learning.

INFORMATION INTERWEAVE™ (DIABETES) (TC9): THE BULLET I WAS ALWAYS AFRAID OF

Introduction

This is a 55-year-old man who has recently been diagnosed with type II diabetes and whose mother died at age 56 of complications of diabetes. His primary care physician has referred him for health coaching to help alter his lifestyle not only because of the new diagnosis but also because this man suffers from several other chronic conditions (osteoarthritis of hip and knees and cardiovascular disease). He has not been making use of evidence-based information the physician repeatedly has given to him. In the Introduction of this book you were asked to review videos of only the patient's opening statements and then to speculate on your choices of response and strategy. Now that you have read about the updated model, here are the options that this clinician chose during her interview with him. Time designations are located on the left side of the page and should correspond to the audio and video track you access via the link.

The text below contains an annotated processing of the entire interview (from a triple perspective—inside the patient, inside the clinician, and the dynamics between them) that draws your attention to strategy and tactics heard and seen in the video.

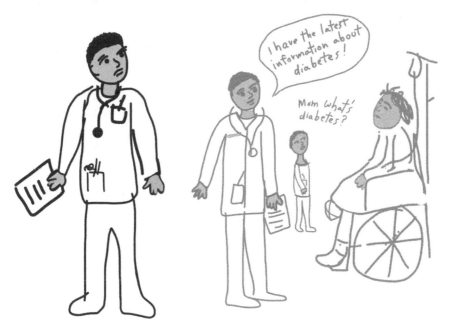

MEMORIES ACTIVATE CLINCIANS

This video may be accessed at http://goo.gl/idFlS9

Annotation

This clinician has gone through TC1, Step II, from Chapter 8, on previous occasions after interviewing patients with the same condition. In this interview demonstration you are observing an experienced clinician who does not use Step I vigorously since it is almost organic for her to help her parts to remain in the background of her mind so she can pay attention, be quiet, and wait, as needed (TC2). If *you* were the clinician in this case, you would use TC1, Step I, to take care of your personality parts that become activated so they do not take the lead during your interview, including feelings about diabetes, being video recorded, and doing a good job. The timeline is on the left side of the page in seconds. The numbers (TC1–TC10) used throughout the interview refer to the Key and corresponding descriptions of tactical competencies in Chapter 8.

Key: Tactical competencies used in the interview

TC1:   Using Step I of clinician emotional self-care
TC2:   Paying attention, being quiet, and waiting
TC3:   Mirroring and validating
TC4:   Helping patient to locate and/or identify and become aware of bodily sensations
TC5:   Helping patient find words for emotions, distinguishing between emotions, thoughts, and body sensations
TC6:   Extending empathy—both components
TC7:   Noticing, exploring, and enhancing awareness of the set of emotions, thoughts, body sensations carried by each personality part, especially the presenting part
TC8:   Enhancing awareness of each personality part that is involved in a polarization (a pair of opposites) and prompting the patient to tolerate having both in awareness simultaneously
TC9:   Interweaving information when patient is ready and shaping it to fit the interview process
TC10: Asking periodically for feedback (emotions, thoughts) from patients of what they heard and its impact; also, checking on influences coming from family and other clinicians

C = clinician, J = patient (Joe)

This experienced clinician is able to start in TC2. You would start with TC1. See line drawing page 171 about inner reactions of clinicians to diabetes.

The interview

0:00–3:10
Note: This is an introduction by Dr. Livingstone about communication and information transfer. The interview starts at time mark 3:11.

3.11 (Affective connection and reason for the meeting; notice how somber he seems at first.)
C: Comments that she understands that he has been given a lot of information—**I'm wondering how that is sitting with you—you're thinking about it and feeling about it?** She gives him an option between *thinking and feeling,* giving an opening to whatever presenting part is activated within him (TC5).

J: **I'm upset that I have it—going to require for me a very difficult life change, eating, social habits, as far as drinking—it's going to be a major transformation.** Not with emotion. He talks about it—*analyzing and thinking* is his presentation. The information he has heard is not integrated with his emotions.

C: **Uhuh, uhuh—so you have been thinking about the hugeness of this.** (TC3, TC7) Beginning exploration of presenting part: a mirroring back his presenting parts, words as "thinking," not "feelings." Notice, she does not draw attention to "upset." She is waiting for a more solid platform to develop with him, letting him make the choice of how he is thinking.

4:18

J: **Of course, have family history; my mother got it in her 40s and it was so severe—long time ago—they didn't have what they have today—essentially that's what killed her, died at 56—the bullet I was always afraid of—ya know, ya know.**

C: (TC2)

C: **OOH—wow.** She responds to the emotions beginning to come through—the fear. Notice how soft and connected her empathy is, but she does not pull for more. **I'm hearing you have a family history of a real tragedy—very young—the death of your mother and that you also are aware that there have been improvements in the ability to control—not only medications but changes you can make in your own life.** (TC3, TC6, TC9) C wants to find out what he already knows about reducing the risk factors of his diagnosis. **—am wondering what it's like holding together the experience you had with your mother and your awareness that there are many more things available for your health today?** (This creates space for TC7, TC8, TC9). Notice she does not go deeper into feelings about his mother's death as he is already using a major protector (a "program" for himself is the solution) to shield himself from too much feeling (scared? helpless? memories of his mother?) and C is also beginning to use the word "and" to name possible polarities between personality parts. It is subtle but a very purposeful choice by the clinician. (TC8)

J: **I guess I need a program, I've read up—exercise and things like that—need someone to put the program together for me—once I have it, eventually I have to get the discipline.** He identifies his presenting parts' approaches: "Thinking/knowing about a program" and probably a separate part that conducts the "trying." The clinician knows she needs to relate to his thoughtful and trying parts that are dominant at this point.

C: **This is great that your thinking about it in this way.** (She's in tune with his presenting parts' approach and acknowledging it with the intention of extending it, TC7.) **That's my role, is to help you get a program**

together—one that really fits you. (TC7) She already senses that putting together a program for him will probably not work. This feels like a compliant part that could easily lead a clinician into giving information that won't be integrated by parts that carry his emotions. She senses this because his body language is solid and nonmoving as he talks about what he needs to *do*, and his language is about outcome, not process. She uses his words and shifts them slightly to make it more personal—"to help you," "that fits you"—and opens room for more parts to emerge (TC3, TC6, TC7). **It is very complicated; can't do this on your own—and you have to do one step at a time—not take on all the different factors at once** (exactly what his thinking part has already done). **You're aware that exercise is one of them, right? Dietary might be another, and medication. Those are good places to start.** (He nods.) **How does that feel to you?** (TC5, TC8)

J: **Very difficult, major transformation.** (TC7)

    (Three items of information he already knows and asking him to focus on these three and hold them together in her presence, to tolerate awareness of all three and see what comes up (preparation for TC9).

J: **Am going to have to start** (his "trying" part comes up) **following them— my mother died—not only that but strokes—and I want at least to have a life.** Here is a vulnerable part emerging and talking with a tone of feeling and concern—"at least." C will want to acknowledge this part (TC7) and also his compliant part that tries to protect him from feelings by getting him to follow a program.

07:14

C: **Yah and yah—a quality of life, yah—yah.** (TC6, TC7) Acknowledging the emergence of a vulnerable part by her tone and body language, she begins TC9, an information interweave by linking the information to his stated concern about strokes and wanting at least to have a life and his wish to do it with a "program" (TC9). She mentions two programs and adds the relationship piece he identified that he needs to support beginning a program.

C: **So you know from personal experience that diabetes starts to pose hazards to the circulatory system, your kidneys—. Those are the things the doctor wants to keep a check on and this includes checking on cholesterol, blood sugar, blood pressure.** (TC9, interweave) **He can help with those guidelines; and I can help you put together a program that enables you to make some healthy life choices to support your health.** (Both are being imaged as *programs* with the help of two clinicians. The clinician is *interweaving* the information regarding monitoring of blood pressure, cholesterol, etc. with both his presenting part's desire for a "program" and another part's desire to have a "quality of life." She deliberately uses the words "healthy life choices."

08:00

J: **Uhuh—That is something I would definitely be interested in.** This response indicates resonance with the clinician. He is interested in this because she has linked it to several of his personal concerns for a quality of life—"at least." It is in this context then that evidenced-based information, some he has already heard and read, will be assimilated and used to promote behavior change (TC9).

08:05

C: **That's great—so, you've done some reading.** (TC7) **So have you tried to initiate any of these?** Now she is helping him explore for parts that are in **opposition** to the part that wants to improve his health (TC8).

J: **I've been eliminating alcohol—, but I try to watch myself—my food intake—watching my carbs—eating less! You know.**

C: **Uhuh, uhuh. So, you're looking at what causes a spike in your blood sugar** (TC9, interweave) **and not giving you nutrients—help you have energy** (TC9 interweave) **and function at the level you want to function at** (have a life)—**right? We have a dietitian who—can look at food and their glycemic—but I think you could start by thinking about the way you eat right now—with what you like and start there! And see how we can add healthier things so that you're not just giving things up. I heard that you gave up alcohol—was that hard to do?** Loss is always part of behavior change and it can block information transfer unless processed. C is helping him become more aware of the feeling parts associated with changing his diet (TC8). If he can be in relationship to these parts, they are less likely to sabotage his program of change.

J: **Not as difficult as I thought—cause—.** (TC6) He's beginning to smile just a little about trade-offs between drinking and food, and the clinician is mirroring this and being with him. She has started with focusing on what he likes and also his experience was with his feelings when giving up alcohol (TC3, TC7). **I'd rather have the food!**

C: **Wow that's great; did you know that you were this focused on it?** She giving him lots of credit for thinking about and remaining "focused" on his program (TC7).

J: **No—It's not going to happen overnight—until "I can control it—until I can fully come around."**
Note a heavy sigh, an expression of a feeling in addition to the part that is being expressed verbally. C notices it. (TC6, TC8)

C: **So what does "fully coming around" mean to you?** (TC7—exploring traits of his parts) **What's your vision of that for yourself?**

J: **A good exercise regimen—I do no exercise now at all! And my food intake.**

C: **So—when you say exercise—you know that exercise is part of a healthy life choice—but you say you do none at all.** Note C's tone and body language. (TC3, TC6)

J: **That's right.** He agrees with her feedback (TC10).

10:50

C: **So if you just allow yourself to be with what you just said, I'm wonder-ing what you notice about that?** (TC8) C, having heard the sigh, is opening the space for his feelings about a health program to enter more consciously. C did not challenge his compliant part. His compliant protector needs to feel safe enough in this relation-ship with her to soften. She is extending curiosity (TC3, TC6, TC8) to enhance his awareness: A pair of opposites is emerging: *know-ing about healthy life style*, and the parts involved in his *doing no exercise*—parts ill-defined to him and her. She will want him to hold both in consciousness, simultaneously expecting that he will become more aware.

J: **My energy level isn't what it should be** (mood looks down); **everyone tells you—When I do something physical, I feel it the next day.**

C: **You feel it?** (TC3)

J: **I'm sore.**

C: **Oh, Oh.** (TC6)

J: **Not using my muscles the way I should.**

11:29

C: **So then, how do you react to the soreness?** Again, opening space for all the parts that are activated by behavior change (TC7).

J: **I do nothing until the soreness goes away.** The first humor comes through about his behavior and in a trusting fashion with C.

C: **And then you are back at the start again?** (TC8) C is safely enhancing his awareness of the barriers to his "fully coming around." **That's one of the things I'd like to work on with you—to just be able to have an experience of learning how to exercise in a way that enables you to—start feeling—better—afterward. So—are there exercises you enjoy doing?**

J: **Stationary bike—no pounding on my joints—can do it for a long time—but the credit card goes to the gym.** Notice the increasing personal affective interchange. It is a sign of a shift and his increased sense of safety and trust in the rela-tionship is enabling him to identify and explore more vulnerable feelings.

12:32

C: **Did you know the majority sign up** (normalizing his behavior and under-cutting any shame); **so there is a part of you that has the desire 'cause you put the money down, but then what happens?** (TC8)

J: **So easy—wake up—"I don't feel like going today."** (Another part with feelings comes in.) **Have a neighbor who has a workout partner.**

C: **Super idea; also there are personal trainers, every other day, not over-doing it—an amount of bike without getting yourself stressed and sore.** C became aware that the exercising part of him does not feel what is inside his body. Overdoing it contributes to his not doing it again.—**exercise partner**—(TC8, TC9)

J: **Exercise partner. 45 min or half hour.**

C: **So what about half an hour and every other day? And not overdoing it. We can check at our appointment next week. Expectations— experiment with it?** (TC9) C is making room for the balance of these opposites, even though they are not fully known by J yet. (TC8, TC9)

J: **Easy enough start.** Evidence of resonance—he is willing to start, has softened from his focus on outcome.

C: **Anything at home that would get in your way of getting to gym.** Welcoming other parts that might be polarized (TC8, TC10) and checking environmental influences.

J: **No.**

C: **What about the food piece? What comes in the way of that?** (TC8)

J: **Quantity—pasta; have to cut back; yeah!** He is telling her what "**you gotta do**," scales etc.

C: **So wait a second—I'm also hearing a "yeah"; what is that voice about—the "yeah"?** (TC5 and TC8)

16:40

C has waited until she has more of a relationship with J's parts that have less emotional valence than the food part before she focuses on it. We do not know what eating has served historically in his life—but emotions around it usually drive the behavior. This is going to be important and not solved by a program.

J: **When you love food** (C mirrors, TC3) **best part is going back up there. Dieting is hard; the best part is when I work my way back up again.**

16:53

C: **So there is a part of you that goes through the deprivation of giving up the lots** (of food) **and going with these little amounts, but then there is your going back there again; that's going to be fun. That's the yo-yo that everyone talks about.** Notice the lack of shaming and judgment. C is relating to the two opposing parts with acceptance and openness (TC6, TC8).

J: **That's right! That can also cause problems with sugar.** Interesting: *He is now interweaving* with these opposing parts information that he already knows.

C: **I'm wondering if you could be with the part of you that loves eating and the part of you that knows it can cause problems—not to have one negate the other—to hold them both—they are both true—right?** (TC8)

J: **Uhuh** (resonance).

17:37

C: **So what comes up for you—what are you thinking about as you say that?** (TC8) C relates to his presenting part first, his thinking part, she does *not* ask him how he feels about it.

J: **I don't know—I have to pick a starting point** (his thinking part) **like diet—dealing with my mind I never thought in terms of diabetes. Right now, I'm in the acceptance stage of this.** (He's relating to the reading he has done in a personal way now—another interweave of his own.)**—the dieting—about pounds—now gotta play games with your mind—coming up with a program.** His protector (TC7), but with a slight shift in that he is owning his need to come up with a program of his own—rather than being given one—the way he stated the interview.

18:46

C: (C follows J's lead and continues with the process of change.) **So, you're in a phase with this diagnosis which affects your life and you know what a big impact it has when untreated—to be in a phase of just accepting it! Acceptance** (TC3, TC5, TC6, TC7)—**what does that feel like—with your just accepting it right now?** (TC8)

J: **Maybe with a program of exercise and dieting, I could back-off on the drugs—can control it without the drugs.** Here, he is just beginning to express what would motivate him, and his mood looks down.

C: **You're really open to thinking about all aspects—I'm just noticing it is depressing for you to have this as a diagnosis.** (TC5 and TC8) Now she has named the mood which she noticed earlier and which through as the relationship feels safer to him. **Can you say more about what is depressing for you?** (TC5 and TC8) C is *not* asking him to go deeper into the *feelings of depression*; she is asking him to speak for what is depressing for him.

20:05

J: **It's depressing—that you gotta deprive yourself of something, you can't do what you want to do—you're restricted!** His compliant part is smiling, but the feelings are different from that.

C: **So it's depressing to have anything from the outside saying you can't do want you want to do, what you feel like doing on the inside.** (TC3, TC6, TC8) His compliant part asked again for a program from the outside.

J: **Yes, yes.**

C: **Yah, Yah** (TC6). **So, I'm wondering as you say that, that is that you can't do what you want to do, I'm also hearing that another part of you wants to have a quality of life.** (TC8) This is the important polarity for the awareness work at this point.

J: **You got it!** (resonance)

20:44

C: **So what is it like to be able to hold both of those? The truth—that it is depressing to have a constriction on—and the experience and knowledge you have about this particular illness and that you chose to have a quality of life, not to have the illness control your life.** (TC8, TC3, TC7—a subtle reframe of polarity with his illness constricting his life, not the diet.)

J: **That's it—I gotta find that balance.**

C: **I'm here to support you in finding that balance. The truth is, when you can find that balance for yourself** (not by yourself), **it's not going to be a deprivation or something you're trying to do, or a mind game** (C purposefully mentions the concerns of his main personality parts), **it's going to be the way you feel, but it is a process to get there!** (TC8 and TC9) **You're already on that path—do you realize that?** (TC7) He has already started in the process of change by exploring all of this in this context. (TC8, TC9)

J: **If you say so—you're the expert.** C saying, "You're already on that path," has triggered his presenting part to come back in, so it must have felt too vulnerable for him to be seen this way.

C: **Just listen to what you're saying—you've been thinking a lot about this.** This allows his protective part to soften and allow the feeling to come in (TC7, TC8).

J: **More seriously—I have (been thinking a lot about this) since I got the diagnosis.** Now he looks more worried, with a down mood.

C: **So, you know you are in a phase of acceptance right now** (TC3, TC7) **and as you can more fully accept it** (emotionally and the meanings) **then you'll be ready to start a program. Support from the outside—.** C is not getting ahead of where he is. That would increase his vulnerability and bring in more protectors. She mirrors what he had said about where he is!

Notice that she is not launching into giving him a program that his presenting part asked for or referring him to one.

22:28

C: **So, wondering—during this phase of acceptance—can you say any more about what you are feeling about it or thinking?** (TC5, TC7)

J: **Right now, it's all I can think about—what my future's going to be—with this disease—trying to process all this—trying to accept it to be honest with you—a big shock to me.**

C: **Right—unh huh, right.** (TC6)

C: (TC9) **As you're processing this, it is a condition of your body** (the metabolic aspect of the disease, and the ABCs—A1C, Blood pressure, and Cholesterol as main items)**—this is what we now** know—following these factors like exercise and healhtly diet, low glycemic—not a lot of sugar in your system, and your blood pressure. Those are things that offset the disease process of diabetes. This we know now. Those levels (again she lists the ABCs), they make you feeling better and people actually don't put on weight. It is to serve you, not deprive you—and it is to keep the disease process contained, that's what you want to be constricting—not the things you love—right? (J chuckles) Interweaving the ABCs, again and again, and in step with his knowledge and with how things have changed since his mother's time (TC9).

C: Sounds like a good beginning. You're willing to look at an exercise program, your diet and working with your doctor to decrease you medication. So lets start with one thing at a time. (TC6) Space for feelings that have come up and slowing it down so he can learn to regulate feelings.

C: I heard you say you'd be willing to experiment—gym 30 minutes and day off—check for a buddy; we meet next week; pay attention to what you really like to eat and don't think about anyone taking it away from you. (TC9)

26:29

C: And then you're going to keep your appointments with your doctor—he did say that you were missing some of them? (TC8, exploring a polarized part)

J: (joking discomfort) You know.

C: I know, it's hard (TC6). I want you to be thinking of what you want to learn from your doctor instead of thinking he's telling you about a disease (TC9). You now know that your blood pressure, your blood sugar and your cholesterol are really indicators of how well you're doing. You want to know that—right? Nodding, talking to his quality of life part that knows this. She keeps mentioning these ABC items—A1C, Blood pressure, and Cholesterol—purposely as a repeating interweave into his cognitive and emotional process so she stays in relationship with him.

C: So how does this feel to you? (TC5 and TC7)

J: Most constructive thing I found—

C: Oh—so glad to hear that. (TC6)

J: Rather than having a doctor more or less scolding you.

C: (TC7) Could you just say a little bit more about how it was constructive? She wants to enhance his awareness more, by verbalizing where he stands with himself.

J: Not giving up anything, including exercise, basically not giving up anything just modifying things, inclusion of exercise, a basic lifestyle change but not so dramatic as to be in a different world! (TC9) He's assimilating and beginning to integrate opposites in a process that will be continued.

C: **I want to support you with your program;** not anyone else's. My notes are to be e-mailed (etc.). **See you next week. And, if you can do the exercise piece and observe what you're eating—that would be great. And make an appointment with me on your way out.**

Possible takeaway

This demo unfolded as both an information interweave and behavior change process, a common occurrence. The goal of one serves the goal of the other.

Joe already had been told and had been reading, but it served to activate his thinking and trying parts that were not getting him any closer to taking charge of monitoring the factors that mitigate the disease or to making lifestyle changes he already knows in his head (weight, activity, nutrition, and smoking). *He possessed a lot of knowledge that had not been integrated on the inside.* He had turned to the methods of his protector parts: thinking, trying, talking, overdoing, and quitting, and he was victim of a parts-dynamic in relation to food—deprivation, desire, and reward.

The clinician respected his presenting part's wish for a "program," but she did not respond by giving him one or referring him to one. Instead, she kept partnering with him to hold opposite personality forces he was experiencing and *kept repeating pieces of medical information only when it was in-step with the parts available in the conversation.* She did not go deep into emotion-laden issues such as the loss of his mother. This helped him remain in control of his emotions and to focus on his plan of being in control of the diabetes disease process and keeping a quality of life, rather than being deprived and scolded and having the disease be uncontrolled. It was a key strategy that she helped this patient realize and accept that he is in an early emotional acceptance process about the diagnosis and its meanings to him. The repetition of evidence-based information, discovered since his mother's onset (within the context of an increasingly open and engaged conversation with a clinician aware of personality parts) is what Information Interweave is about in this case. You may have noticed many features of interest to you that we have not mentioned.

MEDICAL DECISION MAKING (BREAST CANCER TREATMENT DECISION): WANT TO PUT THIS DECISION BEHIND ME

Introduction

This is the first interview between a hospital outpatient oncology social worker (C) trained in relational science (health coaching) and a patient (K) who, five days before, heard she has breast cancer. Her physician has already given her evidence-based information about her illness and treatment choices.

The text below contains an annotated processing of the entire interview (from a triple perspective—inside the patient, inside the clinician, and the dynamics between them) that draw your attention to strategy and tactics heard and seen in the video.

This video may be accessed at http://goo.gl/EEv770

Annotation

This clinician has used TC1, Step II, on previous occasions after interviewing patients with the same condition. In this interview demonstration you are observing an experienced clinician who does not use Step I vigorously since it is almost organic for her to help her parts to remain in the background of her mind so she can pay attention, be quiet, and wait, as needed (TC2). If *you* were the clinician in this case, you would use TC1, Step I, to take care of the personality parts that become activated within you so they do not take the lead during your interview, including about breast cancer, being video recorded, and doing a good job. The timeline is on the left side of the page in seconds. The numbers (TC) used below refer to the Key and corresponding descriptions of tactics in Chapter 8.

Key: Tactical competencies used in the interview

TC1:   Using Step I of clinician emotional self-care
TC2:   Paying attention, being quiet, and waiting
TC3:   Mirroring and validating
TC4:   Helping patient to locate and/or identify and become aware of bodily sensations
TC5:   Helping patient find words for emotions, distinguishing between emotions, thoughts, and body sensations
TC6:   Extending empathy—both components
TC7:   Noticing, exploring, and enhancing awareness of the set of emotions, thoughts, body sensations carried by each personality part, especially the presenting part
TC8:   Enhancing awareness of each personality part that is involved in a polarization (a pair of opposites) and prompting the patient to tolerate having both in awareness simultaneously
TC9:   Interweaving information when patient is ready and shaping it to fit the interview process
TC10: Asking periodically for feedback (emotions, thoughts) from patients of what they heard and its impact; also, checking on influences coming from family and other clinicians

C = clinician, K = patient (Karin)

The interview

0:00–2:45
Note: This is an introduction by Dr. Livingstone about medical decision making. The interview starts at 2:47.

C: (This experienced clinician is able to start in TC2. You would start with TC1.)

2:47

Notice that when the clinician (C) introduces herself, it is preceded by eye contact, smile, calm, warmth (an affective connection) with Karin (K), whose face looks tense. Notice that C acknowledges to her that she knows she has received information and has a decision to make, the agenda of agreement about the meeting. K starts right in.

K: **Met with Dr. Hill five days ago and haven't slept since then—but she was wonderful in giving me all the medical information.**

> After K tells the increasingly pressured story of all that she has heard from her doctor and the **"lose–lose"** sense of it and describes herself as being **"all over the place,"** the first thing C does is to find some words acceptable to K, which verbalizes the felt state K is in.

C: **This sounds really big** ("big" (TC3) is validation of the sense of overwhelming and urgency she's picking up from K) **and I appreciate the lack of sleep.** (TC3, TC6) K nods in agreement and feels invited to elaborate further and identifies that she's been racing and her heart's been racing. (The need to make a decision often includes two polarized protective parts and a third part that carries anxiety and a sense of urgency.)

> C's first strategy and tactic: Taking her cue from K's fast speech, train of racing thoughts that she feels in her body, and K's resonating with C's saying that this is really big, she asks K (tactic) if she could join her (K) in **"slowing this down and just be with all that is happening"** (TC6, TC7, fostering unblending and regulation). The theory is that K's presenting part (her inner pusher) senses the high vulnerability and has been strongly activated and blending with her (**"want to put this decision behind me"**). The strategy for C is to help regulate both the presenting part of K's personality (a pusher) and her flooding vulnerability (fear for her life) by forming an attuned relationship with both. This requires interviewing tactics. C chooses to say what you hear below.

4:36

C: **So how about slowing down a little bit right now—yah.** They breathe together—a basic regulatory maneuver.

> Notice that C is not in judgment of the rushing, nor is she taking the tactic of sorting information K may have received.

4:57

C: Reflects back her sense of what K has said and checks. (TC3) C is making an initial affective connection with K and is mirroring and validating the concerns of her presenting part.

C: **It helps to take a deep breath**. (C's strategy is to deepen the engagement. She reflects back in K's language what she has said so K can hear it again and also know that C is getting it). **So much information and a push to make a decision**. (C decides to help normalize K's intense experience with receiving a lot of information from her doctor.) **Trying to make the right decision always triggers anxiety**. (TC6)

K: Feeling enough trust to continue, K reports awareness of her body. **My heart is racing a million miles per hour**. K is tuned in to her body (TC6).

5:29

C: Works with K to slow her breathing even more. **Recognize your heart is trying to keep up with all the information—. Be *with* it for a minute**. (TC6 and TC8) C offers a distinction between what is happening in K's body (heart racing) and the agenda of their meeting—"all the information" to sort to make a decision. (TC8) *These are two different parts, and C is beginning the process of helping K become aware that there are two parts—as she helps her regulate by asking her to "be with" what her bodily sense is.* C does this two-part awareness work rather than saying something about either the one part carrying anxiety or the other part that wants to sort information and push to "put the decision behind." K is quiet for a bit; notice C does not interrupt with questions or provide information. "Be with it" fosters separation from the part as compared to "being it," which is being bended (Glossary). She is facilitating K's psychological separation from her anxious part and her pusher–protector within the direct supportive attunement of the relationship.

K: **Wish I knew that this was possible five days ago**. C hears this as an increasing sense that K is beginning to separate from the parts that have been blended with her and that she is ready, without getting overwhelmed again, to explore her presenting part, slowly.

5:48

C: **So did you feel pressure to make a decision right away?** (TC7) C is starting to explore K's presenting part and sort with K the outer sources of decision pressure as distinguished from inner sources of rushing.

5:56

K: Explains that Dr. Hill said that she had a **very aggressive type of cancer**, and goes on anxiously sharing that she is age 50 and wants many more years so wants to make the **right decision**. So C understands that K's protective pusher part was triggered by her doctor's words of "very aggressive" C does not yet know what K means by "right decision."

K: Goes on to let C know that she already realizes that the decision issue for her is not only a "medical decision" (meaning treatment statistics); it **involves lots of emotions.**

C: Going with this awareness—**And how are you with the emotions coming in?** (TC5, TC6) C is checking K's sense of her ability to identify and cope with the emotions. This is felt **as empathy** by patients without saying empathic phrases.

K: **Like a roller coaster.**

C shows her acknowledgment in eye and head nod (TC6).

C: **Is it OK to just name the emotions, to be with them? It helps to recognize, identify and name them** (TC5).

6:33

K: **Fear, anxiety, don't know if I can make the right decision—overwhelming.** The personality parts that are invested in the "right decision" and "rushing" are trying to protect her from survival anxiety but are not successful, especially at night.

6:50

C: **It sounds like slowing it down would help with the overwhelm— Because fear is** (mirroring K's words strengthens attachment) **big when it is life or death. When you want to make the right decision for your life there is always anxiety attached to it—let's be with it.** (TC3, TC6)

Remember when C says "let's," it is felt by K as "let us," a *you and me* relationship of being *with.*

7:12

C: In tune with K—**But trying to push through it too quickly always makes people feel overwhelmed by the process, and you want to be with the process—right?** (TC6 and TC9 psychological information establishing an agenda to work with parts)

7:25

K: **This is new information—cause I thought if I pushed through, it would be behind me.** More medical information at this point would only further overwhelm her system. What K needed is this new connected relationship both with an outside person and with her core self—one that fosters emotional regulation of the decision stress and discovery of information stored in her own system about her past.

7:45

C: **I really suggest that you be with the decision and have it be a thoughtful decision that feels right to you**—you know because the fear is here—because of the diagnosis. (TC3, TC6) Notice how C rocks her head as if talking to the young child part of K but without a tone of voice that patronizes K. Notice the nodding and synchrony in the respectful connection.

7:53

C: **But of the options presented to you, what are you feeling about them—what is your gut response to them?** (TC8) Notice C moves not to what K is thinking but what she is feeling at a gut level because that is K's core response and where the regulation is needed. K's bodily response needs to be accepted and identified by K.

K: (First response is a *thought* voiced in an anxious tone, not verbalizing the feeling word.) **Neither is a good choice.** (TC8, thinking, sorting)

8:10

C: **OK, so that's a place to begin—neither is a good choice. Can you say more about the choices?** C just heard K's protector of her feelings—a thinking part—so she joins with this protector to befriend it and find out more about it. This is awareness enhancement and is felt by patients to be empathic and attuned. C sits quietly and listens attentively to K's story about what the doctor said about the management schedule if she chooses lumpectomy. She thinks her knowledge of herself has taught her it would result in an unacceptable lifetime of worry.

K: **On the other hand, losing my breast doesn't seem like a good way to live.**

8:53

C: (TC8) C prompts K to explore this more because this statement reflects an opposite part in the decision process, opposite to the part with which K is more familiar—that would just carry worry, and it has not yet been explored. This allows K become more aware of this part that is operating in her decision process.

9:05

K: **Umm** (in an anxious tone) **I nursed two babies—it's part of me, and has ramifications not only for me but also for my husband. As I said neither feels like a good choice.**
(TC2, TC6) Notice how calmly and tuned in C's listening is to K's torturous dilemma and uttering **"uhuh"** as a way of staying attuned and acknowledging what she's saying. C would do this even if she disagreed with some fact that K might bring in. It is not a cognitive-fact-driven conversation; *it is attunement.*

9:18

C: (TC8) **So, I'm just getting that one thing also coming into this is that there is a part of you that doesn't even want to have to make one of these two choices.** (K is nodding her head yes.) **So just acknowledge that. That's important.** One part wants to rush through the decision "so it will be behind me"; another part doesn't even want to make the decision. This consciously identifies K's ambivalence and makes it normal and acceptable.

9:32

K: **I know that running away and not doing anything—is a death sentence.** Another part of K of which she fortunately is aware that sometimes takes over other patients no matter what facts they are told.

C: (TC8) Responds by recalling with K the part of her that counterbalances the running away part. **Because you also have the fear of dying—You want your life and I am also hearing you want quality to your life, and with these two decisions** (alternatives) **you're articulating what will happen to the quality of your life.**

9:53

C: (TC8) **So, what if we held both of those decisions for a couple of minutes so you can just be with them. You could say: on the one hand there is the lumpectomy with the monitoring and the way that would make you feel, radiation possibly; and the other is to have a mastectomy—and imagining what that would feel like—living your life without your breast.**

At this point, within the safety of the relationship with both C and within herself, K is able to simultaneously experience and tolerate these two alternatives with *their corresponding emotions.* You will see the value of this increased capacity for awareness and emotion tolerance in a moment.

C: (TC8) **So, what happens if you're with both of those decisions** (choices) **at the same time and feeling into them—just looking a them and feeling into them?** (Rather than pushing herself to choose between them) This gives K the possibility of a way of coping differently from having her pusher part running the show—and it should reduce her anxiety level. K could not be doing this without the "container" of the attuned relationship with C.

C: (TC2) Gives K plenty of time to be inside herself to try this. This helps her reprogram her system.

10:30

C: **So what happens as you are with both?** (TC8, This is a crucial tactic.)

K: (Sitting quietly) **Want to explore that, but if I had to make a decision this minute, I'd go with the mastectomy, but having said that, it doesn't feel totally right either—so—**(K continues doing some shifting back and forth, as one would be expected.)

11:08

C: **OK, so you do not have to make a decision right this minute** (some reality for K's pusher part), **and I know it is urgent** (TC6, TC7, addressing the concern of the part pushing her and carrying the urgency), **but** *what* **doesn't feel quite right to you about this choice of the two?** (Continued deeper exploration of each side of her ambivalence)

11:26

K: Had a hip replacement—have a prosthetic hip—and it took me a year to get used to that—it's internal but could feel it and sense it; and considering bilateral mastectomy, I would have reconstruction; but I don't know if I'd ever get used to fake breasts—to feel like me. I think about my hip—it became part of me—how it didn't and then it did. (TC8, an interweave of information from the inside of K by K, as memory)

12:20

C: (TC6) So you do now have the experience that the hip does feel like a part of you even though it is prosthetic?

K: I don't feel any different—do feel it is part of me.

12:32

C: So I am wondering what it is like letting that information into your body. (TC4, TC5)

C is allowing time for an integration of this internally generated information from K's experience of her hip replacement, which is different from K's sense of what reconstructing her breast would be like.

K: I hadn't even thought about it until we started talking. (K closes eyes and takes in the information that is new to her decision process.)

13:06

K: I guess it's a little affirming because I had done it, and I wasn't conscious it happened. Last time I thought of my hip it was years ago.

C: (TC9) So great—just let yourself be with that information again—this is not about your hip, but it is not unrelated to one of the choices you have available to you—right? (TC8)

13:40

C: Believing that K may now be ready for more information, this time from outside her own system, she asks whether K has ever met anyone who has had that kind of constructive surgery, anyone who would know about what it is like for a woman.

K: Focuses instead on a meeting with a plastic surgeon in the next week to go through it.

C: Goes with the association K has to this question to find out more of what is coming up for her.

C: (TC9) Sounds like having that meeting and asking for more information would be helpful, right?

K: Right.

14:21

C: (TC8) So can you let that racing heart and anxiety know you are in the process of making a decision and there is more information to get? Without being explicit about personality parts, C is speaking to the parts in K, the ones carrying her emotions and body sensations. She does this to boost K's psychological differentiation from them while C extends to them *directly* the relational connection needed in order to regulate the emotions driving them.

14:31

K: **Actually since we started talking, my heart has slowed down considerably—feels like I'm just listening to it.** Notice the flow back and forth between K and C, the mirroring, the checking as whether the communication is sound. Notice that there is an engagement with the parts involved in the decision conflict. *Engagement* here means an attuned, exploratory and therefore empathic relationship with the parts involved, as if they are distinct people—each with their distinct emotions, beliefs, bodily sensations.

14:46

K: **It's hard.**

C: **It's really hard.** (TC6) Hear the vulnerability and the flow of empathy from C on a feeling and thinking level.

14:56

Notice that K returns her attention to work with each side of her decision conflict focusing on the quality of her life.

15:27

C: (TC8) Acknowledges this. **It sounds like that aspect is important to factor in because this is not just about saving your life but living your life. Right?**

K: **Right.**

C: **Do you think that would get better over time?**

K: **No—I think if I had the mastectomy, that would get better over time. The other option of frequent mammograms goes on forever.**

16:06

C: (TC5, TC8) **Just let yourself be with what you just said so you can feel it a little bit more.** C can feel that K's thinking system is playing a role and is facilitating her other, more emotionally filled parts not to be left out of her process. K is quiet for a while, and C is letting her be inside, without interrupting. (TC2)

16:40

K: **I feel a shift. am able to look at them independently—they were all one big muddle.** (Notice the body language of her past, more muddled, anxious state.)

C: **Am so glad to hear that. It's important for you to hang on to looking at this choice as two possibilities that you can *be with* each of them to weigh them *for yourself*** (emotionally and cognitively).

17:04

C: (TC10) **Also when you mentioned the mastectomy choice, you mentioned your husband. I'm wondering if your relationship with him will come into the decision making** (TC5).

K: **He's a wonderful husband and support. He says whatever I decide, he'd love me with or without a breast. But I feel that is what he thinks he should be saying, and it may not be true. I worry about that.**

Be aware that her husband also has different parts of him that each may have different feelings and views of her choices. How aware he is of himself will make a difference, because if he inadvertently identifies with wanting to please her, he might live with remorse about not speaking up before the final decision. But, if he becomes one of his parts rather than to speak for them, the relationship between them over the decision is likely to be taken over by a parts-to-parts dynamic. The latter feels disconnected and lonely for both partners. C will try to avert that and assist K in being aware of his reaction as coming from his parts and her reactions to his as coming from her parts. This way K can keep herself centered on making a decision that is best for her and also expect that her husband will do the work he needs to do on his own psychology. What works for her will ultimately work for them as a couple.

17:49

C: (TC8) **So let yourself be with that. So there's a part of you worried about his reaction to your choice, whichever one you make.**

K: **It's hard.**

C: **It's very hard.** (TC6) C is maintaining support for the attachment and empathy and reading K's intensity ("very") from her body language.

18:09

C: **So what would help you with the relationship—with your husband's part of this?**

K goes on to tell C that she has been really helpful, that is, she trusts her, and wonders if it is possible for her husband to come in with her. C strengthens the commitment to be *with* K through this until she's made a decision **"which settles in best"** for her. And, replies she's glad to see them both. K expresses she thinks he'll be more honest with C than he will with her and expresses that she needs him to be OK with this. C acknowledges, **Of course you do—you need to trust that in your body and your gut.**

Notice how K expresses her emotions in the lower part of her face, cheeks, and lips. C is tracking that and gets the sense that K is holding in her emotions.

19:17

C: **You know it's OK to let those feelings out; you don't have to hold them in. It's normal. You are in a really, really hard place right now.** (TC6 and TC8) C is tracking emotions bubbling up, which are different from anxiety and overwhelm, and gives K the opportunity to express them directly, rather than hold them in. This helps with identification and awareness of the most conscious parts of K that are present. C believes that K has more separation (is unblending) from her presenting part and that her system can be **with** the emotions—instead of feeling overwhelmed.

K: Does not let out more emotions but mentions the people who say they are being supportive and tells C that talking with her has been a wonderful experience. There seems to be some sadness. The gratitude feels genuine.

C: (TC6a, TC8) Acknowledges K's openness to processing her choices and goes on to say, **They are not great choices but they are your choices that you believe will save your life—and you want the life you want to have, so it has to feel right to you.** This acknowledges again the different parts presented by K, which C lets her know she has understood—basically in K's words.

    This is an important felt moment of understanding and empathy between these two people.

K: Another part—inner critic—comes forward: **Part of me that thinks I'm making too big a production out of all this.** C takes the opportunity to speak directly to this part of K—a part that would block her from connecting to her core feelings about this choice.

20:35

C: **I want that part of you to hear from me that it is not a big production—that a careful and thoughtful decision is going to help you get through what you have to do, whichever choice you make—you don't want to rush into it—you really want to feel in your bones about these two choices, neither of which you want to have. I get that; that it is the best choice for you, and that you will have the support of your husband behind you. That's where your focus needs to be, not with what other people have to say or even what a part of you might be saying about this. Because actually, Karin, being with your feelings is going to help your anxiety and your sleep.**

K: Sighs with relief.

C: (TC7) **It's when you try to push them all away, especially when you have such a big decision to make, that they keep coming up, especially at night.** Addresses the concern of the inner critic part, which just came up. Saying she is making a "big production" of this is not really working to protect her from her feelings.

K: **What we are doing here is just the opposite of what I thought I needed to be doing. I thought I needed to push through; I'd be strong and I'd just go for it.** A style this woman has used often to shield herself from anxiety; and although it has worked fairly well for discrete, time-limited situations, it does not work well for a decision crisis with this level of vulnerability.

21:42

C: (TC7) Valuing the presenting part again. **Well I know you have that part obviously and it's great as a resource but that's not the way to process a decision that so personally affects your body and your life. You have to be with it, right?** This honors a major protector part of K, which was clear at the outset and has helped her cope in the past. For cancer decision making, C is facilitating and teaching K on an experiential body level to be **with** the vulnerable parts of her that carry her emotions—all sides of her ambivalence at once. This allows an organic decision process to move ahead and be tolerable for K with C facilitating.

K and C: Mutual head nodding.

K: **So you're going to be there.**

C: (TC9, TC10) **Yes, until you feel you've made a decision that feels best to you and until you have processed it with your husband, and until you have gotten more information from the plastic surgeon, and then set up another meeting with you; and I don't know if you want your husband to come into that meeting or—.**

K: Says that the more he (husband) is exposed to this, the better, and agrees to include him on their next meeting.

22:51

C: Also wonders with K if she wants to meet with a nurse practitioner about medication for anxiety or sleep. (TC9)

K: **I'm not a med person.** C accepts this comment from a part in K, but has noted it within herself. They can return to this in a subsequent meeting. K sounds unaware that *her pusher is speaking* for her. Any clinician would need to work with this part of her to be certain she gets the assistance from medication she might need, especially for pain after a surgical procedure. Right now, if anxiety got very high and became a barrier even with this relational approach, C would help her use medication not as a substitute for the personal work but to enable the interpersonal process of decision making for which there is no substitute.

C: (TC6) Leaves it with an invitation for K to call her—reemphasizing how important sleep is right now. She asks K, **What else needs to happen for you now to feel OK with our meeting today?**

23:30

K: **Permission not to make a decision in haste—the biggest thing.**

C: (TC6) Agrees that is really important and they she's glad that K gets that.

K: **It was all in one big ball. I now have some separation—could do it on my own, too.**

24:10

C: (TC9) Explains that K could write down the pros and cons of the choices, on the one hand and on the other. But reminds her that it is *not only the facts*; she needs to sit with them and *feel* her reactions and what comes up with each decision—to take the time to do this. It's how she feels in her body about each one as well—so she gets used to being with the two decisions and feeling them.

24:30

K: **I haven't been going there at all. Could you say that again?**

C: Explains about being with the two sides of the decision and feeling them; about having her body be part of the process. (TC8)

K: Taking it in, replies, **That has not been included at all.**

C: **You want to change that. It's not going to feel good, but I want you to feel that it is the right** (TC7) **decision you make, for your life going forward and your relationship with your husband; but most important is that it is right for you and your body.** (TC6 and TC8)

K: Thanks C, and there is an agreement that she will call.

Possible takeaways

All three aspects of medical decision making are illustrated: the cognitive (rational thinking, informational), emotional (affect regulation), and relational aspects (safe attunement with clinician and respect for spouse). It is taking place in an interactive system within the patient, within the clinician, and between them, and between the patient and her husband. The dialogue sounds seamless, and yet is totally strategic on the clinician's side. The patient presents *both* a protector part and her vulnerable part.

This clinician demonstrates the essential value of mirroring and empathy and the resulting attunement that facilitates affect regulation and emotional safety for this patient to become more increasingly aware of and psychologically separate from the two parts of herself that participate in **stressful internal conflict**—to be "with them" instead of "being them." The clinician is hearing K's opening presentation as experiencing **emotional overwhelm** triggered by the diagnosis, the information she has already heard, and **a need to rush** to save her life and a need to **make the right decision**. Although K is calling it anxiety, it is not clear yet what aspects of K's personality have gotten triggered and by what. C does know that emotions coming from parts of the patient are blending with her, that there is too little space between K and her racing emotions. C's first tactic is to bring a relational connection to whatever personality parts or conflict between parts are contributing to K's overwhelmed state. The tactic she uses is asking Karin to join her in slowing things down and being with the bodily state she is experiencing and to breathe into it. C models that for K, and K picks it up. C's strategy is to build the best attuned relationship she can with K and also help K to internally build one with several parts most in the foreground of her decision process. C help K's affective overwhelm from the start by being quiet and asking K to be with what she notices in her body, heart racing, etc. There is acknowledgment between them that it is "big" and there is lack of sleep. This is the beginning of an attuned relationship that K needs for her parts that may be younger than she is.

Author's comment

The clinician knows that if Karin continues to process and becomes aware of what within her gets activated by others (her husband and her doctors), a good-enough decision that belongs to her will be an outcome of her process. C will be her facilitator, continuing to maintain a relationship that we view as the meaning of Shared Decision Making in the context of Patient-Centered Care. Not only is Shared Decision Making the cognitive sharing between clinicians and patient of evidenced-based information about illness and treatment options—the latter being a necessary aspect—it is also the sharing of emotions, beliefs, bodily sensations, historical memory from all the sides of ambivalence that come up around the medical facts, and it takes place in the context of an attuned relationship with a clinician who has learned a self-awareness process and who is able to foster regulation of intense emotions and the assimilation of information. The clinician needs to understand that decision conflict is an internal matter within the patient's personality and often involves at least two distinctly different personality parts rather than primarily being a matter of the patient's reaction to conflict about pieces of information coming from the outside.

10

A learning tool to sequence strategies and tactics: **S**elf-aware **I**nformational **N**onjudgmental interviewing in **H**ealth **C**are (SINHC®) ("synch")

INTRODUCTION

This interviewing model is offered as a guide for trainees and faculty mentoring. It helps with the understanding of the sequencing of the strategies and tactics of an interview. Synch, however, is not meant to be followed in a linear, rote fashion, since the decisions of the interviewer, although within a framework, are heavily determined by what is happening in the moment. It may be helpful at some point for you to have both this model and the annotations of Chapter 9 in front of you during one of your viewings of the videos.

While mentoring trainees, we assist them briefly to take care of what is activated within them so that they can become open enough to focus on more than the content of what is being said by their patient and the concrete diagnostic and/ or treatment tasks at hand. The student or trainee is facilitated to observe body language and notice emotional cues in patients, to help patients label their own affects in single words, to provide genuine compassion and empathy, to check the readiness of the patient's emotion and belief systems before trying to convey information, to appreciate that patients normally present their protective personality part in the beginning, which shields a more vulnerable emotional part, and eventually to help the patient identify their different personality parts that are involved in conflict over decision and behavior changes. Often, the presenting part is a protective part (controlling by talking, extreme pleasing, etc.) that is "in the foreground" and is shielding a more vulnerable part carrying emotions (such as fear, hopelessness, and trauma anxiety). Trust is gained by slowing down the interviewing process enough to leave space for identifying and relating to *both* the protective parts as well as the vulnerabilities. Sometimes gaining an understanding of what the protector part is trying to do for the patient helps the clinician appreciate and relate to the part.

For example, when a protector (like "I'll do it my way") starts to promote avoidance of a change in diet, it is often found that it is trying to protect the patient from feelings that have been too much to bear (in the patient's emotional history) such as grief associated with the diagnosis or with loss (of their youth, autonomy, health). Sometimes loved ones collude with the patient's protectors because they have one that is similar.

If the clinician understands the role of the protector part, for example, of his diabetic patient, he/she will "befriend" it, rather than "resist" it with rational data and information. Data and information may only increase the strength and agenda of the protector part. The clinician's genuine curiosity in relationship with the protector—acknowledging what is being said, identifying the general tone associated with statements such as "sounds very important to you" or "you seem determined to keep your diet unchanged"—tend to soften the intensity of the protector. Then more information or different parts can emerge. This is now an empirically validated pathway for patients to become aware of and to tolerate emotions activated by a diagnosis or treatment, and it opens the door to behavior change and assimilation of new information. All of these tactics require that clinicians establish and maintain interpersonal attunement, which means they need to keep themselves centered as well.

It saves time when clinicians are able to make a nonjudgmental and empathic relationship with both a patient's protective system and their vulnerable personality parts, as they become activated within the patient *in their office*. Attunement to this process lessens resistance and noncompliant behaviors that happen *outside the office*.

Here is one model of interviewing we developed for medical care (for physicians and nurses) based on what is known. During its development, certain aspects were research tested, as we have explained earlier, and are empirically validated. This is the only model at this time, of which we are aware, that is based on the past and updated knowledge accumulated for this book.

SELF-AWARE INFORMATIONAL NONJUDGMENTAL HEALTH CARE FOR PATIENT-CENTERED CARE SINHC® ("SYNCH")

This model seems to be the first theory-based strategic and tactical model developed for the relational side of health care. **It synchronizes the power of attending to emotions, beliefs, and bodily sensation with the power of medical knowledge.**

Already stated several times, this is not presented as the only path to making use of the advances in psychological and neuroscience over the last two decades. This is one way that we have found that works and is grounded in available science. It can be tried, taught, and compared for efficacy with other models that may be developed. An adherence scale tool and research manual is being created so that this model can continue to be reliably researched for educational feasibility, patient outcome, and cost containment.

This tactic of interviewing can sound like ordinary conversation to the outside observer.

Getting started

Clinicians, before starting and throughout the contact, make use of Step I of clinician self-care (Chapter 8) to become mindful of their own emotions and thoughts that are activated by their task and/or the patient's condition and behaviors. The clinician starts by greeting and connecting affectively and by beginning to track the relational triad (Chapter 8). He or she listens for the feelings and beliefs of the patient's presenting personality (aka "presenting part").

Although usually leading with a protector, people sometimes are flooded with emotions and lead with a lot of vulnerability, which needs stabilization and regulation via relational attunement. The clinician must be willing to start making a relationship with whichever part shows up first. This is the patient's psychic survival mechanism and cannot be sidestepped. You will discover that if you try, the presenting part will keep getting even stronger and you will think you're at a standstill. You are.

Throughout the SINHC® process, while remaining within the patient's comfort zone, the clinician will engage the patient's presenting part with interest and concern but will not offer alternative beliefs, feelings, or advice. It is helpful to assess with curiosity the values and emotions of the presenting part. This personal assessment is the first step in connection and relationship building. It overlaps "history-taking" about the health condition, and it may overlap into physical examination and reviewing technical and radiographic data together. If the clinician can engage both his/her right-brain and left-brain functions, this is helpful.

One tactical approach is to invite the patient to share: "Would you be willing to share what is most important to you?" This type of inquiry can pull for the concerns of the protector or the emotions of the vulnerable part, if it is ready to show up. The clinician continues to notice reactivity with themselves that may be activated by the patient's responses. The clinician (without editing) mirrors, and appreciates the values, beliefs, and goals that are voiced. These are the characteristics of the patient's presenting personality. This is building the attunement of a relational foundation, which guides all remaining contacts. The presenting personality, usually a protector, may soften back and allow a more vulnerable emotional aspect to come up. Shifts in personality can be felt and observed in the patient's, eyes, face, and voice tone. If this should happen, the patient is probably ready to have you make a relationship also with their more vulnerable aspect, *while also maintaining your relationship with their presenting protector(s).* This is a favorable sign. Now you can connect with your patient's vulnerable part by tuning in with compassion and empathy (both aspects) to the emotions, thoughts, and memories that come up from this vulnerable side. This means you need to be comfortable responding to your patient's emerging emotions and the protectors that periodically cover them (as well as your own) (see Chapter 8).

For example, if the patient says he feels angry and scared about the diagnosis, the clinician may respond, "I am hearing that one part of you is feeling angry and another part is feeling scared about the diagnosis. Does that sound accurate?" If appropriate, the clinician may introduce *parts* language, but this it not necessary. He could say he's hearing two "feelings," knowing that it is more complicated than that. The clinician normalizes the feelings of being confused by new information and experiencing ambivalence and possibly conflicting agendas when making medical decisions and changing behavior. The clinician takes the temperature of the relational connection between him and whatever personality of the patient is dominant in order to assess readiness for new information to be taken in. Asking the patient periodically for what information they might want or believe they need is one component of checking readiness. When the patient appears ready, the clinician communicates evidence-based information in a manner that connects to the language, pacing, and cognitive style of the then-dominant personality. In a nonpatronizing fashion, the clinician checks and rechecks what the patient has heard. The clinician can always say some version of, "So that I know I have been clear and so can repeat if need be, could you give me some idea of what you heard me explain?" As the clinician hears the patient's version, he or she should repeat the more accurate version and adjust it—rather than correct the patient's version with a "no, what I said was—," which could shame the patient. Impatient and rushing personality parts within clinicians need help to soften back (Clinician Self-Care, Chapter 8). It saves time to take the time to take care of yourself.

By using your personal version of the above approach to *getting started* we hope you will be more prepared to be mindful of the three psychologically based systems and seven clinical tasks illustrated in the diagrams in Chapter 8. We hope that both you and your patient stay in relationship as your patient's needs are revealed.

Sequencing of interview strategies and tactics

The SINHC protocol is not a linear interviewing process. It guides the interviewer to start by connecting with the patient's presenting affect and exploring the concerns of the activated parts rather than focusing right away on medical facts, such as the importance of continuing on beta blockers. It creates a road map between clinician and patient, which helps them stay connected as the patient's needs are revealed. The interview may briefly move beyond medical concerns and parts to other relevant factors, including difficult economic and environmental circumstances and the insensitive behaviors of relatives or care providers. Your initial goal, in addition to feeling open and grounded, is to establish a connection with the patient's parts(s) while moving toward diagnosis and treatment planning. The clinician accepts all vulnerability with compassion and grounding, and models regulation of emotions, as needed.

In the initial contact, he/she offers empathic containment of emotion to help the patient from being overwhelmed. The clinician tracks the patient's internally generated conflicts as well as those activated by family or medical providers or by conflicting information available. To increase the patient's self-awareness, you would expresses curiosity about the meaning of your patient's emotional tone, sighs, pauses, and any storyline contradictions. When opportunity arises, *the clinician encourages the patient to identify his feelings and activated parts but may not call them "parts."* Rather than providing him with answers, she stays affectively connected, follows clues, and explores his parts' concerns. Emotional readiness for more information tends to emerge after parts have been acknowledged and met with understanding and compassion. As discussed in Chapter 8, Tactic #9, the clinician interweaves information by offering small chunks and checking how it was heard by the patient (Information Interweave™). You will have opportunity to observe this process in the demonstration videos linked to Chapter 9.

The following table shows a typical interviewing sequence using SINHC, and it served as an invisible roadmap for the clinician in the audiovisual demonstrations. Although the interviews appear to be ordinary conversations, they are fully strategic. It is one choice for interviewing patients, and currently seems to be the only contemporary tactical model available. Hopefully, additional models will be designed that will also incorporate unfolding advances in multiple fields.

Process of SINHC®

Internal within clincian (a–e) (before starting and throughout)	Interpersonal with patient (1–11) (leading priorities)
a. Connect with a sense of openness/relaxation in mind/ body and hold intention to maintain this as you hold the territorial map of seven tasks and three spheres to track (Chapter 8).	1. Make affective, open connection with the patient and a relative if present.
	2. Build attuned connection with patient's presenting parts and find words for emotions and concerns.
	3. Begin tracking emotions, content, and agendas of the different parts.
b. Be aware of the agendas (goals/internal purposes) and be in relation to your healthcare parts and the agendas of patient's parts while noticing where connections can be made to join these agendas.	4. Establish clarity with the patient about the agenda of the meeting. Integrate the above priorities of attunement, clarifying emotions and concerns of patient's parts until there is a sense of agreement between you and the patient about the focus and tasks of your contact.

(Continued)

(*Continued*) Process of SINHC®

Internal within clincian (a–e) (before starting and throughout)	Interpersonal with patient (1–11) (leading priorities)
c. Notice your internal reactions to the patient's specific illness, attitudes, and choices.	5. Create an opening for and acceptance of the patient's vulnerability; name it without editing it or going deeper. (Used in Flexible Order as Indicated by Diagnostic and Treatment Needs and Patient's Process.)
d. Be open with curiosity and compassion to the dual awareness of your internal system and that of the patient.	6. Interweave credible information guided by the readiness of the patient.
e. Notice any internal reactions that signify that part of you has been activated by what the patient is saying about their relatives and care providers.	7. Invite identification and limited exploration of beliefs, emotions, responsibilities of opposing (polarized) personality parts within the patient, particularly when they get activated during the interview.
	8. Invite identification and some exploration of opposite priorities generated by relationships with care providers and family.
	9. Identify and explore factors and competencies supporting internal motivation for specific behavior changes and decision making.
	10. Identify and explore cultural, economic, and environmental influences.
	11. Establish agreement with each of the patient's personality parts on an action plan, on follow-up contacts, and referral to others, as appropriate.

A *second viewing* of all videos is suggested using companion annotations. We suggest you make note of your questions, keeping both right- and left-brain functions engaged.

11

Referring to behavioral health professionals

The process of referring patients to a mental health professional or a behavioral health clinic evolves from the same set of interviewing skills and "felt sense" of what is happening inside the patient, as in all the previously mentioned interventions that facilitate behavior change, decision making, or information interweave.

WHY REFER?

If you believe that significant psychological dynamics might be blocking your patient's progress toward health behaviors and decision making and/or that he or she is suffering from emotions or other symptoms that need attention and are beyond your expertise, a referral to a mental health specialist might be indicated. Or, if the patient specifically wants to work more steadily with a behavioral health specialist, this is a reason to refer to mental health for evaluation as there may be issues that the patient doesn't wish to share with you. The more competent you become with interviewing, the more you can engage the patient in the decision process about a mental health referral. And, the more you can engage in self-care and extend respectful curiosity toward the patient, the more clarity you will have regarding the need for a referral. Reasons for clinicians to *consider* a referral appear in our video demonstrations.

At one point the clinician mentions the option of a referral for "evaluation," basically for what is being called depression. In any case, she does not propose a referral for psychotherapy, as that is not within her expertise, can be confusing and upsetting to patients, and is premature without an evaluation first. A clear period of mental health evaluation, which provides increased understanding and agreed-upon goals, helps the patient gain clarity about the issues and treatment options.

There can be a second and third health coaching visit to bring the issue forward if the clinician hears material that supports her sense from the first interview. Even when a patient repeatedly uses the word *depression*, the clinician can explore what is meant by that word, and might inquire about bodily manifestations of depression such as weight loss, loss of interest, and sleep troubles. This helps determine the need to recommend an evaluation. The patient's experience can be labeled as "depressing," without a clinical depression being present.

The referring clinician would explore the patient's reactions (what parts get activated) to the idea of a mental health evaluation, including feelings about any previous experiences with mental health services. A referral to a behavioral health specialist often activates all kinds of meanings and emotions within patients, some of which you will need to process with them for the referral to be effective. You need to be willing to listen to the negative side of their ambivalence about a referral without trying to talk them out of their hesitation and to supply information requested. Being with both sides is essential. It is better to ask them to "check out" whatever mixed thinking and feelings they may notice. This is done because you would not want hidden negative feelings to be behaved as a failure to follow through or as a disruption in the trust you have built in your relationship. Health coaching usually needs to continue parallel with a referral. Also, even if the patient makes an appointment for evaluation, this action may be coming from a part of them that wants to please you, the patient may behave another part that experiences the referral quite differently. If your patient does follow through, you may suggest that they process any reservations about seeing a specialist with that specialist at the beginning of the evaluation.

You may refer because of concern about your competency to work with the emotions and conflicts within your patient. That is probably a part within you that needs your attention so that you can proceed with courage to use what you are learning in this textbook. This book is a guide. Your ability to be present and explore *with* your patient is initially the most normalizing and supportive strategy. You can make another appointment to see how their inner experience and reactions are progressing.

When you still have clear concerns about the scope of your ability to be psychologically helpful to your patient within a general medical context, this would be a time to offer additional help from a mental health specialist in ways that do not blame them for having something "wrong" or being "difficult." The latter may be their emotional conclusion because of their own history and will be validated if you communicate the referral in any kind of negative way. Nothing is "wrong" with them (or your ability and desire to help). The present situation is activating parts of their psychological system and memories of the past in ways that would be helped by the skills of a psychotherapeutic specialist.

TO WHOM TO REFER?

Several different licensed professionals are similarly trained in diagnostic evaluation and in verbal therapies about emotions, beliefs, and behaviors and are called behavioral or mental health professionals: licensed clinical social workers, clinical psychologists, psychiatric nurses, adult psychiatrists, child and adolescent psychiatrists (a subspecialty within psychiatry), and licensed marital and family therapists. Medical social workers (in contrast to clinical social workers) are variably qualified to evaluate the need for a mental health intervention.

Clinicians in each of these professions tend to possess other specialized skills unique to their scope of practice: Clinical social workers also know about community resources and tend to work well with parents and families. Clinical psychologists also conduct diagnostic cognitive and personality psychological testing. Nurses know daily patient care, teamwork, holistic approaches, and are sometimes trained in psychotherapy and/or prescribe psychoactive medications. Psychiatrists know clinical medicine including neurology, have expertise with psychoactive medications, and are often trained in psychotherapy of adults. If you are working with children or teenagers, be aware that child and adolescent psychiatrists have trained an additional two years in child development, diagnostic evaluation, and psychotherapy with children, teenagers, and their parents. They prescribe medications to children and youth, when needed, and work collaboratively with pediatricians and school staff.

Many otherwise qualified psychotherapists from all these professions may not be conversant with the strategies and tactics of brief interventions to facilitate medical care. We have come to view medical interviewing as a unique domain, requiring a specialized body of knowledge and particular skills—the ones described in this text. You could contact the mental health clinician, even if it is a referral to a clinic, and ask about their training and experience to see if their skills match your patient's needs.

PART **5**

For Faculty and Others

PART 5

Practicality and Curiosities

12

Pathways in education and training

For students and practitioners to bring their behavior into alignment with the Core Values of holistic nursing and primary care doctoring will require learning psychologically-based strategies of relationship relevant to shared decision making and life-style change.

Roy L. Simpson, PhD, RN, FACP
Vice President Nursing Informatics, Cerner Corporation, 2013

INTRODUCTION

Your students and trainees can be confident that the strategies and interviewing tactics presented in this text are linked to theoretical hypotheses in neuroscience and relationship psychology. The hypotheses are in various stages of evidentiary validation, and they are far enough long to be worthy of the effort it takes to master them. They are either *well-established*, or *probably efficacious*, or *empirically validated*, or *evidence-based*. Applying them in these stages of validation is more likely to improve patient outcome and clinician well-being than the unintegrated potpourri of models from the past. We have included valued methods from the past and have integrated them with the newest findings.

Education in doctoring and nursing has changed from the old days of "Watch one. Do one. Teach one." Faculty members are expected to be clinically competent in their area of teaching and also to be skilled as educators. This dual skill set is often hard to attain. There are too few opportunities for faculty to gain significant training in principles of adult education and in advances in interviewing. We appreciate how "full" the education and training curricula in doctoring and nursing already have become. Relational science and clinician self-care needs to be integrated into the entire curriculum, not as silos of independent topics. This saves time.

Becoming an educator in the subject of behavior change and medical decision making requires an integration of right-brain learning with the left-brain cognitive paradigm. It is a courageous process for students and trainees to become conversant with both the rational, doing side of their personalities, and the feeling, sensing side of their personalities that use self-awareness, emotions, intuition, and relational cues. We can't imagine effective care of a patient without at least one member of a patient's team, in an Accountable Care Organization (ACO), for example, being conversant in both. Today, patient care requires that clinicians stay abreast of vast amounts of knowledge and maintain technical skills, while also being competent in navigating the territories of responsibility, risk, and emotional vulnerability of others and of themselves. The personal side of patient care also requires both right- and left-brain processing by faculty members to be effective teachers and mentors, and also requires them to stay abreast of new learnings in this fact-evolving domain. We are also familiar with how it is hard to teach psychologically-based skills that have not already been mastered by a faculty member. The interpersonal interviewing skill is one of the least-well-mastered areas in medicine and in other fields. For example, I am asked to consult to MBA human resource managers about how to interview executives. Since the science of interviewing has only recently been articulated, it is not yet a vigorously known and taught topic in schools of business or medicine.

Faculty members at the medical schools where I have worked (Harvard and Brown) are finding that lecturing alone is no longer enough for this aspect of learning. It is now necessary to observe students interacting with their patients and to understand what is going on within them, and also in the dynamics between them and their patient, in order to help them integrate the skills of diagnosis and treatment with their emerging interpersonal skills. This is a relatively new challenge for faculty, which cannot be passed off to someone else, for example, to traditional behavioral health professionals, most of whom are sparsely knowledgeable and experienced in this area. Through multiple exposures to the audiovisual demonstrations in this book, it is possible to experience what it looks like and sounds like to put theory and strategy into practice in encounters with patients. We hope that the description of tactical competencies and the demonstration of these skills in audiovisual form make it possible for you to teach skills more effectively.

The bias that we hear about adding this to the curriculum is lack of time and room for an additional dimension, "when there is so much to learn in medicine today." From observations while teaching at several medical schools, I find it is a not matter of room or time. It is a matter of having a textbook and reducing fear by having a process with which to practice the skills. The topic is neither complicated nor does it develop from experience alone. Establishing faculty with competency in the skills is a necessity. In the past, the tendency has been to divide physician from nurse education, and science learning from patient-related learning; that is, the basic science years from the clinical years. When exposure to the science of patient care is inserted from the start of medical and nursing schools, the hands-on clinical and the basic sciences still may become integrated topics. For example, students can learn a great deal about functional neurobiology and relational psychology from their general patent care experiences, but this would require simultaneous faculty-team teaching, rather than teaching in tandem.

The knowledge is assimilated only as the personal experiences of talking with patients and learning to listen and make interview choices unfolds. This, of course, is also true regarding the theoretical hypotheses and strategies of clinician self-care. The latter is always needed and is pertinent for students to practice for as many years as possible before postgraduate clinical responsibilities. I believe it is better to weave the new theoretical knowledge into all encounters with patients, not as a course but as a highly mentored, integrated learning of theory, strategy, and demonstrated interviewing tactics. Done in this way, it is fun, empowering, and growth-enhancing. This is non-silo approach.

Integrating the interpersonal skill of tracking the patient and attunement to what information is needed within a process of clinician self-care is a skill that must be learned by faculty and mentors. Without a recorded final assessment of the learner's interviewing skills and establishment of minimum standards, the program cannot be evaluated and improved.

Stephen Klasko, Thomas Jefferson Health System president, when dean at Morsani College of Medicine, said, "Medical schools typically select and educate students based on standard testing and science grade, not on empathy and communication skills, and clinicians learn in silos." A 2012 study from Boston University, published in *Medical Teacher: The International Journal of Education in Health Services*, found that medical students self-reported more empathy in their preclinical years than after they had advanced in their training. Likewise, the British study in the March 2012 issue of the *American Journal of Pharmaceutical Education* found that nurses became less empathic as they completed their studies, but pharmacists became more empathic. We hypothesize that the differences in the degree of vulnerability (exposure to illness and suffering) experienced by students from each specialty contributed to a difference in personal access to empathic abilities.

Empathy and compassion for patients does not need to be taught as "things to say" nor does it need to be left to inherent talent. There is a third pathway. We find that it is a matter of *releasing the empathy from within*, which is possessed by most clinicians but has been covered over by layers of protection from their personality parts. When the empathy from within can feel welcomed and safe in a medical/nursing educational environment, these protections soften. Being empathic includes the self-directed inner self-care we have described, and it supports attunement to a patient's personality parts.

Earlier in my career as a faculty instructor, I was fortunate to be offered a year-long weekly course in medical school curriculum design and implementation. Despite my 12 years of experience as a medical student, resident, and fellow, and then, several years afterward, becoming the teacher as a medical school faculty instructor, this course increased my competency as a medical educator. Robert Mager's *Preparing Instructional Objectives* (1962) was used in the course. Below, in the section "A generic framework for curriculum design" I have shared a generic method of curriculum design that has been useful for me and others.

MEDICAL SCHOOL AND RESIDENCY TRAINING

For young doctors and nurses to gain specialized relational skills, it is clearer now that it involves their learning specific knowledge content, studying interviewing demonstrations, and having their interviews recorded and mentored by appropriately trained faculty. Also, it includes training to conduct self-directed work within their personalities. From clinical observation and evidence-based research we believe there is good evidence that the ingredients of how clinicians relate to their patients impacts the mind, brain, and body of their patients and probably of themselves as well, although the latter remains unstudied.

In some centers, there is an ongoing concerted effort to include the interpersonal domain in the curricula. It is called *behavioral medicine*. The curricula tend to be outdated, and the time devoted to behavioral medicine is too brief and destined to be disappointing as has been medical school education about pain and its management (Foreman, 2013). Much of the focus is on old-fashioned methods of behavior change for the addictions—alcohol and smoking, cost factors in health care, and the focus of liberal funding. This narrow focus is a loss for the health behavior change field and effective interviewing, which are relevant throughout health care. All chronic conditions are cost factors in health care.

The principle proponents of medical school and other post-graduate programs about interviewing are handicapped by a plethora of disease-related research funding (for example, the addictions or diabetes management) and by the lack of a unifying modern theory, strategy, and tactic for facilitating behavior change, decision making, information, assimilation, and clinician self-care.

There are also institutional barriers to fill curriculum redesign. Our previous chapters and the research publications cited show the futility of efforts to bypass interpersonal forces. Patient's emotions and reactions remain operative whether heath care has time for them or not. We have found no evidence that interpersonal factors can be bypassed or substituted for through the use of manuals, changing the patient's cognitions, and improved information and technology.

Skill acquisition on this topic requires left-brain functions plus right-brain functions. At this writing (May 2015), we have located many writings that talk about these topics, but we have not found programs that train faculty in the relational interviewing skills to apply good intentions. If faculty were to have access to significant continuing education experiences in this subject, it would be possible for them to lead the learning of students while continuing to hone their own interviewing skills.

We are sharing some of our experiences as faculty. Dr. Livingstone had an opportunity recently to observe and participate as faculty in behavioral medicine programs for advanced medical residents at Harvard Medical School–affiliated Beth Israel Deaconess and also for second-year medical students at Warren Alpert Medical School, Brown University. The Harvard program was focused on how to interview "difficult" patients and was too brief. The Brown program was too brief committed to training their students to interview patients when the goal is behavior change for issues like smoking cessation and diet. Although the students learned protocols like Motivational Interviewing (MI), they had difficulty applying the protocol face-to-face with patients for two reasons. Talking with some of them revealed that they were having inner emotional reactions that blocked their best functioning, and that they understood too little theory and strategy about the role of emotions and relationships and how to work with them in a behavior change process. To be learning an interpersonal process rather than a technique would have been helpful to them.

In the programs focused on behavior change that I have witnessed (health coaching, home care, medical schools, residencies and post-grad nursing), clinicians felt frustrated and patients were identified as being "resistant." We believe the addition of two items into the curriculum of the programs with which we are familiar would improve medical and nursing student training and patient outcome: clinician emotional self-care and affect labeling as part of being empathic. A comparative study could be designed after implementation. This research would add to Frotin's work on assessing the teaching of interviewing (Ellman and Frotin, 2012).

NURSING EDUCATION

Some insights from our teaching experiences of groups of nurses from several programs are offered here. The programs were in the health coaching industry and in the home care outreach program of a large health plan.

The nurses had already been trained in and were using the following models: Motivational Interviewing, Stages of Change, Shared Decision making, and many of the practices from holistic nursing (Dossey, 2009; Bark, 2011). Neither the underlying nursing education or their contemporary in-service training had included learning the knowledge and skills necessary for enhancing their self-awareness and regulating their emotions or for helping their patients to regulate emotions or process internal conflicts that were activated by behavior change and medical decisions.

We used contemporary science to enhance the nurses' work in health coaching. They were health-coaching a heterogeneous population of patients covered by many health plans. In collaboration with their faculty and administration, we designed a year-long, twice-a-month program that taught them new theoretical and strategic content in a series of lectures, workshops, and discussions. Then we added a series of live demonstrations of interviewing, and they participated in role-playing of interviews. Lastly, there was a six-month segment of periodic mentoring of their daily clinical work as they began to integrate the new strategies and tactics into their other clinical competencies. These programs in the early and mid-2000s were ahead of their time and now are in concert with expanding roles of nurses in health care including primary care, home care, palliative care, and prevention (Roberts Woods Johnson Foundation, 2015). Because of the favorable educational and patient outcome research findings, we were asked to train groups of faculty so that they could train other nurses in the new interviewing approaches.

The programs therefore had two levels of education and training—nurse health coaching for practitioners, and training of their faculty about mentoring relationship-based interviews and designing curriculum in health coaching. It was nursing postgraduate education.

For training practitioners, we developed a manual from which we ran workshops. For mentoring their recorded encounters with patients, it was decided, after trial and error, to mentor in stable groups of four nurses in three-hour sessions over many weeks. This way each learner's skills reach competency by reviewing with the mentor their interviews of several very different patients and by hearing the interviews of three other learners. The mentoring sessions covered a large spectrum of clinical situational territory. The learner, whose recorded work was being used, was asked to enhance listening skills, to comment on what they are hearing, to stop their recording, to go back and relisten, etc. We fostered safety in learning in each group.

Key features of creating psychological learning safety were as follows: (1) The other three, each of whom also had a turn with their own material, are requested not to critique the other's person work. They are asked to enhance their listening skills of the interview, to listen to the mentors' approach to the mentoring, and to comment on what came up for them (their own reactive thoughts and emotions to a similar situation). For the observers of the colleague, these were exercises in self-awareness and critical listening of patient dialogue. (2) Each was asked to make a commitment that *nothing that is said or that happens in the teaching sessions leaves the room*. (3) Our interactions with each of them modeled respect for the inner vulnerability inherent in learning and in processing recordings of their own work.

During the review of their own recorded sessions, the learners reported as most helpful (1) to renotice the characteristics of the presenting personality part of the patient and how they related to that part first; (2) to notice choice points in their interview and to understand what went into their choices—to get curious about what their choice was and observe what happened; (3) to note when, where, and what the rationale was for providing information; and (4) to watch how the mentor worked with one of their group colleagues.

After a period of group mentoring, each trainee in one of the programs was offered individual telephone mentoring over an extended period of months. They sent audio recordings ahead to the mentors and made appoints to review. Here is where some self-awareness could be fostered in a safe environment.

Take-aways from the earlier nurse training programs

Several conclusions were taken away from this early experience as faculty. The content taught in the workshop presentations was fully assimilated only after (1) interview demonstrations and a Q&A involving faculty, and (2) a role-playing by the learners. Competency in a variety of patient care situations was gained only via small group or one-on-one mentoring of recorded material. The latter was an essential aspect. The mastery of skills by faculty, however, needed to be high. The separate training program for the future faculty trainers of nurses (training of trainers) required observing their workshops with the trainees and processing recordings of their mentoring sessions. It was mentoring of their mentoring, and was found to be invaluable to them. Both the clinical trainees and the faculty trainees responded positively in each program and commented on the subjective increase in their observational powers (patients and themselves) and a decrease in personal daily tension. The unexpected take-away was that nearly every trainee, none of whom had experience in psychotherapy, became an increasingly competent interviewer in less than a year, with a full range of patients as assessed by testimonials and confirmed in one program by a blind comparative (before and after training) education research study. Also, team teaching (a duo) increased effectiveness. What one faculty member doesn't pick up or address, the other one will. Having two faculty means they can demonstrate the interviewing process with each other modeling the skills for the learners early in their learning curve. (At that time when these programs took place, early 2000s, the strategies and tactics of clinician emotional self-care, Steps I and II, had not been developed.)

We expect that teaching with the new SINHC® Model will give you, as faculty, an opportunity in real time to train your students in emotional self-care. For example, if one of your learners should get activated during a practice interview, what was found to be effective with athletes is to put the interview on hold for about 1 minute and to facilitate that student to notice the shift in their demeanor that just "popped up," and ask him or her **to be with** (See "Being With" in Glossary) what they notice. It is best to notify the learners that this is going to be part of the learning exercise and to help the participants be OK with it, since reactions are often the same for many in the group. The actual content of what came up inside does not have to be shared. This facilitation in affect regulation and asking activated parts to soften-back is briefly conducted in front of the others in the group as a model of what they can do for themselves for the rest of their years in practice. Anyone who does not wish to participate can opt out without prejudice and meet with the instructor at another time. The instructor needs to help the student go inside to observe and to inquire with curiosity (not judgment) as to what he or she noticed—a thought or a feeling. The point is for the student to practice not burying their interior experiences but to get curious and non-judgmental about inner shifts, to be with them and breathing into whatever they notice is coming up for them. This strengthens their clinical skills with patients. This real-time training of your students in emotional self-care during the vulnerability of learning is something new in professional schools. It carries over to their direct patient care. Instructors need to have experience working quickly with their own personality parts activated when teaching their students.

A GENERIC FRAMEWORK FOR CURRICULUM DESIGN

Create five vertical columns on a large piece of paper or on your computer using the headings below. Start at the left and keep filling in each column across the page while keeping a correspondence between the five categories. You will end up with a grid of items related to each other horizontally. Creative ideas will occur to you as you go along. Try to keep the first edition on one or two pages.

Then you can rearrange and deepen sections of it in separate outlines. Here are the five categories adapted from Robert Mager's work (1962):

- Responsibilities (student's future responsibilities and tasks)
- Knowledge (knowledge content needed to fulfill each responsibility)
- Skills (skills needed to apply each piece of knowledge)
- Methods (method of education-training for each piece of knowledge and skill)
- Evaluation (methods to evaluate efficacy of the curriculum)

To assess the efficacy of the curriculum, you could decide in advance at what point and how you wish to monitor efficacy of various aspects of your instructional program—so that you can redesign it based on fact. For example, in one of our programs we used a written exam that tested the knowledge learners had acquired from the manual, presentations, and discussion, and a separate test for skill acquisition using the submission of audiotapes of a full session of their direct interviewing of at least two different patients.

13

Health coaching

HEALTH COACHING: WHAT IS IT, WHO DOES IT, AND WHERE IS IT GOING?

The topic of who will learn the interpersonal skills of patient care, how will they learn them, and who will have the time to take a major responsibility for this domain is increasingly discussed in national-level meetings of physicians, nurses, and nongovernmental organizations. Whether this is within the scope of health coaching is another question. If yes, then who would be best suited for health coaching? Is it those who already are licensed health professionals (nurses, physicians, physician assistants, allied professionals) who could learn a set of theories, strategies, and tactics that would define the modality of health coaching, or is it to be a group of professionals called "health coaches" who have acquired a free-standing credential from a certified training program and who would not be required to practice within a health care licensure? The answers to these questions continue to be debated.

Could there be two routes and two practices of health coaching that include both of these options? Both routes could require training and examination in the theories, strategies, and interviewing skills that are specific to health coaching. Because of pivotal differences in underlying education and health service experience, the expectations of performance that would be warranted by each of the two routes are likely to be significantly different. It is reasonable to expect that consumers of health coaching, both the public and sectors of the health care industry, would need to be informed of the difference and distinction between the training and experience of each type of health coach. The National Consortium for Credentialing of Health and Wellness Coaches (NCCHWC) wrestles thoughtfully with these issues. This organization has a leadership board of which I am a member, and the consortium has a membership of individuals and entities, many of whom are licensed in health care, and some who are not. The Appendix includes a list of the leadership group. The goals of the NCCHWC make sense to us when they include deepening the professionalization of a domain of health service, defining parameters and core competencies of practice, and creating guidelines for education and training at an affordable cost in various U.S. sites. Because health coaching for many years has been loosely defined and practiced by people who may or may not be licensed in a recognized health profession in their state (for example, a fitness coach or a life coach), the double task of ensuring scientific and ethical integrity, while also being sufficiently inclusive of existing talent and practice, has been a challenge for NCCHWC.

Ruth Wolever, from Duke Integrative Medicine, one of the founders of NCCHWC with a PhD in clinical health psychology, and David Eisenberg, MD, from Boston's Beth Israel Deaconess, published "What Is Health Coaching Anyway?" (Wolever, 2011). We suggest that you read this article. Also, Wolever, one of the creators of Integrative Health Coaching (IHC), led a review of 284 full-text articles on health coaching (76 percent empirical) and found that, despite past diversity, there is a growing consensus that "health coaching is a patient-centered process based on behavior change theory and delivered by health professionals with diverse backgrounds" (Wolever et al., 2013).

Health coaching has been one of the main users of the various health-psychology models discussed in Chapter 3. The training includes learning the knowledge, for example, of Motivational Interviewing and Shared Decision Making, and then applying it. As you have read in previous chapters, we found gaps in theory, strategy, tactics and the training process in the specific health coaching programs to which we have consulted. Our increasing awareness of additional health coaching programs through my work on the board of NCCHWC and my discussions with the president of the International Coaching Federation, Magdalena Mook, confirm the worldwide intention to address gaps in training. Please see the Appendix for a list of people involved nationally in health coaching.

Meg Jordon, RN, PhD, of the California Institute of Integral Studies, and I wrote an article on the overlaps, dissimilarities, and opportunities for collaboration between health coaching and psychotherapy (Jordon and Livingstone, 2013). We listed red flags that alert trainees that a client's underlying condition might mean that a psychiatric assessment may be a best next step. Some of these are mentioned in Chapter 11, "Referring to behavioral health." In the article, Jordon and I described that, although both modalities may draw from some similar basic relational approaches, psychotherapists have been trained to deeply explore and to work for multiple sessions to relieve symptoms of diagnosable conditions such as depressive illness, posttraumatic stress disorder, and generalized anxiety, and to reduce dangerous behaviors such as violence, suicidal behaviors, eating disorders, and the addictions. Psychotherapists are expected to be available for urgent matters between sessions and in off-hours. Health coaches accomplish goals involving health behaviors and decisions, wellness maintenance, stress management, exercise, nutrition, and adherence to a medical regimen. Affects are noticed, acknowledged, and appreciated, but not deeply explored. Diagnoses are not offered, but further evaluation elsewhere is invited, as needed. It is a health coaching responsibility to talk with clients in a manner that does not trigger intense affects, backlash, and action behaviors. We posited that the depth of psychological self-awareness and self-care needs to be greater when conducting psychotherapy than when doing health coaching. Also, we posit that health coaching is more than health education, but includes it.

Margaret Moore, MBA, CEO of Well Coaches School of Coaching, is also associated with McLean Hospital and one the founders of the NCCHWC with a business background. For the NCCHWC website, she described our earliest model of health coaching as follows:

> Livingstone and Gaffney have recently adapted the Internal Family Systems Model (of RC Schwartz, PhD) to health coaching. They developed a model called SINHC™, which stands for self-aware informational nonjudgmental health coaching. It starts by prompting coaches to notice when their own personality "parts" become activated before and during a coaching session and to give them some attention. For example, impatience, judgment and fear may cover over the coach's Self presence and connection to their client and their ability to listen accurately. Coaches work with their inner reactivity to help it soften (and to be addressed later) so that they can attune with compassion to what is really going on inside their client around their health issues and relevant relationships. The coach's own "parts" activation is kept out of the way so that she can remain attuned toward her client's personality presentations, especially as vulnerability is shared. The coach and client in relationship may explore pertinent emotions and beliefs of the client's different personality parts but not so deeply as to overwhelm. They explore options of behavior change and health decision making. Health information is only supplied in tune with the client's psychological readiness. More than it is a process of following a protocol of steps, the SINHC™ coaching process is guided by tracking the client's personality parts and by the coach's awareness of their own parts, their awareness and respect for vulnerable parts in their client, and understanding of strategic principles of un-blending from parts (psychological separation) and self-regulation, the sine qua non of IFS.

Moore's generous statement describes only the first aspect of our approach, the establishment of the initial relational foundation for health coaching. We wish to add that, after establishing a relational foundation, the clinical effectiveness of health coaching that embraces "synch" derives from the clinician's skill to help the patient simultaneously attend to the opposing and polarized personality parts that normally become activated by behavior change or decision situations. It heavily embraces Interpersonal Neurobiology (IPNB) and the multiplicity paradigm (see Chapter 4). This is saying that specific skills to help people make shifts in their personality are required in health coaching that are different from health education, traditional psychotherapy, and behavioral medicine as currently conceptualized.

The more holistic and even spiritual side of health coaching is reflected in the work of Linda Bark, PhD, RN, a winner of a 2012 *American Journal of Nursing* Book of the Year award in Professional Development for her book *The Wisdom of the Whole* (Bark, 2011). She teaches integral and holistic coaching in Alameda, California, informed by philosopher Jean Gebser's model of structures of consciousness, that now has support from Anna Wise's work in EEG biofeedback. Bark finds that her multidimensional health coaching approach "helps clients move more quickly and easily, with greater authenticity, often eliminating false starts and saving time and energy." Her coaching academy teaches this model in a 60-hour program for application in healthcare, management, and other fields (Bark, 2011; Gebser, 1986; Wise, 2002).

Our experience as curriculum designers, faculty, and practitioners in health coaching has taught us that health coaching also is significantly different from all other coaching, for example, from coaching athletes and executives to communicate, lower stress, and collaborate with colleges. When applied in the health arena, coaching usually is focused on preserving health, managing chronic conditions, making treatment decisions, conveying information more effectively, and facilitating integration of care. The distinguishing combination of features in health coaching are (1) a uniquely high degree of vulnerable emotions within the client/patient, (2) the necessity for patient/client to assimilate complex information in the presence of these strong emotions, and (3) a high level of life-determining responsibility carried by the professional. These features determine the type and strength of the personality reactions that emerge within the people involved and the level of expertise needed to work with interpersonal dynamics. There is no way to side-step these relationship-related facts. In our view, training must reflect these realities and the reality that the modality of health coaching currently fills a significant relationship-based gap in health care for chronic conditions such as diabetes and arthritis and for decision-sensitive illness such as coronary artery disease, prostate or breast cancer, and herniated disc (Wennberg et al., 2010; Wolever, 2011; Livingstone and Gaffney, 2013).

Some believe that one route into the field should not require a professional health license (state licensing board) but that it should require minimal training requirements and a certification exam. This route is more inclusive in the face of a growing need. Others tend to believe that an unlicensed route would make standards of competency harder to define and regulate, and may make it harder for consumers and medical personnel to have accurate expectations. The quality of state oversight of health licensure in the United States, however, varies from state to state and is not a perfect guarantee of integrity and professional competency.

Nevertheless, the activity of health coaching has been found to enhance patient outcome. Ruth Wolever conducted a randomized trial at Duke of health coaching for patients with type II diabetes (Wolever et al., 2013). The Wennberg RCT involving more than 174,000 patients has already been discussed in Chapter 4 (Wennberg et al., 2010). Our controlled comparative clinical research in 2007 on nurse telephonic health coaching was discussed in our 2013 publication (Chapter 4). The core competencies for any type of coaching that are embraced by the International Coaching Federation's *Code of Ethics* are available on their website (2013).

The most relevant question, to us, is how will the combination of requisite knowledge and effective skills be learned and who will learn it? Currently, competency in the SINHC® model, our contribution to health coaching, is within the scope of a small number of nurses, allied health professionals, and health psychologists who call themselves health coaches, but it is not within the scope of most doctors, physician assistants, and medical social workers. For the foreseeable future, there is just too little opportunity to train. We believe once the modality is more deeply understood and defined, perhaps a significant number of doctors and nurses, and others such as medical social workers who already are credentialed health professionals, will choose to add health coaching as specialty training. That might give an already growing modality a well-defined boost and encourage others to expand the field. Being a health provider or a health educator does not automatically make one a health coach. On the other hand, to practice health coaching, it may be best for that individual to have experience as a licensed health provider.

Some workers call the interpersonal and intrapersonal processes of health behavior change and shared decision making "Health Coaching in Primary Care." Others call it Integrated Health Coaching. Recently, what is being called Lifestyle Medicine seems to be including health coaching as a modality within medicine and offered a two-day continuing education course at Harvard Medical School in May 2015 to "physicians, physician assistants, nurse practitioners, registered nurses, fitness, nutrition and wellness professionals, health care executives, health coaches, exercise physiologists, physical therapists, occupational therapists, psychologists, social workers, residents and fellows." Organized by Edward Phillips, MD, founder and director of the Institute of Lifestyle Medicine in the Department of Physical Medicine and Rehabilitation at Harvard Medical School, the underlying theory and strategies about relationships and behavior change processes that inform their teaching are not clarified in their publicity (Phillips, 2015).

Whatever it may be called or by whom it is practiced, the advances we have presented in this text fill gaps in skill-teaching and patient care. Many physicians and nurses could now gain the knowledge and acquire the skills, but our experience tells us that it will definitely take more than a continuing education course or two. Our hope is that this text will facilitate robust teaching of a science of health coaching, at least as a modality, throughout the primary education and training of doctors and nurses and will also be made accessible as a specialty certificate curriculum for attending registered nurses, physician assistants, family practitioners, practicing primary care physicians, and others. There is some hope that such training programs would receive funding from government agencies and foundations such as Roberts Woods Johnson and Gates. Otherwise, it is hard to picture how the national vision of effective Patient-Centered Care and Shared Decision Making could be realized in the foreseeable future.

14

Future research

To turn the hypotheses stated in this text into researchable hypotheses is a first step. It is the same challenge as it is in any behavioral health field in which different levels of evidence need to be embraced, not only the random controlled trials. The latter is a sparsely used format in this field because of the complex and uncontrollable variables operating in behavioral research involving emotions and relationship factors, just as they could not control many variables in the research on whether smoking causes lung cancer and on whether human activities cause global warming.

In recent years, the randomized controlled trial (RCT) has been placed above nonrandomized trials as conveying level of proof and certainty. Although this may be a reasonable assumption when the topic is about medication effects, it can only apply to research that lends itself to comparing single discrete treatments against placebo. This is not possible when human behaviors are involved. To discard methods that are well established and empirically validated (but not evidenced based by RCT standards) would ignore work relevant to actual practice that is scientifically sound and statistically no less certain to be effective than those methods that lend themselves to RCTs. Wachtel (2010) discussed this issue and pointed out that behavioral methods are inherently filled with uncertainty—a condition that "dogmatically embracing only evidence-based research does not solve." This is similar to trying to get a study to fit a specific lens, rather than developing a lens that fits the study.

By this point in the text we hope you are appreciating the need for multispecialty team research in this field. Without a team effort that covers the major parameters of relational psychology, brain biology, doctoring, nursing, and behavioral research design, it seems unlikely that the research could be valid enough to inform definitive education curricula change and health care policy planning. For example, imagine that the Wennberg study (2010) of more than 174,000 random patients, rather than it having been a retrospective study, could have been a prospective random controlled study that compared patient care inclusive of the skilled relationship-based nurse health coaching outlined here—fidelity checked by recording and analyzing interviews—*with* patient care that excluded nurse health coaching services. The costs and research infrastructure of such research would have been significantly higher and the design quite complex.

Such a design, however, would have provided specific information for clinical education and training and for service system design. Such a study would have indicated pivotal elements at the interface of clinician and patient that might lower costs and improve outcomes. Our sense is that this type of research and smaller, more limited studies, are needed to balance the current emphasis upon research and solutions that omit the contemporary science of relationship in patient care.

In the field of neuroscience research, we anticipate that looking for neural activity that corresponds with psychological observations will continue using existing and new measurement tools. All the parameters have not been exhausted, for example, comparing neural reactions to decision making in a solo situation with those taking place between people in relationships. Baseline fMRI studies of relationships have barely begun. Montague et al. (2002) used fMRI to study social interaction but not with people face-to-face. The search for improved measurement tools that record events at the speed of synaptic responses would be helpful. Correlations between observable neural activity and observable personality phenomenon are important. They stimulate development of new clinical hypotheses, but do they not replace evidence of efficacy derived from carefully designed clinical research.

A main feature in clinical research involving human behavior we have found is the gap in the fidelity checking of the interpersonal aspect of the intervention—both in the intervention and control cohort. We view this as a challenge of research in this field. Perhaps some researchers, for lack of measurement tools in this area, have tried to step around it by using reliability-tested questionnaires with both clinicians and patients. These approaches appear to pose significant problems for validity while solving ease of measurement. On the other side of this issue, however, is the challenge to design a format for assessing interpersonal interviewing that is both valid and reliable. A research team with which we are associated has been developing an intervention adherence tools that will be useful to all of us. The new adherence tools have been compared to unstructured assessments of the same recorded clinician–patient interactions and have also been found to have high interobserver reliability, provided that the observers/scorers fall within certain definable backgrounds and training parameters.

The strategies and concrete tactics outlined in this text we hope will take us and others further toward creating assessment tools for checking the fidelity of the interpersonal interactions of facilitating behavior change and decision making. There is a need for small, carefully designed comparative pilot studies that track both the intervention and the control side of the interpersonal domains. What has yet to be done is a blind outcome study comparing an intervention using a monolithic frame with an intervention using multiplicity frame (working with personality parts), which includes recordings of the actual encounters to check fidelity to discover common features and differences, and which uses a valid instrument to assess short-term outcome.

Domains of research in relational aspects of patient care include (1) feasibility studies in the education and training of clinicians, (2) patient outcome studies, (3) patient satisfaction studies, and (4) clinician satisfaction studies—sense of competency, desire to continue primary care practice, recruitment to primary care, and reduction of burnout.

As a researcher, if your goal and financing necessitates studies in a disease-related fashion, we suggest that you review in the Appendix a list of clinical topics that have drawn sufficient attention for several companies to warrant the expense of producing Patient Decision Aids (PDAs). You may also wish to return to the beginning of this text to review the Framework for assessing scientific status.

Glossary

Many terms associated with the psychological and social sciences are used with a meaning different than the colloquial one. Our intention, rather than to define, is to be clear about what we mean. Although some readers may differ with how we use the terms, we have made an effort to be consistent in their use, and are not claiming them as a standard of usage.

Anger: A body-based feeling/emotion that has many modifiers, levels of intensity, and synonyms: pissed, furious, enraged. Sharing your label for an angry feeling with someone verbally is a different process than behaving the anger by verbally calling them names or inflicting flesh wounds or property damage, all of which hurts other people.

Attunement: An interpersonal, brain-to-brain state that is deeper than affective connection. The clinician is resonating inside him- or herself with the emotions, body language, and thoughts within the patient, and doing so with nonjudgmental separateness and curiosity.

Attuned relationship: A term from attachment theory meaning an interpersonal relationship characterized by resonance between people on an emotional and body-language level. It requires perceiving the other person as psychologically separate, and having emotional regulation of, and separation from, one's own activated personality parts. It does not necessitate agreement with the thinking and beliefs.

Behavior: Can consist of verbal behavior and physical action. Calling someone "stupid" is *verbal behavior*. Saying, "I think your behavior was stupid," or even better, "I felt hurt by your behavior" is sharing verbally and is not an action. The impact on the other person is different.

Being with: Being aware of a part of one's own personality as a separate division and being nonjudgmental toward it.

Blended and unblended: Refers to whether a personality part is in a state of "being the person" or "blended with" or "identified with" as compared to "being with" the part as a psychologically separate identity and energy. There are degrees of being blended with a part. If someone is completely "blended" with one of their parts, their core self is not available to help regulate the emotions carried by that part. They "ARE" the part.

Clinician emotional self-care: The strategies and tactics clinicians use within themselves to sooth emotion and other mental activity so as not to let their abilities to focus on their patients get covered over by personality parts within them. Prevents clinician burn-out and compassion fatigue.

Compassion: The emotion of caring and warmth within one person *toward* another, with a sense of separation, and not requiring actions or agreement. Self-compassion can be extended to parts of oneself. Schwartz describes it as loving-kindness, witnessing, and wishing to alleviate suffering for which the witness may feel connected to the sufferer, but through the common bond of humanity, rather than overly personalized or self-centered emotions.

Connection: In the context of relationship, an interpersonal state of being in eye contact and with a flow of affect. *Rapport* is a word that is often used. This is a relatively superficial state compared to attunement, compassion, and empathy.

Consistent: When referring to a theory, means a theory without internal contradictions.

Continuum model: Conceptualizes a process through time with elements that do not need to occur in linear stages in order to reach the defined goal.

Decision support: A dual process of providing external clinical and research information in any form (including printed or recorded patient decision aids) and also providing the patient with a nonjudgmental relationship for processing their internal conflicts activated by the health condition and the decision issues.

Decision conflict: Inner conflict of an affective and cognitive state of normal distress that occurs *within* the person's personality in the process of making a health care decision. Contributions to conflict often originate simultaneously from the person's personality parts dynamics and as reactions to the medical information received.

Education: The cognitive-based learning of a body of knowledge, and learning how to think and problem-solve.

Emotion/feeling: A body-based experience for which feeling-words can be used to label the felt emotion. *Emotion* and *feeling* are often used synonymously, although some use the word *emotion* to refer to the bodily aspect. Words for emotions/feelings are usually single words such as: happy, sad, fearful, mad, disappointed, and confused. Saying, "I feel that—," is not verbalizing a feeling; it is verbalizing a thought, even if the tone of voice is carrying some unverbalized emotion.

Emotional arousal: An internal physiological and psychological state that varies in its intensity, in the degree to which it is conscious, and in the way it is shown (body language, voice tone, verbalizations, or actions).

Emotional regulation: A psychological, neural, and physiological process of reducing the intensity of an emotion.

Empathy: *The awareness* of another's thoughts, ideas, beliefs (not necessarily agreeing) and *the briefly felt experience of* other's emotions, experienced by standing briefly in their shoes (without becoming the other person). It is both an affective and cognitive personal experience.

Guilt: A feeling/emotion that goes with thinking you have *behaved* badly.

Heuristic: An experience-based technique (tool, aid, or method) for problem solving, learning, and discovery by themselves. A theory, hypothesis, strategy, or set of tactics can be a heuristic. It does not imply proof.

Hypothesis: Not synonymous with a theory, which is a set of proven hypotheses. It is an explanation *framed to enable testing* based on observations that have not yet reached the validation level that warrants it being called a theory.

Implicit: A feeling, thought, or memory in variable states of unconsciousness capable of being understood from something else, though it is unexpressed—as compared with **explicit.**

Informed choice: *Updated definition*—A choice made by a person who has accessed, understood, and integrated the valid information relevant to the choices via the process of Information Interweave™, which includes receiving information from their internal system of parts. *Traditional definition*—The person has been told or given in writing the evidence-based relevant information; may include a Q and A opportunity.

Intersubjectivity: The psychological realms of relationships between people.

Mindfulness: An intentional and nonjudgmental focus of one's attention on the emotions, thoughts, and sensations occurring within oneself and others in the present.

Model: A set of hypotheses and/or theories *and* their respective strategies in any state of validation that are designed to guide some process or procedure and are simplified versions of the real world, dealing with a limited amount of detail.

Monolithic view of personality: A hypothetical assumption that normally the human personality is organized and can be perceived as one entity (one mind) with one set of many emotions, beliefs, memories, and behavioral tendencies, all mixed together and functioning to motivate behavior and to defend them from vulnerability—the assumption being that there is a division of function, but not organized as internal, separate, full personalities.

Multiplicity of personality: A hypothetical assumption based on observation that normally the human personality is organized into distinctly separate, functional, full personality clusters (parts/subpersonalities/selves), each of which carries a separate set of emotions, beliefs, memories, behavioral tendencies, and a functional role within that person's internal system, and each of which can be in relationship with one aware, nonjudgmental core aspect within that person ("Self," Schwartz; "Aware Ego," Hal and Sidra Stone).

Part: A natural division of personality with a distinct constellation of emotions, beliefs, body sensations, memories, and behavioral tendencies, and with a specific role within that person's personality. Each part is capable of being interviewed as a separate individual, either by an outside person or from within by the aware core of that person. Parts are classified by function into those that protect the person (a protector part) from experiencing too much emotion and those that carry the emotions and vulnerability, often from childhood years (a vulnerable part).

Protector: *see* Part.

Patient-Centered Care (PCC): *IOM definition*—Providing care that is respectful of, and responsive to, individual patient preferences, needs, and values, and ensures that patients' values guide all clinical decisions. Now used as a broader concept than the original IOM definition to include shared decision making, health behavior change, and transfer of evidenced-based information to the patient. *Our updated definition*—Includes four interpersonal tasks—facilitation of health behavior change, facilitation of shared decision making, Information Interweave™, and clinician emotional self-care—with the integration of all four into the tasks of prevention, diagnostic assessment, and treatment.

Patient Decision Aids (PDAs): User-friendly information in multimedia forms about the illness, diagnostics, treatment, and outcomes. Material is focused on options and their pros and cons from evidence-based science, with specifics about what is not yet known. Companion audiovisual presentations include presentations by specialist clinicians and may include testimonials by patients. Please see the Index for a list of existing PDAs and international standards for their production.

Polarity or polarized parts: A set of personality parts with conflicting opposite emotions, beliefs, and behavioral tendencies that is in a variable state of consciousness within the personality. Another word used is *internal conflict*, but this term does not indicate so well that opposite parts are involved.

Processing: An integrative mind operation (like that of a computer) of enhancing perception, awareness, understanding, and regulation of whatever is coming up from within the mind and body of that person, including polarized and opposing personality parts and physiological responses.

Relationship: Can be either an interpersonal relationship or an internal relationship within the person (intrapersonal relationship) with parts of him- or herself. It involves connection and attunement with the other, and the perception that the other is a separate entity.

Self: (called "Aware Ego" by Hal and Sidra Stone) A natural function within all human minds that has the traits of calmness, curiosity, and the ability to be in a consciously aware, compassionate, and nonjudgmental relationship *with* other people and *with* all the parts of that person.

Shame: A feeling/emotion that goes with thinking, "I am a bad person"—as contrasted with *guilt*, which is driven by "I have behaved badly."

Shared Decision Making: *Trademarked version* (SDM®)—A free-choice-promoting process of sharing evidence-based information that also considers the patient's stated personal values (as if there is *one* mind). The strategy and tactical processes involved in communicating the information and for discovering the patient's values are not specified. *Emotion-imbued Decision Making* (Lerner et al., 2015)—Similar to the above, but enhances it by considering the patient's emotions as well as their values. *Updated definition*—An interpersonal facilitative process that promotes free choice in a multiplicity-of-mind paradigm by helping the patient to assimilate evidence-based information and to become aware of, and tolerate, their own conflicts/polarizations coming from their different parts that have been activated by having to make that decision.

Softens, or softens-back: A personality Part begins to become less intense, unblended, or psychologically a separate identity from the person within whom it exists; a process of conscious awareness that the Part is a part of them, not all of them, and that the person can be *with* their own Part rather than *be* the Part.

Space: An opening in awareness and inner experiencing (cognitive and emotional) of psychological phenomenon within.

Stable decision: A decision that does not change or swing, despite continuing conscious awareness of opposing forces, and that has the characteristic of tolerating, but not behaving, the emotions which arise. There are few surprises since most of the contingencies have been preprocessed cognitively and emotionally by the patient and loved ones. It does not mean that continuing concerns are not given a voice, but decision-remorse is not a high risk.

Stage model: Conceptualizes a process through time, in this case, behavior change, as occurring in discrete stages or steps that need to happen in linear order to reach the defined goal.

Strategy: A high-level plan of action designed to achieve specific goals under conditions of uncertainty, for example, an interview with a patient. Strategies can be based upon either hypotheses or theories, and are tools used in interviewing and testing scientific validity. The set of planned and systematic actions coordinated in time to be carried out to achieve a specific purpose.

Substantive (logic): A word or phrase without substance that is meant to function *only* as a noun in syntactical expression and, therefore, cannot be discovered as a *substantive physical entity* such as a region of the brain.

Sympathy: Although the authors rarely use the term, it means having a feeling similar to and in agreement with someone else's. It sometimes means to feel sorry for another.

System (systems theory): A person's *personality system*, the dynamic, interdependent, and interactive community of personality functions that operate in the mind. It also refers to the system of interactions between people which operate on the principle that if one aspect changes, others aspects must also shift.

Tactics: A specific set of verbal or action behaviors or methods or maneuvers designed to apply a certain strategy (and often the theory underlying it) to meet its goal.

Testable: Something that can be proven false. For a theory to be good for something, it must be possible to falsify that theory.

Theory: A well-substantiated explanation of some aspect of the world that is acquired through the scientific method and repeatedly confirmed through observation and experimentation. As with most (if not all) forms of scientific knowledge, scientific theories are inductive in nature, synthesize knowledge, and aim for predictive power and explanatory force. They may be in different degrees of validation. Psychological theories, similar to theoretical physics, remain potentially untestable for a long period of time because the farther the theory departs from everyday experience, the more effort has to be made to design suitable experiments. This is why researchers are always looking for "good hypotheses." Internal consistency of a theory, although reassuring, does not establish its validity. The common usage of the word *theory* implies that something is a guess: "Nice theory you've got there."

Tracking: The conscious following of the elements of some process through time.

Training: A process of skill acquisition based upon knowledge.

Verbal: Spoken words; can be used as *verbal sharing* with another person ("I feel hurt by what you did," "I feeling angry enough to burn this place down"). In contrast, *verbal behavior* is used *toward* other people ("You are an idiot," "Let's you and I burn down this place"). The difference between *verbal behavior* and *verbal sharing* (the latter being protected by the First Amendment) is pivotal to the impact on the other person. These two aspects of verbalization are often confused by the media and the law. Verbal behavior is not protected and is sometimes considered to be a crime; for example, verbal abuse, inciting a riot, racial slurring.

Vulnerability or vulnerable part: *see* Part.

References

Adolph K, Kretch K. 2012. *Gibson's Theory of Perceptual Learning.* New York: New York University. //psych.nyu.edu/adolph/publications.pdf

Affordable Care Act. 2010. Compilation of Patient Protection and Affordable Care Act, Section 3506. Washington, DC: U.S. Department of Health and Human Services.

Ajzen I. 1991. The theory of planned behavior. *Organ Behav Hum Dec* 50:179–211.

Alcauskas M, Charon R. 2008. Right brain: Reading, writing, and reflecting: Making a case for narrative medicine in neurology. *Neurology* 70(11):891–894.

Assagioli R. 1975. *Psychosynthesis: A Manual of Principles and Techniques.* London: Turnstone Press (originally 1965, New York: Viking).

Associated Press. 2014. *Overtreating Medicare Patients Costs $8 Billion. Associated Press*, May 16, 2014.

Badenoch B. 2008. *Being a Brain-Wise Therapist: A Practical Guide to Interpersonal Neurobiology.* New York: Norton.

Badino L et al. 2014. Computational validation of the motor contribution to speech perception. *Top Cognitive Sci* 1–15:1756–8765.

Baldwin C et al. 2008. Evidence-based holistic nursing practice. In *Holistic Nursing: A Handbook for Practice.* Dossey B and Keegan A (Eds). Burlington, MA: Jones and Bartlett.

Bandura A. 1997. *Self-efficacy.* New York: Freeman.

Bark L. 2011. *The Wisdom of the Whole: Coaching for Joy, Health, and Success.* San Francisco: Create Space Press.

Barrett LF. 2017. *How Emotions Are Made: The New Science of the Mind and Brain.* Boston: Houghton Mifflin Harcourt.

Barry MJ, Edgman-Levitan S. 2012. Shared decision making—the pinnacle of patient-centered care. *N Engl J Med* 366:780–781.

Bartol G, Courts N. 2009. The Psychophysiology of Body-Mind Healing. In *Holistic Nursing: A Handbook for Practice.* Dossey B and Keegan A (Eds). Burlington, MA: Jones and Bartlett.

Bekker H. 2010. The loss of reason in patient decision aid research: Do checklists damage the quality of informed choice interventions? *Patient Educ Couns* 78(3):357–364.

Black S. 2013. *Affect Labeling as an Emotion Regulation Mechanism of Mindfulness in the Context of Cognitive Models of Depression*. Dissertation. Shimrit K. Black, Temple University, August 2012.

Blalock S et al. 1996. Osteoporosis prevention in premenopausal women: Using a stage model appropriate to examine predictors of behavior. *Health Psychol* 15(2):84–92.

Bolby J. 1969. *Attachmènt and Loss*. 2nd edn. New York: Basic Books.

Braddock CH. 2010. The emerging importance and relevance of shared decision making in clinical practice. *J Med Decision Making*. 30(Supplement 1): 5s–7s.

Bradley E, Taylor L. 2013. *The American Health Care Paradox: Why Spending More Is Getting Us Less*. New York: Perseus.

Braten S. (Ed.) 2007. *On Being Moved: From Mirror Neurons to Empathy*. Amsterdam: John Benjamins.

Braten S. 2009. *The Intersubjective Mirror in Infant Learning and Evolution of Speech*. Amsterdam: John Benjamins.

Bretherton I. 1992. The origins of attachment theory: John Bowlby and Mary Ainsworth. *Dev Psychol* 28(5):759–775.

Brown B. 2010. *The Gifts of Imperfection: Let Go of Who You Think You're Supposed to Be and Embrace Who You Are*. Center City, MN: Hazelden.

Brown B. 2012. *Daring Greatly: How the Courage to Be Vulnerable Transforms the Way We Live, Love, Parent, and Lead*. New York: Gotham.

Brunero S et al. 2010. A review of empathy education in nursing. *Nurs Inq Mar* 17(1):65–74.

Burklund LJ et al. 2014. The common and distinct neural bases of affect labeling and reappraisal in healthy adults. *Frontiers Psychol* 5:221.

Carabetta M et al. 2013. Implementing primary care in the perianesthesia setting using a relationship-based care model. *J PeriAnesthesia Nurs* 28(1):16–20.

Caress A-L. 2003. Giving information to patients. *Nurs Standard* 17(43):47–54.

Carey B. 2015. Learning to see data. *New York Times*, Sunday Review, March 29, 2015.

Charon R. 2001. Narrative medicine: A model for empathy, reflection, profession, and trust. *JAMA* 286(15):1897–1902.

Chen Y et al. 2010. Correlated memory defects and hippocampal dendritic spine loss after acute stress involve corticotropin-releasing hormone signaling. *Proc Natl Acad Sci USA* 107(29):13123–13128.

Connolly C. 1944. (Palinurus: pseudonym) *The Unquiet Grave*. London: Hamish Hamilton.

Coy P. 2015. A way out of the vaccine wars. *Bloomberg Bus* February 9–15:12–13.

Cozolino L. 2010. Healing the social brain. In *The Neuroscience of Psychotherapy*, 2nd edn. New York: Norton.

Cozolino L. 2013. *The Social Neuroscience of Education: Optimizing Attachment & Learning in the Classroom*. New York: Norton.

Craig AD. 2009. How do you feel now? The anterior insula and human awareness. *Nat Rev Neurosci* 10(1):59–70.

Cropley S. 2012. The relationship-based care model: Evaluation of the impact on patient satisfaction, length of stay, and readmission rates. *J Nurs Admin* 42(6):333–339.

Damasio A. 1994. *Descartes' Error: Emotion Reason, and the Human Brain.* New York: Penguin.

Damasio A. 1999. *The Feeling of What Happens: Body and Emotion in the Making of Consciousness.* New York: Harcourt Brace.

Deci E, Ryan R. 2002. *Handbook of Self-Determination Research.* Rochester, NY: University of Rochester Press.

Deci EL, Ryan RM. 1985. *Intrinsic Motivation and Self-Determination in Human Behavior.* New York: Plenum.

Deliperi VI. 2011. The neural substrates of mindfulness: An fMRI investigation. *Soc Neurosci* 6(3):231–242.

Diamond L, Hicks A. 2005. Attachment style, current relationship security, and negative emotions: The mediating role of physiological regulation. *J Soc Pers Rels* 22:499–518.

Diamond L et al. 2011. Individual differences in vagal regulation moderate associations between daily affect and daily couple interactions. *Pers Soc Psychol Bull* 37(6):731–744.

Dolcos F, McCarthy G. 2006. Brain systems mediating cognitive interference by emotional distraction. *J Neurosci* 26(7):2072–2079.

Dossey B. and Keegan A (Eds). 2009. *Holistic Nursing: A Handbook for Practice,* 5th edn. Sudbury, MA: Jones & Bartlett Learning.

Drybye LN et al. 2010. Relationship between burnout and professional conduct and attitudes among US medical students. *JAMA* 304 (11):1173–1180.

Dugdale L. 2015. *Your Annual Checkup.* www.nytimes.com 2015/01/18/opinion/sunday/your-annual-checkup.html

Ecker B, Hulley L. 2011. *Coherence Therapy Practice Manual and Training Guide.* Oakland, CA: Coherence Psychology Institute.

Ecker B et al. 2012. *Unlocking the Emotional Brain: Eliminating Symptoms at Their Roots Using Memory Reconsolidation.* New York: Routledge.

Edwards A, Elwyn G. 2009. *Shared Decision Making in Health Care Achieving: Evidence-Based Patient Choice,* 2nd edn. UK: Oxford University Press.

Ekman P. 1989. The argument and evidence about universals in facial expressions of emotion. In *Handbook of Psychophysiology: Emotion and Social Behavior.* Wagner H, Manstead A (Eds). Sussex, UK: Wiley.

Elliott R et al. 2011. Empathy. *Psychotherapy* 48(1):43–49.

Ellman MS, Frotin AH. 2012. Benefits of teaching medical students how to communicate with patients having serious illness: Comparison of two approaches to experiential, skill-based, and self-reflective learning. *Yale J Biol Med* 85:261–270.

Elwyn G et al. 1999. Shared decision-making in primary care: The neglected second half of the consultation. *Br J Gen Pract* 49(443):477–482.

Elwyn G et al. 2012. Shared decision making: A model of clinical practice. *J Gen Intern Med* (10):1361–1367.

Entwistle VA, Watt IS. 2013 Treating patients as persons: A capabilities approach to support delivery of person-centered care. *Am J Bioeth* 13(8):29–39.

Epstein RM. 1999. Mindful practice. *JAMA* 282:833–839.

Erickson MF, Kurtz-Riemer K. 2005. *Infants Todlers, and Families: A Framework for Support and Intervention*. New York: Guilford.

Eslinger PJ. 1998. Neurological and neuropsychological bases of empathy. *Eur Neurol* 39:193–199.

Eslinger PJ et al. 2004. Developmental outcomes after early prefrontal cortex damage. *Brain Cogn* 55(1):84–103.

Fadiga L et al. 2009 . Broca's area in language, action, and music. *Ann NY Acad Sci*, 1169:448–458.

Fagerlin A. 2009. Getting down to details in the design and use of decision aids. *Med Decis Making* 29:409–411.

Fallowfield LJ et al. 2002. Efficacy of a cancer research UK communication skills training model for oncologists: A randomized controlled trial. *Lancet* 359(9307):650–656.

Feldman R et al. 2011. Mother and infant coordinate heart rhythms through episodes of interaction synchrony. *Inf Behav Dev* 34:569–577.

Feshback N. 1978. Studies of empathic behavior in children. In *Progress in Experimental Personality Research*, Maher BA (Ed). New York: Academic Press. Vol. 8, pp. 1–47.

Fisher R. 2011. Mindfulness in psychodynamic psychotherapy (Hakomi). *Therapist* Sept/Oct.

Figley CR (Ed.) 2002. *Treating Compassion Fatigue*. Psychosocial Stress Series. London: Routledge.

Foreman J. 2013. *A Nation in Pain: Healing Our Biggest Health Problem*. New York: Oxford University Press.

Fosha D et al. 2012. *The Healing Power of Emotion: Accelerated Experiential Dynamic Psychotherapy (AEDP)*. New York: Norton.

Fredrickson BL. 2013. Positive emotions broaden and build. *Adv Expl Soc Psychol* 47: 1–53.

Friedberg M et al. 2013. A demonstration of shared decision making in primary care highlights barriers to adoption and potential remedies. *Health Aff* 32(2):268–275.

Gallese V et al. 2007. Before and below theory of mind: Embedded simulation and the neural correlates of social cognition. *Biology* 362(1480):659–669.

Gebser J. 1986. *The Ever-Present Origin*. Parts One and Two. Ohio University Press.

Gerber AJ, Peterson BP. 2008. Applied brain imaging I; What is an image? *J Am Acad Child Adolesc Psychiatry* 47(3):245–248.

Gibson EJ, Pick AD. 2000. *An Ecological Approach to Perceptual Learning and Development*. New York: Oxford University Press.

Gigerenzer G. 2002. *Calculated Risks: How to Know When Numbers Deceive You*. New York: Simon & Schuster.

Gigerenzer G. 2007. *Gut Feelings: The Intelligence of the Unconscious*. New York: Viking Penguin.

Gladwell M. 2005. *Blink: The Power of Thinking Without Thinking*. Boston: Little, Brown.

Goel V, Dolan RJ. 2003. Reciprocal neural response within lateral and ventral medial prefrontal cortex during hot and cold reasoning. *Neuro Image* 20(4): 2314–2321.

Golden A, Djorgovski SG, Greally JM. 2013. Astrogenomics: Big data, old problems, old solutions? *Genome Biology* 14(8):129.

Goleman D. 1995. *Emotional Intelligence*. New York: Bantum Dell.

Goodman DJ. 2011. *Promoting Diversity and Social Justice: Educating People from Privileged Groups* (2nd edn). New York: Routledge.

Green J, Haidt J. 2002. How (and where) does moral judgment work? *Trends Cogn Sci* 6(12):517–523.

Green L, Mehr D. 1997. Heart disease predictive instrument: What alters physician's decisions to admit to the coronary care unit? *J Fam Pract* 45:219–226.

Green L, Yates J. 1995. Influence of pseudo-diagnostic information on the evaluation of ischemic heart disease. *Ann Emerg Med* 25:451–457.

Greenberg LS. 2010. Emotion-focused therapy: A clinical synthesis. Focus, VIII(1):32–42.

Guerlain S et al. 2004. Improving surgical pattern recognition through repetitive viewing of video clips. *IEEE Trans Systems Man Cybernetics–Part A: Systems Humans* 34(6):699–707.

Hagerty BM, Patusky KL. 2003. Reconceptualizing the nurse-patient relationship. *J Nurs Scholarship* 35:145–150.

Hale J et al. 2002. Theory of reasoned action. In *The Persuasion Handbook: Developments on Theory and Practice*. Dillard J, Pfau M (Eds). Thousand Oaks, CA: Sage.

Hammer GP et al. 2003. Low incidence and prevalence of hepatitis C virus infection among sexually active nonintravenous drug-using adults, San Francisco, 1997–2000. *Sex Transm Dis* 30(12):919–924.

Hariri AR et al. 2002. The amygdala response to emotional stimuli: comparison faces and scenes. *Neuroimage* 1:317–323.

Harlow H, Martyn J. 1868. Recovery from the passage of an iron bar through the head. *Publications Mass Med Soc* 2:327–347.

Harper G et al. 2015. Being with the patient: The use of "clinical evidence," reconsidered. From the committee on adolescence, group for the advancement of psychiatry. *J Nerv Ment Dis* 201:813–817.

Hebb DO. 1949. *The Organization of Behavior—A Neuropsychological Theory*. New York: Wiley.

Heekeren HR et al. 2003. An fMRI study of simple ethical decision-making. *Neuroreport* 14(9):1215–1219.

Heekeren HR et al. 2004. Influence of bodily harm on neural correlates of semantic and moral decision-making. *NeuroImage (Berlin)* 24:887–897.

Hendrix H. 1988. *Getting the Love You Want: Guide for Couples*. New York: Holt.

Herbine-Blank T. 2013. Self in relationship: An introduction to IFS couple therapy, in *Internal Family System Therapy: New Dimensions*. Sweezy M, Ziskind E (Eds), London: Routledge.

Herbine-Blank et al. 2015. *Intimacy from the Inside Out: Courage and Compassion in Couple Therapy.* London: Routledge.

Hibbard J et al. 2004. Development of the Patient Activation Measure (PAM): Conceptualizing and measuring activation in patients and consumers. *Hlth Serv Res.* 39(4 Pt 1):1005–1026.

Hibbard J et al. 2005. *Development and Testing of a Short Form of the Patient Activation Measure.* Health Research and Educational Trust.

Hirshberg LM et al. 2005. Emerging brain-based interventions for children and adolescents: Overview and clinical perspective. *Chil Adoles Psychiat Clin N Am* 12:1–19.

Hochbaum GM. 1958. *Public Participation in Medical Screening Programs: A Socio-Psychological Study.* Washigton, DC: Public Health Service.

House JS. 1988. Social relationships and health. *Science, New Series* 241(4865):540–545.

Hughes R. 2011. Overview and summary: Patient-centered care: Challenges and rewards. *OJIN* 16(2).

IFS Psychotherapy Research Adherence Scale. Available at: http://foundationifs.org/index.php/research/adherence-scale.html.

International Alliance of Patient Organizations (IAPO). 2006. *Declaration on Patient-Centered Healthcare.* Available at: www.iapo.org.uk/patient-centred-healthcare. Retrieved Dec. 13, 2014.

International Coaching Federation. 2013. *Code of Ethics.* Available at: www.coachfederation.org/ethics/n.d. (Accessed 2013).

IOM. 2011. *Crossing the Quality Chasm: A New Health System for the Twenty-First Century.* Washington, DC: The National Academies Press.

IOM. 2012. *Best Care at Lower Cost.* Smith M, Saunders R, Stuckhardt L, McGinnis JM (Eds). Washington, DC: The National Academies Press.

IOM. 2013. *Delivering High-Quality Cancer Care: Charting a New Course for a System in Crisis.* Levit LA, Balogh EP, Nass SJ, Ganz PA (Eds). Washington, DC: The National Academies Press. Available at: www.nap.edu.

IOM and NAE. 2011. *Engineering a Healthcare System: A Look at the Future: Workshop Summary.* Washington, DC: The National Academies Press.

Ivy AS et al., 2010. Hippocampal dysfunction and cognitive impairments provoked by chronic early-life stress involve excessive activation of CRH receptors. *J Neurosci* 30(39): 13005–13015.

Janz NK, Becker MH. 1984. The health belief model: A decade later. *Health Ed Q* 11:1–47.

Johnstone T et al. 2007. Failure to regulate: Counterproductive recruitment of top-down prefrontal-subcortical circuitry in major depression. *J Neurosci* 27(33):8877–8884.

Jordon M, Livingstone J. 2013. Coaching vs psychotherapy in health and wellness: Overlap, dissimilarities, and the potential for collaboration. *Global Adv Hlth Med* 2:16–23.

Kabat-Zinn J. 2007. *Full Catastrophe Living: Using the Wisdom of Your Body and Mind to Face Stress, Pain, and Illness.* London: Random House.

Kahneman D, Tversky A. 1979. Prospect theory: An analysis of decision under risk. *Econometrica* 47(2):263–292.

Karmiloff-Smith et al. 1995. Is there a social module? Theory of mind? *J Cog Neurosci* 7:196–208.

Karuza EA et al. 2014. Combining fMRI and behavioral measures to examine the process of human learning. *Neurobiol Learn Mem* 109:193–206.

Kassam K et al. 2013. Identifying emotions on the basis of neural activation. *PLoS One* 8(6):e66032. Retrieved from DOI 10:1371/journal.pone.0066032.

Kelley JM et al. 2010. The influence of the patient-clinician relationship on healthcare outcomes: A systematic review and meta-analysis of randomized controlled trials. *PLoS One* 9(4):e94207.

Keltner DT, Lerner JS. 2010. Emotion. In *The Handbook of Social Psychology*, Gilbert DT et al. (Eds). New York: Wiley. Vol.1, pp. 317–352.

Kim J, Diamond D. 2002. The stressed hippocampus, synaptic plasticity and lost memories. *Nature Rev Neurosci* 3:453–462.

Kirp D. 2014. Teaching is not a business. *New York Sunday Times*, August 16. Retrieved from www.nytJmes.com/2014/08/17/opinion/sunday/teaching-is-not-abusmess.htm

Kreofsky L. 2013. Engaging staff to engage patients: Patient engagement is essential for meaningful use, and studies show it is becoming more definitively linked to consumer satisfaction. *Health Mgmt Technol.* 34(2):12–13.

Kubler-Ross E. 1969. *On Death and Dying*. New York: Macmillan.

Kubler-Ross E. 2005. *On Grief and Grieving: Finding the Meaning of Grief through the Five Stages of Loss*. Boston: Simon and Schuster.

LeBlanc A et al. 2009. Decision conflict in patients and their physicians: A dyadic approach to shared decision making. *J Med Decision Making* 29(1):61–68.

Leibovich M. 2015. Being Hillary. *New York Sunday Times Magazine* July 19: 34–55.

Lenz E, Shortridge-Baggett L (Eds). 2002. *Self-Efficacy in Nursing*. New York: Springer.

Lerner JS et al. 2015. Emotion and decision making. *Annual Review of Psychology* 66:799–823.

Lieberman MD et al. 2007. Putting feelings into words: Affect labeling disrupts amygdala activity in response to affective stimuli. *Psychol Sci* 18(5):421–428.

Lieberman MD et al. 2011. Subjective responses to emotional stimuli during labeling, reappraisal, and distraction. *Emotion* 11(3):468–80.

Lieff J. 2013. *The Limits of Current Neuroscience*. Available at: jonlieff.com/blog.

Lipton BH. 2005. *The Biology of Belief: Unleashing the Power of Consciousness, Matter and Miracles*. San Rafael, CA: Elite Books.

Litvak P et al. 2006. Fuel in the fire: How anger impacts judgment and decision making. *J Behav Decision Making* 19:115–137.

Livingstone J. 1996. *Healthy Communication with Your Child: A Guide for Parents*. Washington, DC: American Academy of Pediatrics.

Livingstone J, Gaffney J. 2008. Outcome study of comparative efficacy using the Hibbard Patient Activation Measure (PAM) of enhanced health coach training (proprietary study awaiting consent to publish).

Livingstone J. 2009a. Medical decision making: Practitioner's curriculum for psychologically based skill building. In *Proceedings: 5th International Conference on Shared Decision Making Conference*. Boston, MA (Onlinelibrary.Wiley.com).

Livingstone J, Gaffney J. 2014. Health-related behavior change and decision making: Survey of relevant theories, methods and research since 1950 (Contact author for unpublished report and see Appendix for Theories and Methods Reviewed in the Design of SINHC.)

Livingstone J et al. 1968. Comprehensive child psychiatry through a team approach. *Children* 16(5):181–186.

Livingstone J et al. (Eds). 1995. *Portraying Enduring Love: Insights into Human Emotions for Creative Professionals*. Washington, DC: Institute for Mental Health Initiatives.

Livingstone JB. 2009b. Medical decision making: Practitioner's curriculum for psychological-based skill building. In *International Conference Informed Medical Decision Making*. Available at: www.isdm.confex.com/isdm/2009.

Livingstone JB. 2013. *Multiple Choice* by Alan Leo. *Harvard Med*. 86(1).

Livingstone JB, Gaffney J. 2013. IFS and health coaching: A new model of behavior change and medical decision making. In *Internal Family Systems Therapy: New Dimensions*. Sweezy M, Ziskind E (Eds). London: Routledge.

Livingstone JB, Wexler R. 2007. Building an enhanced behavior change model. Health Dialogue, Inc. Boston. Available from http://www.healthdialog.com/. Or send request to jlivingstoneservices@comcast.net

Loreg K. 2006. Action planning: A call to action. *J Am Board Family Med* 19(3):324–325.

Lowenstein G, Lerner JS. 2003. The role of affect in decision making. In *Handbook of Affective Science*. Davidson R et al. (Eds). New York: Oxford University Press, pp. 619–642.

Macmillan M. 2000. Nineteenth-century inhibitory theories of thinking: Bain, Ferrier, Freud (and Phineas Gage). *History Psychol* 3(3):187–217.

Mager R. 1962. *Preparing Instructional Objectives*. Belmont, CA: Fearon.

Maizis V et al. 2009. Integrative medicine and patient-centered care. (Commissioned for the IOM summit on integrative medicine and the health of the public.) *Explore: J Science and Health* 5:277–289.

Makoul G, Clayman ML. 2006. An integrative model of shared decision making in medical encounters. *Patient Ed Counsel* 60(3):301–312.

Malberg NT, Raphael-Leff J (Eds). 2011. *The Anna Freud Tradition: Lines of Development*. London: Karnac.

Marchese J. 2014. *How Jefferson's Stephen Klasko Intends to Fix Our Screwed-up Health-Care System*. Available at: www.phillymag/articlke/stephen-klasco-jefferson-future-health-care/.

Mariano C. 2013. *Holistic Nursing Scope and Standards of Practice 2nd edn*. 2013. AHNA and ANA.

Markland D et al. 2005. Motivational interviewing and self-determination theory. *J Soc Clin Psychol* 24(6):811–831.

Mather M, Lighthall NR. 2012. Risk and reward are processed differently in decisions made under stress. *Current Directions Psychol Sci* 21:36–41.

McCaffery KJ et al., Sydney Health Decision Group. 2007. Shared Decision-Making in Australia. *Z Arztl Fortbild Qualitatssich* 101(4):205–211.

McCaffery KL et al. 2010. The challenge of shared decision making among patients with lower literacy: A framework for research and development. *J Med Decision Making* 30(1):35–44.

Meier DE et al. 2001. The inner life of physicians and the care of the seriously ill. *JAMA* 286:3007–3014.

Melnyk BM et al., 2014. The establishment of evidence-based practice competencies for practicing registered nurses and advanced practice nurses in real-world settings. *Worldviews on Evidence-Based Nursing*, 11(1):5–15.

Melnyk BM et al. 2009. Evidence-based practice: Step by step—igniting a spirit of inquiry: An essential foundation for evidence-based practice. *AJN* 109(11):49–52.

Miller WR, Rollnick S. 2002. *Motivational Interviewing: Preparing People to Change*. New York: Guilford.

Miller WR, Rollnick S. 2012. *Motivational Interviewing: Helping People Change*, 3rd edn. New York: Guilford.

Minsky M. 1986. *The Society of Mind*. New York: Simon & Schuster.

Molnar-Szakacs I et al. 2006. Observing complex action sequences: The role of the fronto-parietal mirror neuron system. *NeuroImage* 33(2006):923–935.

Montague PR et al. 2002. Hyperscanning: Simultaneous fMRI during linked social interactions. *NeuroImage* 16(4):1159–1164.

Morelli SA et al. 2012. The neural components of empathy: Predicting daily prosocial behavior. *Soc Cogn Affect Neurosci* 9: 39–47.

Morgan JK et al. 2014. Maternal depression and warmth during childhood predict age 20 neural response to reward. *J Child Adoles Psychiat* 53:108–116.

Mumford E et al. 1981. Reducing medical costs through mental ehalth treatment: Research problems and recommendations. In *Linking Health and Mental Health*. Broskowski A et al. (Eds). Beverly Hills, CA: Sage.

National Consortium for Credentialing Health and Wellness Coaches (NCCHWC). Available at: www.ncchwc.org.

Nishitani N, Hari R. 2002. Viewing lip forms: Cortical dynamics. *Neuron* 36(6):1211–1220.

Nurse.com. 2014. List of 24 competencies helps nurses with evidence-based care. Available at: https://news.nurse.com/2014/01/26/list-of-24-competencies-helps-nurses-with-evidence-based-care/.

Nurses Take on New and Expanded Roles in Health Care. 2015. RWJF Newsletter, January 20, 2015, page 1. Available at: www.rwjf.org/en/library/articles-and-news/2015/01/nurses-take-on-new-and-expanded-roles-in-health-care.html.

NYTimes. 2014. Available at: www.nytimes.com/2014/09/28/opinion/sunday/doctors-billing-practices.html.

O'Connor AH et al. 2003. Decision aids for people facing health treatment or screening decisions. *Cochrane Database Rev.* 2003(2):CD001431.

O'Connor AM et al. 2004. Modifying unwarranted variations in health care: Shared decision making using patient decision aids. *Hlth Aff* October 7.

O'Connor AM, Edwards A. 2001. *The Role of Decision Aids in Promoting Evidence-Based Patient Choice, in Evidence-Based Choice: Inevitable or Impossible?* Oxford: Oxford University Press, pp. 220–242.

Ofri D. 2013. *What Doctors Feel*. Boston: Beacon Press.

Olds J, Schwartz RS. 2010. *The Lonely American: Drifting Apart in the Twenty-First Century*. Boston: Beacon Press.

Osler W Sir. 1892. *The Principles and Practice of Medicine*. New York: Appleton.

Peabody FW. 1927. The care of the patient. *JAMA* 88(12):877–882.

Pennebaker J. 2004. *Writing to Heal: A Guided Journal for Recovering from Trauma and Emotional Upheaval*. Oakland, CA: New Harbinger.

Pennebaker JW (Ed.) 1995. *Emotion, Disclosure and Health*. Washington, DC: American Psychological Association.

Pettinati P. 2002. The relative efficacy of various complementary modalities in the lives of patients with chronic pain. *J US Assoc of Body Psychother* 1(2):6–15.

Phillips E. 2015. *Health Coaching in Life Style Medicine*. Tools for Promoting Healthy Change, Harvard Medical School CME Program, June 2015.

Phillips M, Drevets WC, Rauch SL, Lane R. 2003. Neurobiology of emotion perception I: The neural basis of normal emotion perception. *Biol Psych* 54(5): 504–514.

Porges SW. 2011. *The Theory: Neurophysiological Foundation of Emotions, Attachment, Communication, and Self-Regulation*. New York: Norton.

President's Commission. 1978. President's Commission for the Study of Ethical Problems in Medicine & Biomedical & Behavioral Research. US Dept HHS.

Prochaska J, Norcross J, Di Clemente C. 1994. *Changing for Good*. New York: HarperCollins/William Morrow.

Prochaska JO et al. 2008. Initial efficacy of MI, TTM tailoring, and HRI's in multiple behaviors for employee health promotion. *Preventive Medicine;* 46,226–231.

Rakowski W et al. 1996. Consideration for extending the transtheoretical model of behavior change to screening mammography. *Health Education Research*, 11(1):77–96.

Ramachandran VS. 2011. *The Tell-Tale Brain: A Neuroscientist's Quest for What Makes Us Human*. New York: Norton.

Regehr CD et al. 2014. Interventions to reduce the consequences of stress in physicians: A review and meta-analysis. *J Nervous Mental Dis* 202(5):353–359.

Riess H et al. 2011. Improving empathy and relational skills in otolaryngology residents: A pilot study. *Otolaryngol Head Neck Surg* 144(1):120–122.

Riess H et al. 2012. Empathy training for resident physicians: A randomized controlled trial of a neuroscience-informed curriculum. *J Gen Intern Med* 27(10):1280–1286.

Rinaman L et al. 2011. Early life experience shapes the functional organization of stress-responsive visceral circuits. *Physiol Behav* 104(4):632–640.

Rizzolatti G, Arbib M. 1998. Language within our grasp. *Trends Neurosci* 21(5):188–194.

Roberts Woods Johnson Foundation. 2015. Nurses take on new and expanded roles in health care. *Robert Wood Johnson Foundation Newsletters.* Retrieved from: rwjf.org/en/newsletters/advances.html.

Rosenstock IM et al. 1988. Social learning theory and the health belief model. *Hlth Ed Q* 15(2):175–183.

Rowan J. 1990. *Sub-Personalities: The People Inside Us.* London: Routledge.

Rubenfeld I. 2000. *The Listening Hand: Self-Healing Through the Rubenfeld Synergy Method of Talk and Touch.* New York: Batham.

Rushworth MF, Behrens TE. 2008. Choice, uncertainty and value in prefrontal and cingulate cortex. *Nat Neurosci* 11(4):389–397.

Ruttle PL et al. 2014. Adolescent internalizing symptoms and negative life events: The sensitizing effects of earlier life stress and cortisol. *Dev Psychopathol* 26:1411–1422.

Ryan RM, Deci EL. 2000. Self-determination theory and the facilitation of intrinsic motivation, social development, and well-being. *Am Psychol* 55:68–78.

Sanchez-Reilly S et al. 2013. Caring for oneself to care for others: physicians and their self-care. *J Support Oncol* 11:75–81.

Schore AN. 2003. *Affect Regulation and the Repair of the Self.* New York: Norton.

Schwartz J, Brennan W. 2013. *There's a Part of Me—.* Illinois: Trailheads.

Schwartz RC. 1987. Our multiple selves. *Fam Therapy Networker,* 11(25-31):80–83.

Schwartz RC. 1995. *Internal Family Systems Therapy.* New York: Guildford.

Schwartz RC. 2008.*You Are the One You Have Been Waiting For: Bringing Courageous Love to Intimate Relationships.* Oak Park, IL: Trailhead.

Schwartz RC. 2013. The therapist-client relationship and the transformative power of self. In *Internal Family Systems Therapy New Dimensions.* Sweezy M, Ziskind E (Eds). London: Routledge.

Shadick NA et al. 2013. A randomized controlled trial of an internal family systems-based psychotherapeutic intervention on outcomes in rheumatoid arthritis: A proof-of-concept study. *J Rheumatol.* 40(11):1831–1841.

Shah I. 1965. *The Exploits of the Incomparable Mulla Nasrudin.* London: Jonathan Cape.

Shapiro F. 2002. EMDR 12 years after its introduction: Past and future research. *J Clin Psychol* 58(1):1–22.

Siegel D. 2011. *Mindsight: The New Science of Personal Transformation.* New York: Bantam.

Siegel D, Hartzel M. 2003. *Parenting from the Inside Out,* New York: Penguin.

Siegel D, Solomon M (Eds). 2013. *Healing Moments in Psychotherapy.* New York: Norton.

Sowell N. 2013. Changing the course of chronic illness: The internal family system and adult health. In *Internal Family Systems Therapy: New Dimensions.* Sweezy M, Ziskind E (Eds). London: Routledge.

Spratling M, Johnson M. 2006. A feedback model of perceptual learning and categorization. *Vis Cognit* 13(2):129–165.

Steinbeck J. 1939. *The Grapes of Wrath.* New York: Viking.

Steinbeck J. 1941. *The Sea of Cortez.* New York: Viking.

Steinbeck J. 1945. *Cannery Row.* New York: Viking.

Steinbeck J, Ricketts EF. 1999. *The Log from Sea of Cortez.* New York: Penguin.

Stone H, Stone S. 1993. *Embracing your Inner Critic.* San Francisco, CA: Harper-Collins.

Stone H, Stone S. 2000. *Partnering: A New Kind of Relationship.* Novato, CA: New World Library.

Stone H, Winkelman S. 1985. *Embracing Our Selves: The Voice Dialogue Manual.* Marina del Rey, CA: DeVross.

Stone H, Winkelman S. 1989. *Embracing Each Other: Relationship as Teacher, Healer and Guide.* San Rafael, CA: New World Library.

Strecher VJ et al. 2008. Web-based smoking cessation program: Results of a randomized trial. *American Journal of Preventive Medicine.* 10(5):e36. doi: 10.2196/jmir.1002.

Scherer YK et al. 1998. The effects of education alone and in combination with pulmonary rehabilitation on self-efficacy in patients with COPD. *Rehabil Nurs,* 23(2):71–77.

Stuart-Shor E, Wells-Federman C. 2009. Cognitive therapy. In *Holistic Nursing: A Handbook for Practice,* 5th edn. Dossey B and Keegan A (Eds). Sudbury, MA: Jones & Bartlett Learning.

Stuss DT, Knight RT (Eds). 2002. *Principles of Frontal Lobe Function.* New York: Oxford University Press.

Suchman A, Sluyter D, Williamson P (Eds). 2011. *Leading Change in Healthcare: Transforming Organizations with Complexity, Positive Psychology and Relationship-Centered Care.* Abingdon, UK: Radcliffe.

Sweezy M, Ziskind E (Eds). 2013. *Internal Family Systems Therapy: New Dimensions.* New York: Routledge/Taylor & Francis.

Tanaka JY et al. 2008. Protein synthesis and neurotropin-dependent structural plasticity of single dendritic spines. *Science* 319:1683–1687.

Thompson M et al. 2010. *Focusing on Health Care Value. pwc.com/us/en/view/issue12/focusing on health care-value.jhtml.*

Treadway MT, Lazar SW. 2009. *The Neurobiology of Mindfulness.* New York: Springer.

Tresolini CP. 1994. *The Pew-Fetzer Task Force: Health Professions Education and Relationship-Centered Care.* San Francisco, CA: Pew Charitable Trust. Available at: www.futurehealth.ucsf.edu/pdf_files/RelationshipCentered.pdf

Tronick EZ. 2003. Things still to be done on the still face effect. *Infancy,* 4(4):475–482.

Vaknin S. 2010. *Neuro Linguistic Programming.* Prague: Inner Patch Publishing.

van der Kolk B. 2014. *The Body Keeps the Score: Brain, Mind, and Body in the Healing of Trauma*. New York: Viking/Penguin.

Waal F. 2009. *The Age of Empathy: Nature's Lessons for a Kinder Society*. New York: Broadway.

Wachtel PL. 2010. Beyond "ESTs": Problematic assumptions in the pursuit of evidence-based practice. *Psychoanal Psychol* 27(3):251–272.

West R. 2005. Time for a change: Putting the transtheoretical model to rest. *Addiction* 100:1036–1039,1040–105.

Weisman O et al. 2012. Oxytocin administration to parent enhances infant physiological and behavioral readiness for engagement. *Biol Psychiat* 72:982–989.

Wennberg D et al. 2010. A randomized trial of a telephone care-management strategy. *New Engl J Med* 363:1245–1255.

Williams KD et al. 2000. Cyberostracism: Effects of being ignored over the internet. *J Personality Soc Psychol* 79(5):748–762.

Winsett RP, Hauck S. 2011. Implementing relationship-based care. *J Nurs Admin* 41(6):285–290.

Wise A. 2002. *Awakening the Mind: A Guide to Harnessing the Power of Your Brainwaves*. New York: Tarcher.

Wolever R et al. 2010. Integrative health coaching for patients with type 2 diabetes: A randomized controlled clinical trial. *Diabetes Ed* 36(4):629–639.

Wolever R et al. 2011. What is health coaching anyway? *Arch Intern Med* 2011:171–178.

Wolever R et al. 2013. A systemic review of the literature on health and wellness coaching: Defining a key behavioral intervention in health care. *Global Adv Hlth Med* 2:34–53.

Wolf NS et al. 2001. The developmental trajectory from amodal perception to empathy and communication: The role of mirror neurons in this process. *Psychoan Inq* 21(1):94–112.

Woolf SH, Aron L (Eds). 2013. *U.S. Health in International Perspective: Shorter Lives, Poorer Health*. National Research Council and Institute of Medicine, Washington, DC: The National Academies Press. Available at: www.nap.edu.

Wright B. 2004. Compassion fatigue: How to avoid it. *Palliat Med* (18):3–4.

Wright R. 1986. A better mental model. *The Sciences* 26–28.

Wylie MS, Turner L. 2015. The attuned therapist: Does attachment theory really matter? *Psychother Networker*.

Zald DH, Rauch SL. 2006. *The Orbitofrontal Cortex*. New York: Oxford University Press.

Zikmund-Fisher BJ et al. 2010. The decisions study: A nationwide survey of United States adults regarding 9 common medical decisions. *J MDM* 30(supplement):4S–106S.

Zinker J. 1978. *Creative Process in Gestalt Therapy*. New York: First Vintage.

RESOURCES

Apple LJ et al. 2011. Comparative effectiveness of weight-loss interventions in clinical practice. *N Engl J Med* 365:1960–1968.

Armitage CJ, Conner M. 2001. Efficacy of the theory of planned behavior: A meta-analytic review. *Brit J Psychol* 40:471–499.

Arnold MB (Ed.). 1970. *Feelings and Emotions: The Loyola Symposium of Chicago*, New York: Academic Press.

Berwick DM 2009. What "patient-centered" should mean: Confessions of an extremist. *Health Affairs* w555–w565. Available at: http://www.ncmhcso.org/downloads/berwick-ha-w555.pdf. Retrieved May 23, 2010.

Bird J, Cohen-Cole SA. The three-dimension model of the medical interview. In *Methods in Teaching Consultation-Liaison Psychiatry*. Hale MS et al. (Eds). Basel: Karger. pp. 65–88.

Borland R et al. 2003. The effectiveness of personalized smoking cessation strategies for callers to a Quitline Service. *Addiction* 98:837–846.

Botelho R. 2004. *Motivate Health Habits: Stepping Stone to Lasting Change*, 2nd edn. Rochester, New York: MHH.

Bouton ME. 2004. Context and behavioral processes in extinction 2004. *Learn Mem* 11:485–494.

Bundy C. 2004. Changing behaviour: Using motivational interviewing techniques. *J R Soc Med* 97(Suppl. 44):43–47.

Carrión VG et al. 2010. Reduced hippocampal activity in youth with posttraumatic stress symptoms: An fMRI study. *J Pediatr Psychol.* 35:559–569.

Clerget E et al. 2009. Role of Broca's area in encoding sequential human actions: A virtual lesion study. *Neuroreport* 20(16):1496–1499.

Cole SW. 2013. Social regulation of human gene expression: Mechanisms and implications for public health. *American J Public Hlth* 103 Suppl 1(41):S84–S92.

Coulter A, Collins A. 2011. *Making Shared Decision-Making a Reality: No Decision about Me, without Me*. London: The King's Fund.

Cozolino L. 2012. Attachment and the Developing Social Brain. In *The Neuroscience of Human Relationships*, 2nd edn. New York: Norton.

Cozolino L. 2014. *Attachment-Based Teaching*. New York: Norton.

Efferen L et al. 2012. The case for empathy training. *Health Care News*, June 18, 2012.

Engel GL. 1980. The clinical application of the biopsychosocial model. *Am J Psychiatry* 137(5):535–44.

Epstein RM et al. 2009. Beyond information: Exploring patient's preferences. *JAMA* 302(2):195–197.

Finnegan J, Viswanath K. 1997. Communication theory and health behavior change. In *Health Behavior and Health Education*, 2nd edn. Glanz K (Ed). San Francisco, CA: Jossey-Bass.

Fjortoft N et al. 2011. Measuring empathy in pharmacy students. *Am J Pharm Educ* 75(6):109.

Fortin AH et al. 2002. Teaching pre-clinical medical students an integrated approach to medical interviewing: Half-day workshops using actors. *J Gen Intern Med* 17(9):704–708.

Foundation Informed Medical Decision-Making. Available at: www.fimdm.org/decision_sdms.php.

Frosch DL et al. 2012. Authoritarian physicians and patients' fear of being labeled "difficult" among key obstacles to shared decision making. *Health Aff* 31(5):1030–1038.

Glaser B, Strauss A. 1967. *The Discovery of Grounded Theory: Strategies for Qualitative Research*. Italy: Aldine Press.

Glass DC. 1977. Behavior patterns, stress and coronary disease. In *The Handbook of Emotion and Memory Research*, Christiansen S (Ed). Hillsdale, NJ: Erlbaum. pp. 359–387. (Latest edition of *The Handbook*, 2014, New York: Psychology Press).

Glass J et al. 2005. Memory beliefs and function in fibromyalgia patients. *J Psychosomat Res* 58(3):263–269.

Gordon I et al. 2014. From attachment to groups: Tapping into the neurobiology of our interconnectedness. *J Child Adoles Psychiat* 53:130–132.

Grossmann KE et al. 2005. *Attachment from Infancy to Adulthood: The Major Longitudinal Studies*. New York: Guilford.

Han S, Lerner JS 2009. *Decision Making. Oxford Companion to the Affective Sciences*, UK: Oxford University Press.

Handler JA, Gillam M, Sanders AS, Klasco R. 2000. Defining, identifying, and measuring error in emergency medicine. *Acad Emerg Med* 7(11):1183–1187.

Handmaker NS et al. 1999. Findings of a pilot study of motivational interviewing with pregnant drinkers. *J Stud Alcohol* 60(2):285–287.

Hanson JL et al. 2015. Behavioral problems after early life stress: Contributions of the hippocampus and amygdala. *Biol Psychiatry* 77(4):314–323.

Harre R, Parrot WG (Eds). 1996. *The Emotions: Social, Cultural and Biological Dimensions*. London: Sage.

Hill RW, Castro E. 2009. *Healing Young Brains: The Neurofeedback Solution*. Charlotsville, VA: Hampton Roads.

Izard CE. 1993. Four systems for emotion activation: Cognitive and noncognitive processes. *Psychol Rev* 100(1):68–90.

Kean S. 2014. *Phineas Gage, Neuroscience's Most Famous Patient*. Washington, DC: Slate.

Keltner D et al. 2014. *Understanding Emotions*. Hoboken, NJ: Wiley.

Lazar NA et al. 2007. Statistical issues in fMRI for brain imaging. *Int Stat Rev* 69(1):105–127.

Légaré F et al. 2011. Interprofessionalism and shared decision-making in primary care: A stepwise approach towards a new model. *J Interprofessional Care* 25(1):18–25.

Legare F et al. 2013. Core competencies for shared decision making training programs: Insights from an international, interdisciplinary working group. *J Cont Ed Health Professions* 33(4):267–273.

Leventhal H et al. 1980. The common sense representation of illness danger. In *Contributions to Medical Psychology*, Rachman S (Ed). New York: Pergamon Press. Vol. 2, pp. 7–30.

McCance T et al. 2011. An exploration of person-centredness in practice. *OJIN* 16(2), Manuscript 1.

McCormack B. 2006. Development of a framework for person-entered nursing. *J Adv Nurs* 56(5):472–479.

McMillian M. 2008. Phineas gage-unraveling the myth. *The Psychologist* 21(9):828–831.

Michels KB et al. 2013. Recommendations for the design and analysis of epigenome-wide association studies. *Nature Meth* 10(10):949–955.

Miller WR, Rose GS. 2009. Toward a theory of motivational interviewing. *Am Psychol* 64(6):527–537.

Miller WR et al. 1994. *Motivational Enhancement Therapy Manual*. Washington, DC: National Institute on Alcohol Abuse and Alcoholism.

Miller WR et al. (Eds). 2000. *Motivational Enhancement Therapy: Description of Counseling Approach*. National Institute on Drug Abuse, pp. 89–93.

Park DC et al. 2001. Cognitive function in fibromyalgia patients. *Arthritis Rheum.* 44(9):2125–2133.

Pennebaker JW. 1997. *Opening Up: The Healing Power of Expressing Emotions* (Rev. edn). New York: Guilford.

Pennebaker JW et al. 1983. Disclosure of trauma and immune function: Health implication of psychotherapy. *J Consult Clin Psychol* 56(2):239–245.

Phelps EA et al. 2004. Role of the amygdala and vmPFC. *Neuron* 43:897–905.

Potter J. 2015. Self-discovery: A toolbox to help clinicians communicate with clarity, curiosity, creativity, and compassion. In *The Fenway Guide to Lesbian, Gay, Bisexual and Transgender Health*, 2nd edn, Makadon H et al. (Eds). Philadelphia, PA: American College of Physicians.

Prochaska JO, Velicer WR. 1997. The transtheoretical model of health behavior change. *Am J Health Prom* 12:38–48.

Puetz V et al. 2014. Neural response to social rejection in children with early separation experiences. *J Am Acad Child Adoles Psychiat* 53(12):1328–1337.

Rowan J, Cooper M. 1999. *The Plural Self: Multiplicity in Everyday Life*. London: Sage.

Ruland CM et al. 2013. Evaluation of different features of an eHealth application for personalized illness management support: Cancer patients' use and appraisal of usefulness. *Int J Med Inform* 82(7):593–603.

Salzburg Statement on Shared Decision Making. 2011. Salzburg global seminar. *BMJ* 342:1745.

Sanbonmatsu D et al. 2011. On the importance of knowing your partner's views. *Ann Behav Med* 41:131–137.

Schore JR, Shore AN. 2008. Modern attachment theory: The central role of affect regulation in development and treatment. *Clin Soc Work* 36:9–20.

Sepucha K et al. 2008. Developing instruments to measure the quality of decisions: Early results for a set of symptom-driven decisions. *Patient Educ Counsel.* 73(3):504–510.

Sepucha K et al. 2009. Is there a role for decision aids in advanced breast cancer? *Med Decision Making* 29:475–482.

Shamboliev R. 1992. *The Energetics of Voice Dialogue.* Mendocino, CA: LifeRhythm.

Sharpe L. 2013. Psychological treatment for rheumatoid arthritis works: Now we need to know what elements are most effective and for whom. *J Rheumatol* 40(11):1788–1790.

Stechler G. 2000. Louis W. Sander and the question of affective presence. *Infant Mental Hlth J* 21(1–2):75–84.

Stewart MA. 1996. Effective physician-patient communication and health outcomes: A review. *Can Med Assoc J* 152:1423–1433.

Thevos AK, Quick RE. 2000. Application of motivational interviewing to the adoption of water disinfection practices in Zambia. *Hlth Prom Int* 15:207–214.

Watkins J, Johnson RJ. 1982. *We, the Divided Self.* New York: Irvington.

Weinstein ND. 1988. The precaution adoption process. *Hlth Psychol* 7:355–386.

Weinstein ND et al. 1998a. Stage theories of health behavior: Conceptual and methodological issues. *Hlth Psychol* 17:290–299.

Weinstein ND et al. 1998b. Experimental evidence of stages of health behavior change: The precaution adoption process model applied to home radon testing. *Hlth Psychol* 17(5):445–453.

Wilson SE et al. 2012. Empathy levels in first and third year students in health and nonhealth disciplines. *Am J Pharm Ed* 76(2):24.

Yeates KO et al. 2007. Social outcomes in childhood brain disorder: A heuristic integration of social neuroscience and developmental psychology. *Psychol Bull* 133(3):535–556.

Yourcenar M. 1995. *Memoirs of Hadrian* (trans Fink G.). New York: Modern Library/Random House.

Appendix

SINHC® (SELF-AWARE INFORMATIONAL NONJUDGMENTAL HEALTH COACHING)

Theories and Methods Reviewed in the Design of SINHC

- TTM-SOC (Transtheoretical Model—Stages of Change) Prochaska, DiClemente
- PAPM (Precaution Adoption Process Model) Weinstein and Sandman
- POCM (Perspectives on Change Model) Borland
- STM (Synthetic Theory of Motivation) West
- MVMT (Multiplicity-View of Mind Theory) Stone, Schwartz, Watkins, and Johnson
- PSAE (Psychology of the Selves and the Aware Ego) Hal and Sidra Stone
- IFS (Internal Family Systems) Model RC Schwartz
- HBM (Health Belief Model) Becker and Janz
- SRM (Self-Regulatory Model) Leventhal
- SET (Self-Efficacy Theory) Bandura
- SDT (Self-Determination Theory) Ryan and Deci
- TPB (Theory of Planned Behavior—a modernized Theory of Reasoned Action) Fishbein and Ajzen
- CT (Communication Theory) Lasswell and others
- SM (Social Marketing) and CHC (Consumer-Based Health Communications) Lefebvre, Flora
- MI (Motivational Interviewing) and AMI (adapted MI) Miller and Rollnick
- RSM (Rubenfeld Synergy Method) Ilana Rubenfeld
- VD (Voice Dialogue) and Psychology of the Selves, Based on Mind Multiplicity Hal and Sidra Stone
- MM (Mindfullness in Medicine) Kabat-Zinn
- GI (Guided Imagery) Naparstek
- MHH (Motivate Health Habits) Botelho

- Health Media Research Lab, Strecher
- Weight Watchers Programs
- 12-Step Programs (AA, GA) Shaffer
- ARRM (AIDS Risk Reduction Method) Catania (modification of PAPM for use with AIDS)
- PAM (Patient Activation Measure) Hibbard (for research; applies SDT)
- Hodgins (gambling addiction, applies MI)
- Lorig (applies SET in osteoarthritis)
- Lenz (applies SET in diabetes)
- Thevos (adapted and applied MI and SM in public health)
- EAM (Enhanced Awareness Model) developed by Health Dialog, Inc. and Gaffney and Livingstone
- BE (Behavioral Engagement) and Pure Presence (a relational connection and attachment approach) Donadio
- PD & IH (Psychodrama: based on mind multiplicity and Integrative Health) Lelio Marino

Societies and Journals

Society of Medical Decision Making
  Medical Decision Making, www.smdm.org

Society of Behavioral Medicine
  Annals of Behavioral Medicine, www/springerlink.com
  Translational Behavioral Medicine, www.springerlink.com

Emotions and Decision Making Group: Harvard University
Informed Medical Decisions Foundation: Healthwise
International Society for Evidence-Based Healthcare: Sydney, Australia

Professionals Involved with a Current National Initiative in Health Coaching

1. Michael Arloski (Real Balance)*
2. Linda Bark (Bark Training Institute)*
3. Michael Burke (Mayo Clinic)
4. Robert Crocker (University of Arizona)
5. Margaret Erickson (American Holistic Nurses Credentialing Corporation)
6. Billy Francis (Mindful Coaching)
7. Meg Jordon (California Institute of Integral Studies)*
8. Karen Lawson (University of Minnesota Medical School)*
9. John Livingstone (Harvard Medical School)*
10. Susan Luck (University of Arizona)
11. Linda Manning (Vanderbilt)
12. Magdalena (Magda) Mook (International Coach Federation)
13. Margaret Moore (Well Coaches and McLean Hospital)*

14. Cerrie Phelps (Intrinsic Coaching, YMCA, National Wellness Institute)
15. David Rychener (Whole Health Coaching Course)
16. Linda Smith (Duke Integrative Medicine)*
17. Jim Strohecker (Wellness Inventory)
18. Darlene Trandell (Well Coaches and Mentor Coaching)
19. Cheryl Walker (Maryland University of Integrative Health) Maryland University of Integrative Health
20. Ruth Wolever (Duke Integrative Medicine)*

* Board of Directors member.

INSTITUTE OF MEDICINE (IOM) STATEMENT OF 2012*

A 2012 IOM report on overall US health spending concluded that about 30 percent, or $750 billion, reflects overtreatment, excessive costs, and other problems.

The new study also follows the government's release last month of Medicare billing records for 880,000 physicians and other health care providers, data that consumer advocates and others said might indicate whether some doctors are providing quality cost-effective care or ordering needless services. That data revealed vast differences in Medicare payments, and an agency administrator said Medicare would look into doctors and others who received huge reimbursements, which could suggest overtreatment.

Reasons and Reactions

The authors of *Best Care at Lower Cost*, the 2012 IOM report, said it's not clear why doctors may be ordering needless services, but that sometimes patients may demand procedures they mistakenly think will benefit them.

Doctors also get paid more for ordering more procedures. Fear of malpractice lawsuits is also often cited as contributing to overtreatment.

Policymakers, doctors, and patients should pay attention to the results, the researchers said.

Patients should know they can question their doctors about which procedures are really necessary and whether less invasive and less costly options are available.

PATIENT DECISION AIDS

Library of Shared Decision Making Patient Decision Aid Programs by Health Dialog Services Corporation†:

Acute Low Back Pain: Managing Your Pain Through Self-Care
Chronic Low Back Pain: Managing Your Pain and Your Life

---

* Institute of Medicine: http://www.iom.edu, also www.nap.edu.
† Acquired by Rite Aid in 2014.

Herniated Disc: Choosing the Right Treatment for You
Spinal Stenosis: Choosing the Right Treatment for You
*Managing Early-Stage Knee Osteoarthritis**
*Your Bones: Preventing Another Fracture**
Treatment Choices for Hip Osteoarthritis
Treatment Choices for Knee Osteoarthritis
*Treatment Choices for Torn Meniscus: After Age 40**
Managing Menopause: Choosing Treatments for Menopause Symptoms
Treatment Choices for Abnormal Uterine Bleeding
Treatment Choices for Uterine Fibroids
Breast Reconstruction: Is It Right for You?
Ductal Carcinoma In Situ: *Choosing Your Treatment*
Early-Stage Breast Cancer: Choosing Your Surgery
Living with Metastatic Breast Cancer: Making the Journey Your Own
*Heart Tests: Learning about Your Choices**
Living with Coronary Heart Disease
Living with Heart Failure: Helping Your Heart Day-to-Day
Treatment Choices for Stable Chest Discomfort
*Treatment Choices for Peripheral Artery Disease**
*Treatment Choices for Carotid Artery Disease**
Living Better with Chronic Pain
Living with Diabetes: Making Lifestyle Changes to Last a Lifetime (Spanish
  version available)
Sleeping Better: Help for Long-Term Insomnia
Coping with Symptoms of Depression
Help for Anxiety: Treatments That Work
Colon Cancer Screening: Deciding What's Right for You
Benign Prostatic Hyperplasia: Choosing Your Treatment
Hormone Therapy: When the PSA Rises after Prostate Cancer Treatment
Is a PSA Test Right for You?
*Treatment Choices for Localized Prostate Cancer**
Benign Prostatic Hyperplasia: Choosing Your Treatment
Growing Older, Staying Well
*Advance Directives***
Looking Ahead: Choices for Medical Care When You're Seriously Ill

Additional resource: Ottawa Health Research Institute, A–Z Inventory of Decision Aids. Available at: decisionaid.ca/AZinvent.php (July 15, 2004).
Standards: International Patient Decision Aids Standards (IPDAS). Available at: http://ipdas.ohri.ca/.

PATIENT-CENTERED CARE

The Institute of Medicine (IOM) has set a goal that 90 percent of all patient-care decisions be based on evidence by 2020. The Affordable Care Act calls for reimbursable treatments to adhere to evidence-based recommendations made by the

US Preventive Services Task Force. Despite these efforts, evidence-based practice (EBP) is far from being universally embraced in many health care settings, according to the news release (Nurse.com, 2014).

Don Berwick, formerly of Centers for Medicare and Medicaid Services, defined patient-centered care as, "The experience (to the extent the informed, individual patient desires it) of transparency, individualization, recognition, respect, dignity, and choice in all matters, without exception, related to one's person, circumstances, and relationships in health care."

Patient-centered care supports active involvement of patients and their families in the design of new care models and in decision making about individual options for treatment. The IOM defines patient-centered care as, "Providing care that is respectful of and responsive to individual patient preferences, needs, and values, and ensuring that patient values guide all clinical decisions." Patient-centered care is also one of the overreaching goals of health advocacy, in addition to safer medical systems, and greater patient involvement in healthcare delivery and design. Given that nonconsumer stakeholders often don't know what matters most to patients regarding their ability to get and stay well, care that is truly patient centered cannot be achieved without active patient engagement at every level of care design and implementation.

The application of patient-centered care is often referred to simply as patient engagement or patient activation.

The five attributes of patient-centered care, according to the IOM, are:

- "Whole-person" care
- Coordination and communication
- Patient support and empowerment
- Ready access
- Autonomy

The IOM states that patient-centered care is about much more than simply educating patients about a diagnosis, potential treatment, or healthy behavior. It does not mean giving patients whatever they want; rather, patients want guidance from their care providers, but they expect that guidance to be provided in the context of full and unbiased information about options, benefits, and risks. "Patient-centered" means considering patients' cultural traditions, personal preferences and values, family situations, social circumstances, and lifestyles, as used by the Institute of Medicine and Institute for Healthcare Improvement. A 2001 Institute of Medicine report identified a focus on patient-centered care as one of six interrelated factors constituting high-quality health care. Patient-centered care leads to a higher level of patient engagement. They enumerated five constituent dimensions of patient engagement as follows: communication, provider effectiveness, alignment of objective, information and encouragement, and patient incentive. Engaged patients seem to have better perceived health outcomes.

All these statements and declarations pre-date and motivated the building of the science-based model in this book. (International Alliance of Patients' Organizations [IAPO], 2006. "Declaration on Patient-Centered Healthcare."

Available at: www.iapo.org.uk/patient-centred-healthcare. Retrieved December 13, 2011.)

SEVEN STEPS AND 24 COMPETENCIES OF EVIDENCE-BASED PRACTICE IN NURSING

The seven steps of Evidence-Based Practice (EBP) start with cultivating a spirit of inquiry and an EBP culture and environment; without these elements, clinicians will not routinely ask clinical questions about their practices (see Table A.1). After a clinician asks a clinical question and searches for the best evidence, critical appraisal of the evidence for validity, reliability, and applicability to practice is essential for integrating that evidence with a clinician's expertise and patient preferences to determine whether a current practice should be changed. Once a practice change is made based on this process, evaluating the outcomes of that change is imperative to determine its impact. Finally, dissemination of the process and outcomes of the EBP change is key so that others may learn of practices that produce the best results.

Full report of steps and competencies: Melnyk et al. 2014. http://onlinelibrary.wiley.com/doi/10.1111/wvn.12021/full.

BASICS OF THE INTERNAL FAMILY SYSTEMS MODEL AS PSYCHOTHERAPY COMPARED TO MEDICAL INTERVIEWING

Psychotherapy based on the Internal Family Systems (IFS) Model is listed in the Substance Abuse and Mental Health Services Administration (SAMHSA) National Register of Evidence-based Programs and Practices. A complete outline can be found at www.selfleadership.org/outline-of-the-internal-family-systems-model.html.

1. We recommend that you first read the following books:
   - *Introduction to the Internal Family Systems Model*, Richard C. Schwartz, PhD, 2001, Trailhead Publications.
   - *There's a Part of Me…*, Jon Schwartz and Bill Brennan, 2013, Trailhead Publications.
2. In 2013 The Center for Self Leadership, the home base of IFS, posted a detailed outline of the basics of the IFS Model of Psychotherapy as developed by Richard C. Schwartz and embodied in the certified training programs for psychotherapists worldwide. It can be accessed at: www.selfleadership.org/outline-of-the-internal-family-systems-model.html. This outlines:
   - Details the basic assumptions of this model, defines adaptation and psychotherapy guided by the model
   - Defines observable aspects of the normal personality as a community of personality parts

- Defines a core self-energy capable of self-awareness and curiosity, self-compassion, self-regulation, and relationships with others
- Describes the processes and approaches to a psychotherapy session

3. Behavior change, medical decision making, and information transfer (common features of medical interviewing in health care) are understood differently than in the past when seen through the scientific lens of the IFS Model. People who are in psychotherapy often have health care issues that take precedence. Compared to the brief and limited encounters with a non-therapist in a health care setting, the strategies and tactics of the IFS psychotherapist are similar but geared to work with more intense affects, and the patient is facilitated to take more responsibility for self-awareness. Both medical interviewing and psychotherapy are partnerships between patient and clinician to introduce compassion and nonjudgmental understanding and help regulate affect. The psychotherapist facilitates the patient to take a big responsibility to lead the way, whereas the medical interviewer holds the major responsibility for tackling what is happening within the patient and within himself or herself.

The IFS strategies and tactics for health care issues that arise in psychotherapy are that the clinician:

1. Facilitates the patient to explore and makes a compassionate relationship with the different and often hidden attitudes and motions about a *health behavior change* that one Part of them consciously wants and thereby creates an opening for behavior change to occur. IFS psychotherapists, but not medical interviewers, will also explore sides of the patient (Parts) that carry intense feelings from childhood experiences and will help the patient to sooth and regulate those feelings and to unburden belief systems and emotions that have been stuck in the past. A possibility is established for changes to occur that endure for years.
2. Facilitates the patient to explore and make a compassionate relationship with the many different and hidden ideas, emotions, and memories regarding the *decision choices* in order to normalize and soften the experience of conflict. The patient is helped to slow their decision process so that a decision is not made by only ONE Part of them with the consequence of decision-instability and post-decision remorse. IFS psychotherapists, but not medical interviewers, will also explore sides of the patient (Parts) that carry intense feelings from childhood experiences and will help the patient to sooth and regulate those feelings and to unburden belief systems and emotions that have been stuck in the past. This facilitates enduring change in the patient's experience of themselves.
3. Facilitates the patient to gain perspective or psychological differentiation from parts of their personality that are carrying beliefs and emotions that are blocking the *assimilation of medical information*. The IFS psychotherapist will explore the reactions by other parts of the patient's mind to the information being taken in.

Table A.1 The seven steps and 24 competencies of evidence-based practice

Step 0: Cultivate a spirit of inquiry along with an EBP culture and environment.

Step 1: Ask the PICO(T) question.

Step 2: Search for the best evidence.

Step 3: Critically appraise the evidence.

Step 4: Integrate the evidence with clinical expertise and patient preferences to make the best clinical decision.

Step 5: Evaluate the outcome(s) of the EBP practice change.

Step 6: Disseminate the outcome(s).

24 EBP Competencies

Evidence-based practice competencies for practicing registered professional nurses

1. Questions clinical practices for the purpose of improving the quality of care.
2. Describes clinical problems using internal evidence.* (internal evidence* = evidence generated internally within a clinical setting, such as patient assessment data, outcomes management, and quality improvement data)
3. Participates in the formulation of clinical questions using PICOT* format. (*PICOT = Patient population; Intervention or area of interest; Comparison intervention or group; Outcome; Time)
4. Searches for external evidence* to answer focused clinical questions. (external evidence* = evidence generated from research)
5. Participates in critical appraisal of pre-appraised evidence (such as clinical practice guidelines, evidence-based policies and procedures, and evidence syntheses).
6. Participates in the critical appraisal of published research studies to determine their strength and applicability to clinical practice.
7. Participates in the evaluation and synthesis of a body of evidence gathered to determine its strength and applicability to clinical practice.
8. Collects practice data (e.g., individual patient data, quality improvement data) systematically as internal evidence for clinical decision making in the care of individuals, groups, and populations.
9. Integrates evidence gathered from external and internal sources in order to plan evidence-based practice changes.
10. Implements practice changes based on evidence and clinical expertise and patient preferences to improve care processes and patient outcomes.
11. Evaluates outcomes of evidence-based decisions and practice changes for individuals, groups, and populations to determine best practices.
12. Disseminates best practices supported by evidence to improve quality of care and patient outcomes.

(Continued)

Table A.1 (*Continued*) The seven steps and 24 competencies of evidence-based practice

13. Participates in strategies to sustain an evidence-based practice culture.

Evidence-based practice competencies for practicing advanced practice nurses: All competencies of practicing registered professional nurses plus

14. Systematically conducts an exhaustive search for external evidence* to answer clinical questions. (external evidence*: evidence generated from research)
15. Critically appraises relevant preappraised evidence (i.e., clinical guidelines, summaries, synopses, syntheses of relevant external evidence) and primary studies, including evaluation and synthesis.
16. Integrates a body of external evidence from nursing and related fields with internal evidence* in making decisions about patient care. (internal evidence* = evidence generated internally within a clinical setting, such as patient assessment data, outcomes management, and quality improvement data)
17. Leads transdisciplinary teams in applying synthesized evidence to initiate clinical decisions and practice changes to improve the health of individuals, groups, and populations.
18. Generates internal evidence through outcomes management and EBP implementation projects for the purpose of integrating best practices.
19. Measures processes and outcomes of evidence-based clinical decisions.
20. Formulates evidence-based policies and procedures.
21. Participates in the generation of external evidence with other health care professionals.
22. Mentors others in evidence-based decision making and the EBP process.
23. Implements strategies to sustain an EBP culture.
24. Communicates best evidence to individuals, groups, colleagues, and policy makers.

Index